Neurological Consequences of Nutritional Disorders

Neurological Consequences of Nutritional Disorders

U. K. Misra (0000-0002-7317-957X)
Professor and founder Head, Department of Neurology
Sanjay Gandhi Post Graduate Institute of Medical Sciences, Lucknow, India.

J. Kalita (0000-0002-6141-3592)
Professor, Department of Neurology
Sanjay Gandhi Post Graduate Institute of Medical Sciences, Lucknow, India.

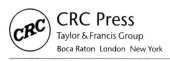

CRC Press
Taylor & Francis Group
Boca Raton London New York

CRC Press is an imprint of the
Taylor & Francis Group, an **informa** business

First edition published 2021
by CRC Press
6000 Broken Sound Parkway NW, Suite 300, Boca Raton, FL 33487-2742

and by CRC Press
2 Park Square, Milton Park, Abingdon, Oxon, OX14 4RN

© 2021 Taylor & Francis Group, LLC

CRC Press is an imprint of Taylor & Francis Group, LLC

Library of Congress Cataloging-in-Publication Data
Title: Neurological consequences of nutritional disorders / U.K. Misra, J. Kalita.
Description: First edition. | Boca Raton, FL : Taylor & Francis, 2021. |
Includes bibliographical references and index. | Summary: "This book
focuses on the impact of nutritional disorders on the nervous system.
Nutritional disorders are caused due to poverty, famine, infestations,
ignorance in the developing world and due to food faddism, isolation,
depression, addictions, and comorbidities in the developed countries.
This book has chapters on various disorders covering basic knowledge,
their clinical manifestations, basis and etiology, laboratory diagnosis,
method of treatment and prognosis. It provides the guidelines to
students and clinicians for dealing with such disorders which are easily
preventable and amenable to treatment whose early diagnosis and
management can avert morbidity and mortality"— Provided by publisher.
Identifiers: LCCN 2020056637 (print) | LCCN 2020056638 (ebook) |
ISBN 9780367313449 (paperback) | ISBN 9780367543068 (hardback) | ISBN 9780429316401 (ebook)
Subjects: MESH: Deficiency Diseases | Neurologic Manifestations | Nervous System—pathology
Classification: LCC RC622 (print) | LCC RC622 (ebook) | NLM QU 246 | DDC 616.3/9—dc23
LC record available at https://lccn.loc.gov/2020056637
LC ebook record available at https://lccn.loc.gov/2020056638

ISBN: 9780367543068 (hbk)
ISBN: 9780367313449 (pbk)
ISBN: 9780429316401 (ebk)

Typeset in Minion
by codeMantra

To the readers who care to read this book and apply to improve the outcome of patients

Contents

Preface

Nutrition is one of the most important requirements of humans, after oxygen and water. Human evolution is closely related to nutrition and aimed at improving **nutrition to meet the high energy needs of evolving brain and body. Globally about 50.5 million children are undernourished, 38.3 million overweight and 20 million obese.** Poverty, war, famine, sanctions and comorbidities are the common causes of malnutrition. Even in the economically developed countries, malnutrition occurs because of food faddism, isolation, depression addiction and prolonged intensive care treatment.

Medical curriculum does not give the desired emphasis on nutrition especially in postgraduate training programs. Malnutrition is one of those disorders for which the treatment is known and available; the question is of awareness and implementation. While organizing neurology training program at Sanjay Gandhi Post Graduate Institute for over three decades, interacting with students and faculty, the need of such a book was felt.

This book begins with a chapter on the role of nutrition in development of the nervous system. Chapters 2–9 are on protein energy malnutrition and vitamin deficiencies. A chapter on fluorosis is added because of its importance in the fluorosis-endemic area. Chapters on deficiencies of iodine, copper and zinc are also included. Fluid and electrolytes are extremely important and are generally excluded from the text of nutritional disorders, but we have included these aspects because of their important role in critically ill neurological patients. The last chapter summarizes the dietary manipulation in various inherited metabolic disorders because of its therapeutic implication.

The authors have tried to simplify the subject by the ample use of clinical photographs, radiological images, schematic diagrams, charts and tables. The emphasis has been on clinical relevance and bedside application. This book will meet the need of medical students pursuing medicine, pediatric, and neurology programs, consultants and faculties.

This is the first edition and may have some shortcomings or limitations. We welcome suggestions that will help in improving a subsequent edition. We sincerely hope that this book would improve the diagnosis and management of patients and help in creating new knowledge in this area.

U. K. Misra
J. Kalita

Acknowledgments

We are grateful to **Mr. Ritesh Butani** of CRC Press for prompting us to commit to this title. We are indebted to Professor **SK Mishra**, Head of Endocrine Surgery, who gave us support and facilities in the telemedicine department to complete this book in this difficult time of the COVID- 19 epidemic. We thank Professors **D. Sharma**, **A. Deka** and **D. Baruah** for sharing clinical and radiological photographs of their patients. Our residents, namely, Drs. **Prakash C. Pandey**, **Sarvesh K. Chaudhary**, **Nikhil A Dongre**, **Abhishek**, **Sachan**, **Mahesh Jadhav**, **Anadi Mishra**, **Ajay Chavan** and **Rabindra Kumar** helped in collecting clinical data and follow-up of the patients. The PhD students, namely, **Abhilasha Tripathi**, **Kamakshi Shukla** and **Ashish Dubey**, helped in collecting references and literature review. We thank Mr. **Shakti Kumar** for secretarial help and Mr. **Anil Kumar** for the cover design. We acknowledge the CRC editorial team **Shivangi Pramanik** and **Himani Dwivedi** for editing this book. We are indebted to our family members for their constant support and encouragement.

About the authors

U. K. Misra was the Founder Head of Department of Neurology at Sanjay Gandhi Post Graduate Institute of Medical Sciences, Raebareli Road, Lucknow, Uttar Pradesh, India, during 1987–2018, and presently is the Director and Head of Neuroscience at Apollomedics Super Specialty Hospital, Lucknow. His teaching experiences of four decades are illustrated by his active participation in national and international educational programs. He has authored 4 books, and his keen interest in research has resulted in more than 468 publications.

J. Kalita is presently working as a Professor, Department of Neurology, Sanjay Gandhi Post Graduate Institute of Medical Sciences, Lucknow, Uttar Pradesh, India. Prof. Kalita is an excellent teacher and clinician. She has an outstanding academic carrier and received "the Best Neuroscientist in India" Award by Carrier 360 based on her number of publications, Hi-index and citations. She is the author of 4 books and has published about 450 papers in peer-reviewed journals.

Role of nutrition in the growth and development of nervous system

INTRODUCTION

Nutrition is essential throughout life, and is especially important during pregnancy, infancy and early childhood for the development of nervous system. Development of brain is related to the development of cognitive and motor functions, and socioemotional skills during childhood and adulthood. Nutritional deficiencies during pregnancy and infancy can affect cognitive and behavioral functions, which predict school performance as well as performance in later life. This chapter highlights the importance of nutrition in different stages of the nervous system development.

STRUCTURAL DEVELOPMENT

The biological time scale of human development requires observation in a large number of individuals. Since it is difficult to accurately decide the time of conception, the gestational age (GA) may not be precise. The average human GA is 40 weeks. In early prenatal life, the chronological and biological scales have special importance. The development in this period is so fast that there is change every day. During infancy, the tempo of development is slower than that in the parental life, but it is faster than that in childhood.

Central nervous system is developed as a specialized ectoderm, called "neuroectoderm". The thickening of neuroectoderm results in the formation of neural plates, which in turn fuse to form a neural tube. The cephalic portion of the neural tube enlarges to form the brain, and the caudal portion narrows to form the spinal cord and peripheral nerves. There are three dilatations in the cranial part: prosencephalon, mesencephalon and rhombencephalon. The prosencephalon differentiates into telencephalon and diencephalon. The telencephalon differentiates into cerebral hemispheres, corpus striatum and cerebral ventricles. The structures develop from the diencephalon are thalamus, hypothalamus and related structures, including the third ventricle. The mesencephalon gives rise to midbrain and cerebral aqueduct. The rhombencephalon has two parts: metencephalon (from which pons, cerebellum and the fourth ventricle develop) and the myelencephalon (which differentiates into medulla and spinal cord) (Figures 1.1 and 1.2). The outer layer of the spinal cord develops into peripheral nerves. The lateral aspects of neural crest and adjacent cells differentiate into dorsal root ganglia, adrenal medulla, sympathetic and parasympathetic ganglia, Schwann cells and neurolemmal sheets. The neural tube with single-cell lining develops into three layers: ependymal matrix, mental and meningeal layers. The neurons are derived from the mental layer.

The development of nervous system is a continuous process rather than a stepwise event. Several functions develop in parallel, and any dissociation is abnormal.

EMBRYONAL AND FETAL DEVELOPMENT

At 3 weeks of embryonic life, there are neuroblastic differentiation, migration and neuronal multiplication, which have a genetic basis. The neuronal

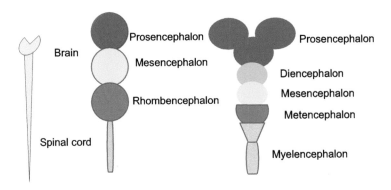

Figure 1.1 Schematic diagram shows the development of different parts of notochord.

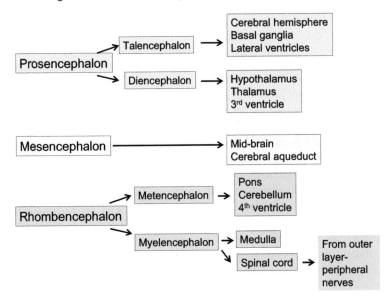

Figure 1.2 Origin of different structures of the nervous system from prosencephalon, mesencephalon and rhombencephalon.

proliferation occurs at an average speed of 250,000/minute for several days to weeks. The neurons become bipolar and migrate to the marginal layer through radial glial cells to form the cerebral cortex. Migration is completed by the fifth fetal month when the cortex contains billions of post-mitotic cells. During the mid-fetal life, cerebral hemispheres develop into a deeply sulcated structure. The major sulci such as Sylvian, Rolandic and calcarine sulci achieve an adult configuration by the fifth month. Secondary sulci develop by 6–7 months of fetal life, and tertiary sulci also develop by 8–9 months. Simultaneously, there is an organization of cortical and neuronal masses. Synaptogenesis and axonal path finding take place

subsequently by 30th week. The cytoarchitectural pattern of the cerebral cortex develops and differentiates neurons of the cortical region, e.g., primary motor, sensory and auditory cortices.

The time scale of myelin development is not as clearly known as that of the neuronal development. By 10th week, spinal roots and nerves are myelinated, which correspond with the reflex motor activity. Subsequently, segmental and intersegmental fibers are myelinated followed by the myelination of ascending and descending tracts that start from the brainstem. By 28th–30th week, vestibulo-cochlear pathways are myelinated; by 37th week, myelination of spinocerebellar and dentatorubral tracts takes place. By 40th week of gestation, the visual system starts myelinating, which is completed by 3 months of postnatal life. The corticospinal tracts are myelinated by 18 months of postnatal life. Posterior frontal and parietal lobes are myelinated by 40th week of gestation, which is followed by the myelination of other parts of the brain. By 2 years, the myelination of the nervous system is complete. The myelination of intra- and interhemispheric fibers continues till 10 years of age or beyond. The density of neurons increases up to 15 months of postnatal life; thereafter, it decreases with increasing dendritic arborization and synaptogenesis. The growth of human embryo and fetus is presented in Table 1.1. The neurons begin to function before myelination. By the age of 12–15 years, the weight of the brain in females is 1230–1275 g and in males 1350–1410 g. The development of brain structure at different time points is shown in Figure 1.3.

REQUIREMENT OF NUTRIENTS IN THE DEVELOPING BRAIN

Growth factors and nutrients play an important role in the development of brain during fetal and early postnatal life. Some nutrients play a greater role, such as protein, carbohydrate, fat, iron, zinc, copper, iodine, selenium, choline, vitamin A, folate and cobalamin. The effects of nutritional deficiency may depend on timing, dose and duration of deficiency. There are three stages of neuronal involvement in malnutrition:

Table 1.1 Growth of nervous system in human embryo and fetus

Fetal age (days)	Length (mm)	Nervous system development
18	1.5	Neural groove and tube
21	3	Optic vesicles
26	3	Anterior neuropore closure
27	3.3	Posterior neuropore closure
31	4.3	Anterior horn cell appears
		Anterior and posterior roots
35	5	Five vesicles
42	13	Primordium of cerebellum
56	25	Differentiation of cortex and meninges
150	225	Primary cerebral fissures
180	230	Cerebral myelination
8–9 months	240	Growth of brain and myelination

1. **Stage 1**: Structure of cell and process may be intact but its function may be impaired.
2. **Stage 2**: Demyelination with an intact axis cylinder.
3. **Stage 3**: Demyelination, destruction of axis cylinder and cell death.

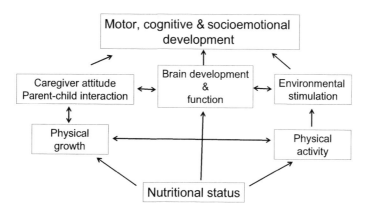

Figure 1.3 Organization of cellular and functional structures at different natal and postnatal periods of life.

Replenishment of nutrients in stage 1 rapidly restores the function. In stages 2 and 3, there may be a permanent deficit. During 24–42 weeks of GA, brain is particularly vulnerable to nutritional deficiency, because myelination and synaptogenesis take place during this period. During the late fetal and early neonatal life, hippocampus, visual, auditory cortex and corpus striatum have a fast pace of development with regard to morphogenesis and synaptogenesis. Hippocampus is the first region to have a cortico-cortical connectivity and becomes functional by 1 month of postnatal life. Myelination may also be affected if there is a nutritional deprivation. Nutrients at a particular concentration may be beneficial at one time, but can as well be toxic at the other time. Iron and certain other nutrients are regulated in a narrow range, highlighting this effect. Deficiency of nutrients in early stage affects the cell proliferation, and at a later stage, it affects differentiation processes such as size, synaptogenesis and dendritic arborization.

Genes of cell proliferation are expressed earlier than those of cell differentiation. Several genes are expressed as regulatory genes from the region-specific development of the brain. To study the spatial and temporal expression of genes, 9955 genes in hippocampus, hypothalamus and frontal cortex were evaluated in rats during four stages of prenatal development and seven stages of postnatal development (Stead et al., 2006). More than 97% of neurally expressed genes showed changes at different time points. There were 20 clusters of transcriptional genes involved in DNA metabolism, nuclear function, synaptic vesicle transport, myelination and neuropeptide hormone activity. There were specific time points for the expression of these genes. The salient findings of this important study are as follows:

1. Two-third of probed genes are expressed in the postnatal period.
2. More than 95% of expressed genes show a change during different time points of the development.
3. More than 85% of genes show a difference in expression in the three regions.
4. The maximum expression of genes occurs in 1–2 weeks of postnatal life.
5. The difference in gene expression is also maximum during 1–2 weeks of postulated life.

6. Less than 300 genes are differentiated in the hippocampus from the frontal cortex at postnatal day, which increase to more than 2000 genes in adult brain. By 2 weeks of postnatal life, the regional differentiation is nearly complete in rat brain (Stead et al., 2006).

Early postnatal life in rats corresponds to late gestational period in humans. These studies underscore the importance of genetic factors in the growth and development of brain.

The nutrients can affect the structure (anatomy), function (physiology, metabolism and signal propagation) and neurochemistry (synthesis of neurotransmitter and receptors, and neurotransmitter reuptake). These also affect the overall neuronal performance. Long-standing nutritional abnormality may result in an irreversible structural damage.

By 24–44 weeks, the bilobed brain and the third ventricle at the beginning of third trimester reach the adult structure in full-term neonates. During this time, there are neuronal growth, differentiation and synaptic connection. There is a formation of experience-based synapse before birth, which explains the anatomical basis of fetal learning. The connectivity of hippocampus to enterorhinal cortex to thalamus to frontal cortex forms the key pathway for memory formation. Nutritional deficiency, therefore, can affect the cognitive and behavioral functions even in the later life if it occurs during the development of this circuit. The important nutrients for the brain development are discussed in the following sections.

Iron

Iron is a transition metal, which has an ability to transport oxygen and transfer electrons, and is a key nutrient for the brain development. Iron acts as a catalyst in various reactions. Brain has a high demand for iron in the last trimester and early postnatal life. Neonatal brain is metabolically very active and consumes 60% of body oxygen compared to 20% in adults (Erecińska and Silver, 1989). Premature infants, on the other hand, have a higher risk of iron deficiency due to early erythropoiesis, rapid growth and low iron store (Choudhury et al., 2015). Iron rapidly accumulates in the last trimester during which it affects myelination, neurotransmitter production and energy metabolism. In the rat model, the biochemical, structural and behavioral effects of iron deficiency have been documented. There are reduced oxidative metabolism in the hippocampus and frontal cortex, increased intra-cerebellar glutamate concentration and reduced striated dopamine concentration (Wang et al., 2019). There is fatty acid and myelin defect globally. Structurally, there are truncated dendrites in the hippocampus and a reduction in neuronal mass.

Behaviorally, there are reduced recognition, procedural memory and spatial recognition. This behavioral abnormality correlates with a reduction of iron in the hippocampus and striatum. Maternal iron deficiency in humans results in intrauterine growth retardation and premature birth. Cord ferritin concentration in infants is related to poor school performance. Infants with low iron also have poor auditory recognition and memory (Wang et al., 2019). Children who develop iron deficiency before 2 years of age show reduced cognitive and school performance at 4–9 years of age (Lozoff et al., 2006). The importance of iron deficiency anemia in infancy and later neurobehavioral functions has been reported in a long-term follow-up study. Those with iron deficiency anemia during infancy when followed up in adolescence revealed lower IQ, social problem and inattention compared to non-anemic counterparts even though they were treated for anemia during infancy (Walker et al., 2007). Maternal supplementation of iron during pregnancy has not shown an improvement in IQ and behavioral performance at the short- and long-term follow-up (Zhou et al., 2006; Parsons et al., 2008). The benefit of iron supplement in infancy, however, has not been confirmed in other studies (Berglund et al., 2013; Christian et al., 2011). To prevent the ill effects of iron deficiency on CNS development, the following steps are recommended:

1. Feed iron-rich food to mother and infants.
2. Provide postnatal services.
3. Encourage mother and infant interaction.
4. Provide learning opportunities.

Iron deficiency should be corrected but taking care to avoid iron toxicity is important.

Copper

Copper is essential for the synthesis of hemoglobin and helps in the formation of connective tissue, blood vessels, bone and tendon. Copper helps in the development and maintenance of myelin, which depends on phospholipids. Synthesis of phospholipids needs cytochrome C oxidase, a copper-dependent enzyme. Copper also regulates ferroxidase activity, which maintains the iron distribution to various tissues (Vashchenko et al., 2013). Premature and low-birth-weight newborns are prone to copper deficiency. The fetus accumulates copper in the last month of gestation, which meets the requirement in the first month of life when the copper intake is the minimum (Harvey and McArdle, 2008). Copper is required for brain energy metabolism and dopamine metabolism, and is also an antioxidant. Copper deficiency results in demyelination of posterior column and cortico-spinal tract of the spinal cord. In rodents, copper deficiency produces cerebellar dysfunction, which manifests with imbalance and incoordination.

Zinc

Zinc is the fourth most abundant ion in the brain and is a cofactor in enzymes of protein and nucleic acid metabolism. Reduced level of zinc is therefore associated with a reduction of DNA, RNA and protein synthesis. Insulin-like growth factor I and growth hormone receptor gene expression is regulated by presynaptic buttons that depend on zinc. Zinc also helps in the release of neurotransmitters. Zinc deficiency results in a reduction of brain mass in cerebellar, limbic and cerebral cortices. Orbitofrontal cortex is also susceptible to zinc deficiency and is associated with a reduction of dendritic arborization. Zinc-deficient fetus shows an autonomic instability in the form of heart rate variability, and there may be a reduced fetal movement. The infants who are zinc deficient have a preferential looking abnormality. In humans, zinc supplementation during pregnancy has not shown any benefit on motor or cognitive abilities during childhood compared to placebo (Gardner et al., 2005). Animal and human studies, however, have shown a reduced activity, poor attention, learning and memory functions (Christian et al., 2010; Tamura et al., 2005; Caulfield et al., 2010).

Zinc supplementation during infancy has not revealed a cognitive improvement (Tamura et al., 2005; Hamadani et al., 2002). In nine randomized controlled trials, zinc was supplemented for at least 6 months within 2 years of age, and was compared with placebo for motor and cognitive effects. None of these studies found a cognitive benefit. In two studies, there was an improvement in motor function (Sazawal et al., 1996; Bentley et al., 1997). In one study, an improvement in motor function was noted when zinc was combined with iron and other micronutrient (Black et al., 2004). A meta-analysis on zinc supplementation revealed no evidence of improvement in cognitive and motor functions; however, the authors felt that studies were small and supplementation was given for a short duration to derive a valid conclusion (Brown et al., 2009).

Fatty acid

Long-chain polyunsaturated fatty acids (LCPUFAs) are essential for the maturation of brain, retina and other organs during the third trimester and neonatal period. LCPUFAs are produced from the essential fatty acids. Docosahexaenoic acid (DHA) is synthesized from linoleic acid, and arachidonic acid is from α-linolenic acid. DHA is needed for neuragenesis, migration and synaptogenesis. It also has an important role in cholinergic, aminergic and GABAergic neurotransmitter systems. There is a preferential accumulation of DHA in fetal retina and brain gray matter. Deficiency of DHA therefore may result in abnormal visual functions and impaired cognitive and behavioral functions. The cognitive and behavioral abnormalities have been attributed to DHA, which is needed for the synthesis of proteins, receptors and neurotransmitters. DHA also helps in synaptogenesis and myelination. In preterm infants, formula feeding enriched with LCPUFA improved electroretinogram, visual acuity and short-term global development (Carlson et al., 1996). Mothers deficient in LCPUFA, if DHA is supplemented, may benefit the neonate because it crosses the placenta and is secreted in mothers' milk. The role of LCPUFA in term infants, however, is not convincing. In a meta-analysis of 38 trials, the effect of n-3 PUFA on visual and cognitive functions in the childhood was evaluated. This study included 13 trials on maternal supplementation, seven in preterm neonates and 18 trials in term neonates. n-3 PUFA supplementation improved visual and psychomotor functions but not global IQ in later childhood (Shulkin et al., 2018).

PROTEIN ENERGY MALNUTRITION

Protein and energy are important for brain development, including intrauterine and postnatal life. Depletion of protein and energy may result in a reduction in DNA and RNA contents, reduced number of neurons, fatty acid synthesis and myelination, which manifest with a reduced brain size. At an ultrastructural level, there is a reduced synaptic and dendritic complexity as well as reduced neurotransmitters, growth factors and structural proteins (Wiggins et al., 1984; Ke et al., 2006). Fetal protein energy malnutrition (PEM) results in intrauterine growth retardation, and PEM during neonatal period results in hypotonia. Postnatal malnutrition is common in preterm infants who have food restriction or food intolerance. Intrauterine growth retardation may be associated with a reduced growth and development in later life. Minimal cognitive impairment, especially verbal and spatial memory, has been reported in 15% of children with IUGR (Cusick and Georgieff, 2016).

OTHER NUTRIENTS

Iodine, sodium, choline, folate and vitamin B6 have a role in the brain development. Iodine and selenium also affect the thyroid metabolism.

Iodine

Iodine is necessary for the synthesis of thyroid hormone. Thyroid hormone helps in neurogenesis, neuronal migration, axonal and dendritic outgrowth, synaptogenesis and myelination. Maternal iodine deficiency results in cretinism, which manifests with mental retardation, facial dysmorphism, deaf mutism and stunted growth. In China, the children in iodine deficiency region had 12.5% IQ point differences compared to their age group (Qian et al., 2005). An RCT on school children, however, did not support this effect (Melse-Boonstra and Jaiswal, 2010). Iodine supplement to pregnant mother, who are deficient in iodine, is the best strategy to prevent cretinism. Two trials in Peru and Congo revealed an increase in 10.2 IQ points in children aged 0–5 years following iodine supplementation to pregnant mothers (Bougma et al., 2013).

Vitamin B12 and folic acid have an important role in the development of fetus. Folic acid

Table 1.2 Role of nutrients in late fetal and neonatal brain development

Nutrient		Part of brain involved	Mechanism
Metal		White matter	Myelin
	Iron	Striatum and frontal	Monoamine synthesis
		Hippocampal – frontal	Neuronal and glial energy metabolism
	Copper	Cerebellum	Neurotransmitter synthesis, glial and neurons energy metabolism, antioxidant
	Zinc	Hippocampus, cerebellar	Neurotransmitter release
		Autonomic CNS	DNA synthesis
	Choline	Hippocampus	DNA methylation
		White matter	Myelin synthesis
		Global	Neurotransmitter synthesis
	LCPUFA	Cortex	Myelin
		Eye	Synaptogenesis
	Protein energy	Global	Cell proliferation, differentiation
		Cortex	Synaptogenesis
		Hippocampus	Growth factor synthesis

deficiency has been linked to the neural tube defect, and its supplementation is recommended for the prevention of these developmental anomalies in children. A systematic review, however, does not support the importance of maternal nutritional status defined by body mass index, micronutrient and macronutrient levels in the cognitive function of the offspring (Taylor et al., 2017). The role of nutrients in the development of the nervous system is summarized in Table 1.2.

ASSESSMENT OF NUTRITIONAL DEFICIENCY IN NEONATES AND CHILDREN

There are several limitations in the evaluation of nutritional effect on brain development in neonates and children (Table 1.3):

1. There are limited methods for evaluating neurobehavioral functions in neonates and infants.
2. Superadded infection may also affect the growth and development.
3. Children may catch up after supplementation, overshadowing the effects of nutritional deficiency.
4. There may be overlapping (similar) effects of different nutrients on the nervous system.

The assessment of neurodevelopment may be done by the following methods:

I. Neurobehavioral and neurological examinations

4 month of age: Cortically dominant behavior may be assessed.

4–6 months: Affect, distractibility, preferential looking task and event-related potential

Table 1.3 Investigative modalities for different parts of nervous system

Techniques	Structure of brain
MRI conventional sequence	Regional and global volume, structural changes
MRI-diffusion tensor imaging	Myelin and tract integrity
MR spectroscopy	Neurochemistry
Auditory brainstem responses (ABT)	Brainstem auditory tract (myelin) and synaptic function
Autonomic function test	Autonomic system

(ERP) are possible. ERPs can assess memory functions.

1 year: Reasoning skills by Bayley Scale of Infant Development.

3 years: Cambridge Neuropsychological Test Battery evaluates strategy, switching, executive functions and working memory.

6 years: Functional MRI, near-infrared spectroscopy and magnetoencephalography.

II. **Brain size:** Head circumference, CT or MRI scan.

III. **Tract size:** Diffusion tremor imaging.

IV. **Electrical activity:** Electroencephalography, evoked potentials.

FACTORS INFLUENCING THE EFFECT OF UNDERNUTRITION

Brain development is not only affected by the nutrition and genetic factors but also affected by the experience and environmental stimulation (Figure 1.4). There are two main experience-based learning methods:

1. **Experience expectant:** In which sensory, visual and auditory circuits are stimulated by the afferent stimuli.

2. **Experience dependent:** Experience-dependent learning refers to the way the brain organizes itself in response to individual stimuli.

Experience-dependent learning is responsible for acquired learning, which continues throughout the life. It helps to adapt and thrive in their respective environment. Nutrient and environment may have an additive, interactive and mediating effect. Environmental stimulation probably has a greater role in the development of motor, sensory, cognitive and socioeconomic effects in children (Grantham-McGregor et al., 1991; Waber et al., 1981).

It has been shown that the children who play with toys, colors, shape and numbers have a higher cognitive and brain development. Children in Costa Rica with iron deficiency anemia from the low socioeconomic background had poor school performance (Lozoff et al., 2006). Children of 12–23 months of age having chronic iron deficiency were followed up at 5, 11–14 and 15–19 years of age. Their cognitive functions did not catch up on iron supplementation compared to those who had the normal iron status. The interacting effect of environment stimulation was illustrated in Chile. Low-birth-weight children from high socioeconomic status who received good environmental stimuli were at a lower risk of poor development

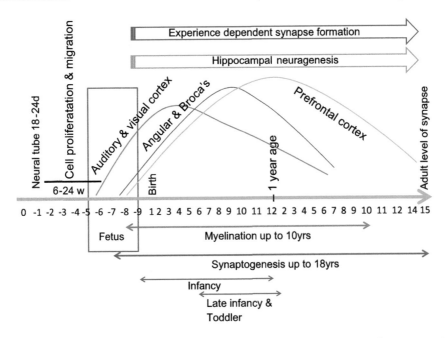

Figure 1.4 Caregiver and environmental influence on the motor, cognitive and socioemotional functions along with nutrition status.

compared to those born in the disadvantaged environment (Torche and Echevarría, 2011). An interacting effect of nutrition and environment was illustrated in a Jamaican study. Infants and children aged 9–30 months received zinc supplementation in one group, and zinc with psychosocial stimulation in the other group. The children receiving both zinc and environmental stimulation had a better cognitive and brain development compared to those who received only zinc supplementation (Gardner et al., 2005).

MEDIATING EFFECT: UNDERNUTRITION AFFECTS PHYSICAL AND MENTAL DEVELOPMENT BY TWO MECHANISMS

1. Caregiver behavior
2. Child's exploration of environment.

Caregiver behavior: (a) The caregiver may treat the child as smaller (younger) than his age, thereby reducing environmental inputs; **(b)** the undernourished child may also have intercurrent infections and irritability, which may render the caregiver unduly protective, thereby reducing environmental inputs; **(c)** the undernourished children may not be able to explore the environment as compared to the well-nourished children. These factors cause a vicious cycle of poor cognitive development and lack of environmental exploration.

RECOVERY FROM NUTRITIONAL DEFICIENCY

Nutritional supplementation and enhanced sensory, linguistic and social interactions may improve the recovery. In a study, undernourished orphans below 2 years of age from Korea were adopted by American middle-class families. These children had normal IQ at school but their IQ was lower than that in the well-nourished adopted orphans (Winick et al., 1974). During World War II, children born in Holland during famine had nutritional deprivation in utero. After adequate health care and nutrition, the IQ at the age of 19 years was normal and was not different from those born out of the well-nourished mothers. This study highlights the recovery potentials of IQ following nutritional supplementation. However,

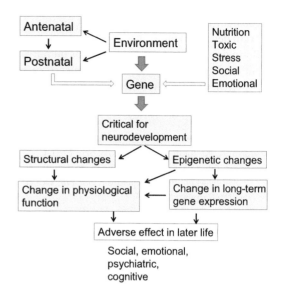

Figure 1.5 Effect of nature and nurture on health and disease.

the children born out of malnourished mothers had higher frequency of schizophrenia, addiction and antisocial behavior (Stein and Susser, 1975). WHO recommends the structured activity to promote cognitive development as a component of treatment of early childhood malnutrition (Ashworth et al., 2003). The protective effects of neurodevelopment and cognitive functions are attributed to high socioeconomic status, cognitive stimulation in early life, increased duration of breast feeding and catch-up growth (Wang et al., 2008). Those results, however, are not supported by some studies from Jamaica, Bangladesh and South Africa (Walker et al., 2010; Emond et al., 2006; Prado and Dewey, 2014). Growth and intellectual development are determined by genetic factors, nutrition at crucial time points and environmental stimulation (Figure 1.5). These factors may result in structural and epigenetic changes leading to the long-term socioemotional and cognitive consequences.

CONCLUSION

1. Central nervous system development is influenced by the nutritional status of the mother and nutrients during neonatal and childhood period.
2. Protein, carbohydrate, fatty acids, iron, zinc, copper, iodine, folic acid, selenium and

cobalamin are especially important for the brain development.

3. Brain development not only depends on nutrients and genetic factors, but also depends on experience and environmental stimuli.

REFERENCES

Ashworth, A., Khanum, S., Jackson, A., Schofield, C. 2003. *Guidelines for the Inpatient Treatment of Severely Malnourished Children.* Geneva: World Health Organization.

Bentley, M. E., Caulfield, L. E., Ram, M., 1997. Zinc supplementation affects the activity patterns of rural Guatemalan infants. *The Journal of Nutrition 127*(7): 1333–1338.

Berglund, S. K., Westrup, B., Hägglöf, B., Hernell, O., Domellöf, M. 2013. Effects of iron supplementation of LBW infants on cognition and behavior at 3 years. *Pediatrics 131*(1):47–55.

Black, M. M., Baqui, A. H., Zaman, K., et al. 2004. Iron and zinc supplementation promote motor development and exploratory behavior among Bangladeshi infants. *The American Journal of Clinical Nutrition 80*(4):903–910.

Bougma, K., Aboud, F. E., Harding, K. B., Marquis, G. S. 2013. Iodine and mental development of children 5 years old and under: A systematic review and meta-analysis. *Nutrients 5*(4):1384–1416.

Brown, K. H., Peerson, J. M., Baker, S. K., Hess, S. Y. 2009. Preventive zinc supplementation among infants, preschoolers, and older prepubertal children. *Food and Nutrition Bulletin 30*(1 Suppl): S12–S40.

Carlson, S. E., Werkman, S. H., Tolley, E. A. 1996. Effect of long-chain n-3 fatty acid supplementation on visual acuity and growth of preterm infants with and without bronchopulmonary dysplasia. *The American Journal of Clinical Nutrition 63*(5):687–697.

Caulfield, L. E., Putnick, D. L., Zavaleta, N., et al. 2010. Maternal gestational zinc supplementation does not influence multiple aspects of child development at 54 mo of age in Peru. *The American Journal of Clinical Nutrition 92*(1):130–136.

Choudhury, V., Amin, S. B., Agarwal, A., Srivastava, L. M., Soni, A., Saluja, S. 2015. Latent iron deficiency at birth influences auditory neural maturation in late preterm and term infants. *The American Journal of Clinical Nutrition 102*(5):1030–1034.

Christian, P., Morgan, M. E., Murray-Kolb, L., et al. 2011. Preschool iron-folic acid and zinc supplementation in children exposed to iron-folic acid in utero confers no added cognitive benefit in early school-age. *The Journal of Nutrition 141*(11):2042–2048.

Christian, P., Murray-Kolb, L. E., Khatry, S. K., et al. 2010. Prenatal micronutrient supplementation and intellectual and motor function in early school-aged children in Nepal. *JAMA, 304*(24):2716–2723.

Cusick, S. E., Georgieff, M. K. 2016. The role of nutrition in brain development: The golden opportunity of the "First 1000 Days". *The Journal of Pediatrics 175*:16–21.

Emond, A. M., Lira, P. I., Lima, M. C., Grantham-Mcgregor, S. M., Ashworth, A. 2006. Development and behaviour of low-birthweight term infants at 8 years in northeast Brazil: A longitudinal study. *Acta Paediatrica 95*(10):1249–1257.

Erecińska, M., Silver, I. A. 1989. ATP and brain function. *Journal of Cerebral Blood Flow & Metabolism 9*(1):2–19.

Gardner, J. M., Powell, C. A., Baker-Henningham, H., Walker, S. P., Cole, T. J., Grantham-McGregor, S. M. 2005. Zinc supplementation and psychosocial stimulation: Effects on the development of undernourished Jamaican children. *The American Journal of Clinical Nutrition 82*(2):399–405.

Grantham-McGregor, S. M., Powell, C. A., Walker, S. P., Himes, J. H. 1991. Nutritional supplementation, psychosocial stimulation, and mental development of stunted children: The Jamaican Study. *Lancet (London, England) 338*(8758):1–5.

Hamadani, J. D., Fuchs, G. J., Osendarp, S. J., Huda, S. N., Grantham-McGregor, S. M. 2002. Zinc supplementation during pregnancy and effects on mental development and behaviour of infants: A follow-up study. *Lancet (London, England) 360*(9329):290–294.

Harvey, L. J., McArdle, H. J. 2008. Biomarkers of copper status: A brief update. *The British Journal of Nutrition 99* (Suppl 3):S10–S13.

Ke, X., Lei, Q., James, S. J., et al. 2006. Uteroplacental insufficiency affects epigenetic determinants of chromatin structure in brains of neonatal and juvenile IUGR rats. *Physiological Genomics 25*(1):16–28.

Lozoff, B., Jimenez, E., Smith, J. B. 2006. Double burden of iron deficiency in infancy and low socioeconomic status: A longitudinal analysis of cognitive test scores to age 19 years. *Archives of Pediatrics & Adolescent Medicine 160*(11):1108–1113.

Melse-Boonstra, A., Jaiswal, N. 2010. Iodine deficiency in pregnancy, infancy and childhood and its consequences for brain development. *Best Practice & Research. Clinical Endocrinology & Metabolism 24*(1):29–38.

Parsons, A. G., Zhou, S. J., Spurrier, N. J., Makrides, M. 2008. Effect of iron supplementation during pregnancy on the behaviour of children at early school age: Long-term follow-up of a randomised controlled trial. *The British Journal of Nutrition 99*(5):1133–1139.

Prado, E. L., Dewey, K. G. 2014. Nutrition and brain development in early life. *Nutrition Reviews* 72(4):267–284.

Qian, M., Wang, D., Watkins, W. E., et al. 2005. The effects of iodine on intelligence in children: A meta-analysis of studies conducted in China. *Asia Pacific Journal of Clinical Nutrition* 14(1):32–42.

Sazawal, S., Bentley, M., Black, R. E., Dhingra, P., George, S., Bhan, M. K. 1996. Effect of zinc supplementation on observed activity in low socio-economic Indian preschool children. *Pediatrics* 98(6 Pt 1):1132–1137.

Shulkin, M., Pimpin, L., Bellinger, D., et al. 2018. n-3 Fatty acid supplementation in mothers, preterm infants, and term infants and childhood psycho-motor and visual development: A systematic review and meta-analysis. *The Journal of Nutrition* 148(3):409–418.

Stead, J. D., Neal, C., Meng, F., et al. 2006. Transcriptional profiling of the developing rat brain reveals that the most dramatic regional differentiation in gene expression occurs post-partum. *The Journal of Neuroscience: The Official Journal of the Society for Neuroscience* 26(1):345–353.

Stein, Z., Susser, M. 1975. The Dutch famine, 1944–1945, and the reproductive process. I. Effects on six indices at birth. *Pediatric Research* 9(2):70–76.

Tamura, T., Goldenberg, R. L., Chapman, V. R., Johnston, K. E., Ramey, S. L., Nelson, K. G. 2005. Folate status of mothers during pregnancy and mental and psychomotor development of their children at five years of age. *Pediatrics* 116(3):703–708.

Taylor, R. M., Fealy, S. M., Bisquera, A., et al. 2017. Effects of nutritional interventions during pregnancy on infant and child cognitive outcomes: A systematic review and meta-analysis. *Nutrients* 9(11):1265.

Torche, F., Echevarría, G. 2011. The effect of birth-weight on childhood cognitive development in a middle-income country. *International Journal of Epidemiology* 40(4):1008–1018.

Vashchenko, G., MacGillivray, R. T. 2013. Multi-copper oxidases and human iron metabolism. *Nutrients* 5(7):2289–2313.

Waber, D. P., Bauermeister, M., Cohen, C., Ferber, R., Wolff, P. H. 1981. Behavioral correlates of physical and neuromotor maturity in adolescents from different environments. *Developmental Psychobiology* 14(6):513–522.

Walker, S. P., Chang, S. M., Powell, C. A., Simonoff, E., Grantham-McGregor, S. M. 2007. Early childhood stunting is associated with poor psychological functioning in late adolescence and effects are reduced by psychosocial stimulation. *The Journal of Nutrition* 137(11):2464–2469.

Walker, S. P., Chang, S. M., Younger, N., Grantham-Mcgregor, S. M. 2010. The effect of psychosocial stimulation on cognition and behaviour at 6 years in a cohort of term, low-birthweight Jamaican children. *Developmental Medicine & Child Neurology* 52(7):e148–e154.

Wang, W. L., Sung, Y. T., Sung, F. C., et al. 2008. Low birth weight, prematurity, and paternal social status: Impact on the basic competence test in Taiwanese adolescents. *The Journal of Pediatrics* 153(3):333–338.

Wang, Y., Wu, Y., Li, T., Wang, X., Zhu, C. 2019. Iron metabolism and brain development in premature infants. *Frontiers in Physiology* 10:463.

Wiggins, R. C., Fuller, G., Enna, S. J. 1984. Under nutri-tion and the development of brain neurotransmit-ter systems. *Life Sciences* 35(21):2085–2094.

Zhou, S. J., Gibson, R. A., Crowther, C. A., Baghurst, P., Makrides, M. 2006. Effect of iron supple-mentation during pregnancy on the intelligence quotient and behavior of children at 4 y of age: Long-term follow-up of a randomized controlled trial. *The American Journal of Clinical Nutrition* 83(5):1112–1117.

2

Protein energy malnutrition

INTRODUCTION

Protein energy malnutrition (PEM) is defined as a prolonged inadequate protein and energy intake with a consequent depletion of body cell mass and body fat. Starvation-induced PEM is also known as "starvation disease", hunger disease or starvation-related malnutrition. Body generally adapts to starvation by reducing energy expenditure and catabolism, which are mediated by hormones and nervous system-regulated changes in the cell metabolism. PEM is associated with a reduced muscle mass. Mild-to-moderate starvation is associated with adaptation but at the cost of lethargy, weakness, hypothermia, muscle and skin atrophy, and functional disability. On clinical examination, muscle atrophy and loss of fat are easily identified. However, in hospitalized patients, these may be overlooked.

Historical background

Malnutrition and its consequences are linked to socioeconomic, political and natural disasters. The description of PEM did not appear till 1865. In 1930s, Cecile Williams described African children with diarrhea, edema and wasting. In local language, it was called as "kwashiorkor" (Williams, 1935). These children were usually between 6 months and 4 years of age when they were weaned from breastfeeding, and were fed maize porridge. These children improved with milk and cod liver oil. Williams considered that amino acid or protein deficiency is responsible for kwashiorkor. In whole of Africa, kwashiorkor was prevalent except in Masai and Batussi tribes who used cow milk for porridge (Brock and Autret, 1952). Kwashiorkor was commonly reported from Central America

and Brazil. In 1949, World Health Organization (WHO) and Food and Agricultural Organization (FAO) conducted investigations of kwashiorkor. In 1952, the experts of WHO and FAO highlighted the malady as protein calorie malnutrition. In 1955, milk was used as a reference protein, and the policy of using locally available food items was advised to overcome malnutrition (Waterlow and Stephen, 1957). Rockefeller Foundation and United Nations International Children's Emergency Fund (UNICEF, 2020) collaborated for research and prevention of protein calorie malnutrition, and highlighted the importance of animal protein, fish and dairy products to prevent and treat PEM. In 1965, UNICEF was awarded Nobel Peace Prize, and the contribution of Maurice Pate was acknowledged (Nobelstiftelsen, 1965). Pate joined Red Cross as Director in 1939. Pate and Herbert Hoover surveyed 38 countries in 76 days, underscored the problem of malnutrition and laid down the concept of UNICEF, which was headed by Pate in 1947 till his death in 1965. Pate emphasized that UNICEF will serve all the children including those from enemy countries without any discrimination regardless of race and politics. UNICEF implemented programs under the leadership of Pate to improve the maternal and child health using low-cost preventive health care measures. In 1971, the United Nations resolved to eradicate protein crisis in the developing countries. Protein calorie malnutrition is related to infant and child mortality, stunted growth, low work output, premature aging and reduced lifespan. Protein advisory group emphasized a dietary improvement by including soy, fish, protein concentrate, peanuts, sesame and sunflower seeds in the diet. Following famine in Bangladesh in 1974, in which 1.5 million people died leading to the concept of quantity over quality, protein gap was no longer acceptable (Waterlow and Payne, 1975). It is estimated that 50% deaths in children have underlying undernutrition, and the cause of death in PEM is diarrhea in 60.7%, pneumonia in 52.3%, malaria in 57.3% and measles in 44.8% (Caulfield et al., 2004). PEM is not restricted to poor and developing countries only, but is also prevalent in economically developed countries because of food faddism, anorexia nervosa, isolation, homelessness, institutionalization and chronic diseases such as renal failure, liver failure, stroke and dementia.

Nutrition is important from the conception to 24 months of age because deficiency during this period may led to the long-term effects on health and cognition. Undernutrition of the mother is reflected by low birth weight. In 2010, there were 15% low-birth-weight newborns especially in low- and middle-income countries, highest in South-East Asia. Asian countries carry 69% of global burden of underweight, 58% of stunted and 70% of wasted children (Kliegman et al., 2019).

Global burden

Malnutrition is a public health problem and is linked to poverty and low productivity. Elimination of malnutrition is likely to reduce the global burden of disease by 32% (WHO, 2020a,b). Malnutrition is a double burden: overnutrition results in overweight and obesity, whereas undernutrition in underweight, wasting and stunting. Malnutrition is prevalent in all the groups of population and geographical regions with an inverse relationship between undernutrition and overnutrition. Overnutrition also contributes to a number of noncommunicable diseases such as diabetes mellitus, heart disease and metabolic syndrome.

The clinical marker of child undernutrition is measured by height and weight against the age-specific standard. Based on height and weight, the effects of undernutrition in children are termed as "stunting, wasting and underweight". It is important to address the problem of PEM by the age of 6 months to 2 years, which is regarded as the window period to prevent or manage acute or chronic malnutrition. Maternal and child malnutrition is responsible for 3.5 million deaths annually (Black et al., 2008). In 2008, the mortality of children below 5 years of age was 8.8 million globally, and

93% of deaths occurred in Asia and Africa (Walton and Allen, 2011). Malnutrition is associated with a series of mental, social, economic and developmental burden. Neonate born out of undernourished mother in a poor family is likely to have a stunted growth with poor neuropsychological development. Malnutrition renders the child prone to poor immunity and infection, leading to a restricted mobility, which in turn results in an impairment of psychological and intellectual development. Studies from Sudan, Bangladesh, Ethiopia and Haiti have revealed multiple causes of malnutrition, including environmental and dietary factors. Diet is the immediate and primary cause of undernutrition. The other factors contributing to undernutrition are household food security, access to health facility, healthy environment and child care practice (Müller and Krawinkel, 2005). Malnutrition in children below 3 years is mainly due to poor feeding practices, education and occupation of parents or caregiver, household income, mother's knowledge about nutrition and residence (Seligman et al., 2010). This study highlights the importance of maternal education. Intervention studies have also shown benefits in terms of development, growth and survival (Bhutta et al., 2013). The global burden of stunting in the children below 5 years of age was 21.3% in 2009, which had declined from 32.4% in 2000. About 199.5 million children below 5 years were stunted in 2000, which reduced to 144 million in 2019. About 40% of stunted children are in South-East Asia, and another 40% in sub-Saharan Africa. Stunting has not improved in West and Central Africa. In 2019, the global burden of wasting in children below 5 years was 47 million, and 14.3 million of them were severely wasted. More than 50% of the wasted children are in South-East Asia, and another 25% in sub-Saharan Africa (UNICEF, WHO 2020).

The global problem of overweight is 5.6%, which is highest in the Middle East and North Africa (11%), Eastern Europe and Central Asia (10.8%), and North America (8.9%), and least in South-East Asia (2.5%). About 1.9 billion adults are overweight or obese, while 462 million are underweight (WHO, 2020a,b). The global burden of malnutrition is shown in Figure 2.1. The percentage of stunting, wasted and overweight is highest in Asia (Figure 2.2). The country-wise percentages of children with stunting, wasting and overweight are shown in Figures 2.3–2.5. In India, the prevalence of

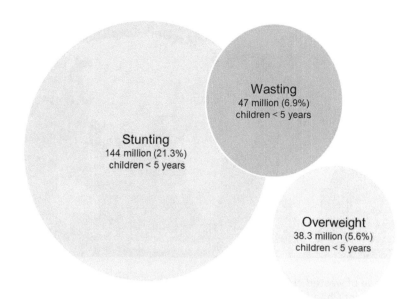

Figure 2.1 Global burden of malnutrition (UNICEF/WHO/World Bank, 2020).

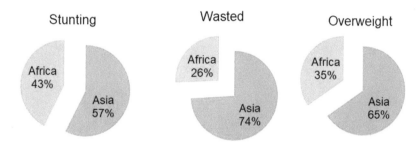

Figure 2.2 Asia shares the highest percentage of stunting, wasting and overweight children under 5 years of age (UNICEF/WHO/World Bank Group – Joint Child Malnutrition Estimates 2020 edition).

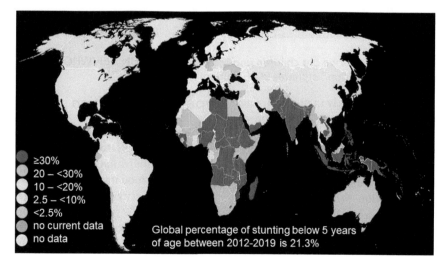

Figure 2.3 Global burden of stunting in different countries during 2012–2019 (UNICEF/WHO/World Bank Group – Joint Child Malnutrition Estimates 2020 edition).

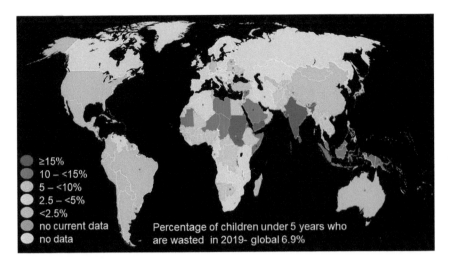

Figure 2.4 Percentage of wasted children under 5 years of age in different countries (UNICEF/WHO/World Bank Group – Joint Child Malnutrition Estimates 2020 edition).

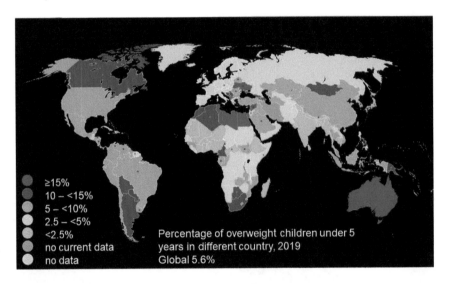

Figure 2.5 Percentage of overweight children under 5 years of age (UNICEF/WHO/World Bank Group – Joint Child Malnutrition Estimates 2020 edition).

child growth failure varies widely in different states and different ethnic populations. In 2017, the prevalence of stunting in different states of India was 21.3%–49.0%, wasting 6.3%–19.3% and underweight 16.5%–42.2% (India State-Level Disease Burden Initiative Malnutrition Collaborators, 2019). National Nutrition Mission of India was launched in 2018 to improve child growth failure and other indicators of malnutrition (India State-Level Disease Burden Initiative CGF Collaborators, 2020). The changes in stunting, wasted and underweight since 2000 are presented in Figures 2.6–2.8.

Types of malnutrition

1. **Uncomplicated protein energy malnutrition or starvation-related malnutrition:** Starvation-related malnutrition occurs due to prolonged inadequate food intake associated with weight loss. The severity of muscle wasting is proportional to the severity of PEM. Sometime there may be edema, which may camouflage muscle wasting. Starvation-related malnutrition is attributable to unavailability of food due to poverty or famine. The hospital cases of

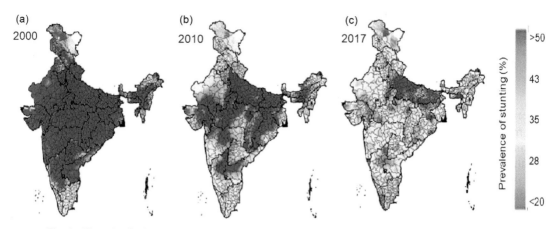

The tertile cut-offs for stunting prevalence were 33.1% and 41.1%, and for its Annual Rate of Reductions were 2.23% and 3.37% from 2010 to 2017

Figure 2.6 The change in prevalence of stunting in different regions in India.

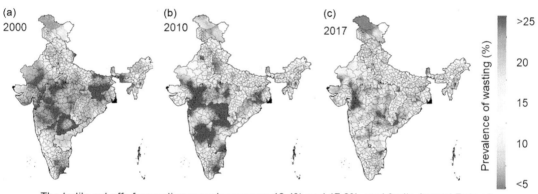

The tertile cut-offs for wasting prevalence were 13.4% and 17.6%, and for its Annual Rate of Reduction were 0.10% and 2.12% from 2010 to 2017.

Figure 2.7 The change in prevalence of wasted in different regions in India.

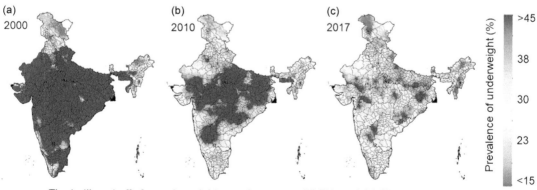

The tertile cut-offs for underweight prevalence were 25.7%, and 34.5% and for its Annual Rate of Reduction were 2.43% and 3.90% from 2010 to 2017.

Figure 2.8 The change in prevalence of underweight in different regions in India.

starvation-related malnutrition are due to physician prescription, depression, anorexia nervosa, nausea, vomiting, dysphagia, and esophageal, duodenal or small intestinal obstruction.

2. **Chronic disease-related malnutrition or cachexia:** Both these terms refer to malnutrition due to systemic inflammation, which is commonly associated with infection, autoimmune diseases, hepatic, renal, cardiac or pulmonary diseases, or malignancy. This group of malnutrition is attributed to an increased catabolism leading to fatigue, weakness and muscle atrophy. In cachexia, there is poor or no adaptation for starvation. The premorbid personality is important in chronic disease-related malnutrition; those who are obese or had good appetite, in them anorexia is less prominent compared to thin and small eaters.

3. **Acute disease-related malnutrition (ADRM):** ADRM refers to specific nutritional condition which results in very high risk severe malnutrition, such as in catabolic critical illness, including severe sepsis and injury. If primary illness is not corrected, then malnutrition will develop in short time.

DIAGNOSIS OF UNDERNUTRITION

The indicator of undernutrition in a society may be measured by underweight, stunting and wasting.

Underweight suggests low weight for the age and may be due to acute or chronic undernutrition.

Stunting refers to low height for the age and suggests chronic undernutrition.

Wasting refers to low weight for the height and suggests acute undernutrition.

The Indian Association of Pediatrics classifies undernutrition into:

Grade I (mild): 70%–80% of standard (reference) weight for the age.
Grade II (moderate): 61%–70% of standard (reference) weight for the age.
Grade III (severe): 51%–60% of standard (reference) weight for the age.
Grade IV (very severe): < 50% of standard (reference) weight for the age (Ghai et al., 2013).

The clinical features of mild-to-moderate malnutrition are growth failure, infection, anemia, reduced activity, and skin or hair changes.

Moderate-to-severe malnutrition manifests with marasmus, kwashiorkor or both. The children with marasmus have severe wasting of proximal muscles. The child appears thin with no fat and has redundant skin and hollowed cheek (Simian faces). The skin of the buttock is loose and saggy (baggy pant) (Figure 2.9). These children are active, do not have edema and have good appetite. With supplementation, they improve better than those with kwashiorkor. The child with kwashiorkor manifests between 1 and 4 years of age and is more prevalent in Africa. Pitting edema of legs and feet which may involve the hands and face later is typical of kwashiorkor (Figure 2.10). Muscle wasting also occurs and may be camouflaged by edema. Skin pigmentation is confluent, flaky and paint-like especially in buttocks and upper thighs (Figure 2.11). Skin may peel off resulting in ulceration, and there may be petechiae. Mucus membrane involvement is associated with glossitis, cheilitis and angular stomatitis (Figure 2.12). There may be Bitot's spot due to the associated vitamin A deficiency (Figure 2.13). Hair are depigmented and lusterless. The nails are brittle and may have associated koilonychias and ridges. Children with kwashiorkor have a multisystem involvement such as gastrointestinal (diarrhea, vomiting, ascites), cardiovascular (cardiomyopathy, heart failure), peripheral vascular diseases, and hematological (anemia) and renal (reduced glomerular filtration rate) dysfunctions. The clinical features of undernutrition are summarized in Table 2.1.

Diagnosis

The diagnosis of PEM is possible clinically by the loss of muscle mass and body fat especially in starvation-related PEM in the community. In acute and chronic disease-related malnutrition, PEM may be overlooked. The nutritional status can be assessed by the measurement of muscle mass, subcutaneous adipose tissue, extracellular fluid volume (ECFV), body mass index (BMI), visual BMI, and laboratory and technical assessments.

Muscle mass: Starvation-related PEM may be easy to diagnose by determining a reduction in muscle mass especially shoulder and pelvic girdle muscles. In hospital setting however, the muscle wasting may be overlooked, which is attributable to disease, old age, high-dose glucocorticoid, endocrine disease or neurological disease. Old age,

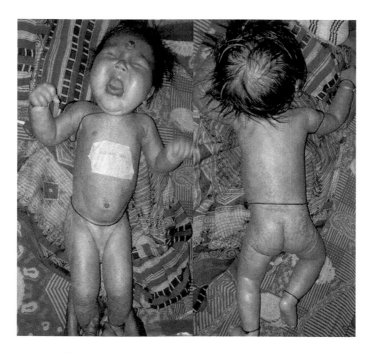

Figure 2.9 A 14-month-old child with kwashiorkor. The child is edematous, irritable with flaky skin lesion on buttocks. (Courtesy Professor A. Deka, Silchar Medical College, Assam.)

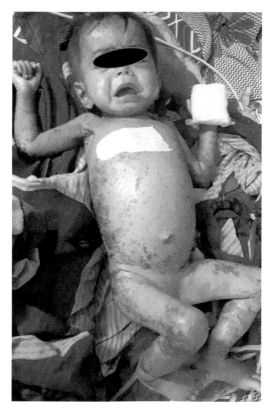

Figure 2.10 A child with kwashiorkor having skin pigmentations that are confluent, flaky, paint-like in buttocks, thighs, legs and trunk. (Courtesy Professor A Deka, Silchar Medical College, Assam.)

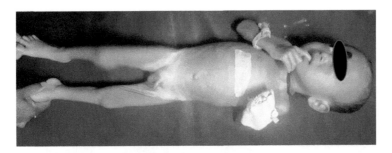

Figure 2.11 A child with marasmus showing wasting of muscles and loss of subcutaneous fat. (Courtesy Professor A Deka, Silchar Medical College, Assam.)

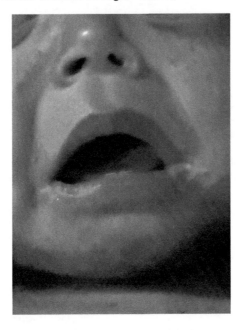

Figure 2.12 A 18-month malnourished child shows angular cheilitis (Courtesy Professor A Deka, Silchar Medical College, Assam.)

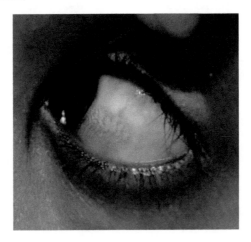

Figure 2.13 A 7-year stunted child having Bitot's spot. (Courtesy Professor A Deka, Silchar Medical College, Assam.)

Table 2.1 Clinical features of malnutrition

1. Facial appearance:
   Moon face in kwashiorkor, Simian face in marasmus
2. Eye:
   Dry pale conjunctiva, Bitot's spot
3. Mouth:
   Angular cheilitis, stomatitis, glossitis, spongy bleeding gums, parotid enlargement
4. Teeth:
   Delayed dentition, mottled enamel
5. Hair:
   Brittle, hypopigmented
6. Skin:
   Loose, and wrinkled in marasmus, shiny edematous in kwashiorkor, pigmentation may increase or decrease
7. Wound healing:
   Poor in keratinization

disease and starvation may coexist; therefore, the reversible cause of starvation should be considered and managed. Muscle disease in ADRM is more serious problem, because internal pool of amino acid from muscle catabolism is not available. Wound healing is also delayed, and reduced immunity predisposes to infections.

Subcutaneous adipose tissue: Measurement of triceps skin fold is a good indicator of fat loss in PEM, but the obese patients on a strict dietary restriction may develop PEM with a relative preservation of fat. In such patients, a targeted examination for muscle bulk may help in revealing muscle atrophy due to PEM.

Extracellular fluid volume (ECFV): Chronic starvation results in increased ECFV and even edema (starvation edema). In chronic disease-related malnutrition, there may be hypoalbuminemia resulting in increased ECFV and edema, which may mask muscle wasting and fat depletion.

Body mass index (BMI): BMI is calculated by body weight in kg/height in meter square

$$BMI = Body\ weight\ in\ kg/height\ in\ meter^2.$$

Normal BMI is 20–25; BMI more than 25 suggests overweight; and BMI less than 20 suggests the loss of muscle mass and body fat. BMI below 13 is incompatible with life, and that below 17 is consistent with PEM. BMI more than 17 does not rule out PEM because BMI may be high due to an increase in ECFV and the presence of fat in the obese person on dietary restriction (Flier, 2018).

Visual BMI may be useful in this situation as an experienced physician could differentiate muscle wasting in an obese and edematous patient. Body fat and protein help the individual to survive in severe malnutrition. In ADRM especially in stroke patients, the survival is better with higher BMI. In a multicenter study in India, the role of premorbid undernutrition was evaluated in 448 patients with stroke. On admission, 27.2% patients were undernourished based on Objective Global Assessment. Older age, hypertensive patients from Andhra Pradesh were more frequently undernourished. Premorbid undernutrition and length of hospital were the independent predictors of 30-day poor outcome (Pandian et al., 2011). In another study, overweight measured by waist circumference was associated with a good outcome in females (Bembenek et al., 2018).

In chronic diseases, frailty is one of the important risk factors for survival. Tuberculosis is endemic in low- and middle-income countries where malnutrition is also prevalent. It has been suggested that undernutrition may impair innate and adaptive immunity required to control *Mycobacterium tuberculosis* infection. Response to BCG vaccination is also affected in poorly nourished children (Sinha et al., 2019). Meta-analysis of six studies revealed that one-point increase in BMI reduces the incidence of tuberculosis by 13.5% (Lönnroth et al., 2010). HIV patients with a BMI of less than 18.5 were at the fourfold increased risk of tuberculosis within 6 months of antiretroviral treatment (Van Rie et al., 2011).

Muscle mass: Muscle mass palpation and power testing during clinical examination is more important than the ultrasound of muscle.

Markers of systemic inflammation: The markers of systemic inflammation differentiate starvation malnutrition from acute or chronic disease-related malnutrition. Serum albumin and C-reactive protein (CRP) are the markers of systemic inflammation, which include anorexia, muscle catabolism and wasting. Hypoalbuminemia occurs after several months of starvation. The intensity of protein catabolism is higher in acute and chronic disease-related malnutrition. Muscle catabolism fulfills the amino acid need and increases nitrogen production, thereby increasing the excretion of nitrogen in urine. Urinary urea constitutes about 80% of urinary nitrogen. The nitrogen loss can be calculated as follows:

$$N \text{ loss (g)} = g\,N \text{ in urinary urea}/0.85 + 2.$$

Muscle catabolism is proportional to urinary nitrogen. In severely malnourished patients, the loss of nitrogen may not be as high as mild-to-moderate malnutrition due to severe muscle weakness. The nitrogen loss data therefore should be carefully interpreted in light of muscle bulk.

Subjective Global Assessment: Subjective global assessment is a cost-effective and easy tool to assess the nutritional status of the patient. This scale includes (a) history regarding the amount of food intake and its composition, weight loss, food faddism and systemic infection; (b) body configuration by examining muscle bulk, subcutaneous fat and signs of ECFV expansion (edema); and (c) functional status of the patient that could be examined by patient's mobility and muscle strength.

Subjective global assessment can clearly define malnutrition as well as severe disease-related malnutrition (Jameson et al., 2018).

PATHOPHYSIOLOGY OF MALNUTRITION

In the early stage of malnutrition, there is a phenomenon of "reductive adaptation" by which body learns to survive with a minimal energy. The body fat store is mobilized for energy production followed by the mobilization of protein from muscle, skin and gastrointestinal tract. The physical activity is minimized and growth is retarded, which reduce the metabolic requirement. In the later stage of malnutrition, the liver becomes less efficient in producing glucose, albumin and transferrin, leading to hypoglycemia, infection and anemia. Low body metabolic rate results in hypothermia, because of reduced heat production, and loss of adipose tissue. Fluid overload occurs due to less-efficient renal functions in excreting fluid and electrolyte. A small heart during the adaptive phase when exposed to high intravascular volume results in heart failure. Hypokalemia occurs due to an increased excretion of potassium in urine. Leaky cell membrane and impaired K+/Na+ pump activity result in the accumulation of intracellular sodium. Muscle catabolism is associated with the loss of copper, zinc and magnesium. Impaired conversion of ferritin results in anemia in spite of high serum iron, and high serum iron produces oxidative stress. As a result of reductive adaptation, there is a decreased intestinal secretion and motility, which increases bacterial growth leading to indigestion, diarrhea and reduced absorption.

Treatment

The treatment of malnutrition depends on severity and underlying disorders. The mode of treatment (oral, enteral or parenteral) depends on urgency of treatment and the underlying cause of malnutrition. In a conscious and cooperative patient without nausea and vomiting, the oral feeding should be encouraged. Enteral feeding is indicated in the patients who are unable to eat because of severe dysphagia, unconsciousness, gastrointestinal motility disorder, anorexia nervosa, severe depression critical illness, and those on mechanical ventilation. Enteral nutrition can be given through nasogastric tube (NGT), feeding gastrostomy or jejunostomy. Nasogastric feeding may be given as a bolus containing 200–400 ml over 15–60 min at an interval of 3–6 hours in an adult. For children, the treatment of malnutrition has been discussed separately. Initially, the feeding is started with 50 ml bolus, which is increased by 25 ml in each feed till the target is achieved. The bolus feeding is not possible in feeding jejunostomy, and the feed is given continuously. If the NGT output is less than 1200 ml daily, the feeding may be continued. NGT feeding is not recommended in the patients with gastrointestinal ischemia, intestinal obstruction, gastrointestinal hemorrhage, coagulopathy, esophageal varices, paralytic ileus and peritonitis. The aim of enteral feeding is to provide macronutrients (carbohydrate, protein and fat). Most feeding formulas also contain standard amount of micronutrients, minerals and electrolytes. In these patients, blood glucose and electrolytes should be monitored periodically. There are several enteral feeding formulas available, some of which are as follows:

1. **Standard polymeric formula:** It comprises carbohydrate for energy and protein (casein, soy, whey). Fat can be added to reduce the volume of carbohydrate. Pancreatic enzymes are important for protein digestion. In this formula, the calorie content is 1000–2000 kcal/l with a protein content of 50–70 g/l, and the remaining is carbohydrate.
2. **Polymeric formula with fiber:** In this formula, in addition to protein and carbohydrate, fermentable and nonfermentable dietary fibers are also added. Fermentable fibers are pectin and guar. These are digested by the colonic bacteria and produce short-chain fatty acid, which is used as a fuel of colonic epithelium. Nonfermentable fibers increase the fecal bulk, thereby improving peristalsis and preventing diarrhea.
3. **Elemental and semi-elemental formula:** This formula is composed of partially or completely hydrolyzed ingredients for the patients with maldigestion and malabsorption.
4. **Immune-enhancing formula:** In addition to macronutrients, some micronutrients are known to enhance immune functions, e.g., arginine, glutamine, nucleotide and antioxidants. This formula is beneficial in the patients with gastrointestinal surgery and head injury, but not in critically ill patients.
5. **Protein-enriched formula:** This formula contains 90 g of protein in 1000 kcal/l. It is used for the treatment of obesity and patients with high catabolism.
6. **F75 and F100 formulae:** F75 formula is used as a starter formula during stabilization, and F100 as a catch-up or rehabilitation formula when the appetite returns. The compositions of F75 and F100 are presented in Table 2.2. These formulae have low thiamine content, which should be supplemented to avoid complications. Thiamine deficiency occurs in the children in precarious communities such as in South-East Asia, Africa and America in whom diet is mainly based on rice, wheat and cassava (Hailemariam et al., 1985; Khounnorath et al., 2011; Tang et al., 1989). The prevalence of thiamine deficiency in hospitalized children ranges between 13.4% and 40% in Laos, Jamaica and Ghana. The majority of infants in Cambodia are thiamine deficient (Coats et al., 2012), and 45% of infant mortality in rural Cambodia is attributed to thiamine deficiency (Kauffman et al., 2011). Rapid initiation of feeding in the malnourished children may increase the requirement of thiamine and may precipitate wet beriberi and cardiac arrest. In F75 and F100 formulae, thiamine is not adequate to avoid these complications. The American Academy of Pediatrics has recommended the administration of thiamine 50–100 mg iv or 100–300 mg po during the first 3 days of feeding (Pulcini et al., 2016).

There are disease-specific enteral formulae such as for diabetes, and renal and hepatic disorders.

Table 2.2 Composition of F75 and F100 feeding formulae

Ingredient	F75	F75 (cereal 1)	F75 (cereal 2)	F100	F100 (cereal)
Cow milk (ml)	30	30	25	95	75
Sugar (g)	9	6	3	5	2.5
Cereal (puffed rice powder, g)	0	2.5	6	-	7
Vegetable oil (g)	2	2.5	3	2	2
Water (ml)	100	100	100	100	100
Protein (g)	0.9	1.1	1.2	2.9	2.9
Lactose (g)	1.2	1.2	1.1	3.8	3.0
Energy (kcal)	75	75	75	100	100

Complications of enteral feeding

Nasogastric and enteral feeding may have the following complications: aspiration, diarrhea, infection, gastrointestinal intolerance to enteral feeding; imbalance of electrolyte, glucose and volume; and inability to achieve nutritional goals. Aspiration is a major complication as it may lead to pneumonia and septicemia. In an adult, if prefeed nasogastric tube output is more than 300 ml, and if there is abdominal pain or distension, NGT feed should be stopped. Diarrhea may be due to disease per se, infection or antibiotics. If these conditions are excluded, diarrhea may be due to enteral formula. The existing formula may be changed to the fiber-containing formula. Diarrhea may be prevented by the use of prokinetics and antiemetics.

Parenteral nutrition

The aim of parenteral nutrition is to provide a complete nutritional requirement through central venous pressure, including dextrose, amino acids, triglycerides, minerals (calcium, phosphorus, magnesium, zinc), electrolytes, and micronutrients. Protein synthesis requires 21 α-amino acids, 9 essential amino acids and 11 nonessential amino acids. The essential amino acids are phenylalanine, valine, threonine, tryptophan, methionine, leucine, isoleucine, lysine and histidine. Six amino acids, namely, arginine, cysteine, glycine, glutamine, proline and tyrosine, are considered conditionally essential. The essential amino acids cannot be synthesized in the body using other amino acid or carbohydrate, whereas nonessential amino acids could be synthesized from the other amino acids as well as from carbohydrates. The parenteral formulation therefore should have essential amino acids and some of the conditional essential amino acids such as arginine, cysteine and glutamine. Carbohydrate is used in the formula as dextrose monohydrate having 3–4 kcal/g. Lipids are used in the form of soybean oil, olive oil or fish oil in different proportion. High lipid content formulations have a possibility of peroxidation leading to oxidative injury. Therefore, the infusion rate should not exceed 8 g/h or 175 g/day in a 70-kg adult man.

These formulations are available in two-chamber bags (dextrose and amino acid bags) or three-chamber bags (dextrose, amino acid and lipid bags) which are mixed just before infusion. A standard amount of electrolyte, vitamins and trace elements are injected into the bag prior to the infusion for maintaining their stability. The requirement of water-soluble vitamins is higher than the oral route because of an increased excretion in urine.

Refeeding syndrome: Refeeding syndrome occurs due to rapid correction during the first week of replacement therapy. Carbohydrate stimulates insulin secretion, which has anti-natriuretic effect, leading to the expansion of ECFV which is compounded by hypernatremia. Refeeding edema can be minimized by a slow introduction of carbohydrate and low sodium-containing diet. Low serum phosphate in refeeding syndrome is due to overactive intracellular glucose 6 phosphatase and glycogen synthase. During parenteral nutrition, the level of potassium, phosphorus, zinc and magnesium should be closely monitored and corrected. An abrupt increase in intravascular volume may result in heart failure, and cardiac arrhythmia may occur due to electrolyte imbalance and wet beriberi. The features of refeeding syndrome in severely malnourished children are summarized in Table 2.3.

MANAGEMENT OF MALNUTRITION IN CHILDREN

Mild-to-moderate malnutrition: Among the malnourished children, more than 80% have a mild-to-moderate degree of malnutrition. These children can be treated in outpatient service advising about the frequency and composition of the diet. The mainstay of the treatment is to provide adequate calorie and protein. The calorie requirement of a child is 150 kcal/kg/day with protein 3 g/kg/day. Protein is given in the form of milk, nuts, soy or nonvegetarian food. A little increase in protein in the diet helps in catch-up. The remaining energy can be prescribed as carbohydrate. Use of oil may help in reducing the amount of carbohydrate and the volume of the diet. The child should be given frequent small feeds every 2- to 3-h interval.

Table 2.3 Refeeding syndrome in severely malnourished children

1. Sodium retention:
   Fluid overload, pulmonary edema, heart failure
2. Hypokalemia:
   Arrhythmia, muscle weakness, rhabdomyolysis, nausea, vomiting, constipation
3. Hypomagnesaemia:
   Arrhythmia, weakness, tremor, seizure, altered sensorium, nausea, vomiting, diarrhea
4. Hypophosphatemia:
   Hypotension, muscle weakness, paresthesia, confusion, seizure, hemolysis
5. Hyperglycemia:
   Dehydration, hyperosmolar coma, hypotension

Severe malnutrition: Severe malnutrition in the children should be managed in the hospital. The attention should be paid to the underlying cause of malnutrition. The death in severe malnutrition increases due to hypoglycemia, hypothermia, electrolyte imbalance, infection and heart failure. The nutritional supplementation should be tailored according to socioeconomic and cultural background. WHO recommends the ten steps for the management of severe malnutrition (WHO, 1999):

1. **Management of hypoglycemia:**
   Hypoglycemia is considered if blood glucose is less than 54 mg/dl. If blood glucose cannot be measured, consider it as hypoglycemia and it should be treated. Asymptomatic hypoglycemia is treated with 10% of 50 ml glucose or sucrose orally or through NGT. This should be followed by formula F75 feeding 2 hourly round the clock. Symptomatic hypoglycemia is treated by infusion of 10% dextrose in a dose of 5 ml/kg. Antibiotic should be prescribed, and hypothermia should be prevented. Once the child is alert, oral or NGT feed should be started as in asymptomatic hypoglycemia.
2. **Hypothermia:** Hypothermia is diagnosed if the rectal temperature is below 35.5°C/95.5°F or axillary temperature 35°C/95°F. The child should be covered with warm clothing including head, and a skin-to-skin contact with mother's chest is encouraged if a warmer or heater is not available. Warming should be slow to avoid a disequilibrium. Usually, hypothermia occurs in association with

infection and hypoglycemia, which should be managed accordingly.
3. **Dehydration:** In a severely malnourished child, it is difficult to assess dehydration. Low osmolar oral rehydration solution (ORS) is used with potassium supplementation, depending on the thirst and output (stool, urine and nasogastric output). Feeding should be started within 2–3 h of rehydration. F75 formula feed and low osmolar ORS should be used alternately. Watch for overhydration, and continue breastfeeding. If there is diarrhea, after each stool low osmolar ORS in a dose of 5–10 ml/kg should be given. Once the dehydration is corrected, F75 formula feed should be started (Ghai et al., 2013).
4. **Electrolyte:** Potassium supplementation of 3–4 mEq/kg/day for 2 weeks should be given. On day 1, 50% magnesium sulfate (equivalent to 4 mEq/ml, maximum 2 ml, thereafter 0.8–1.2 mEq/kg) should be administered daily. Diet should have low salt because serum sodium may be low in spite of high total body sodium.
5. **Infection:** Gram-negative infection is common. The child should be given ampicillin of 50 mg/kg IV 6 hourly for 2 days, followed by oral ampicillin of 50 mg/kg 8 hourly for 5 days. In addition, gentamycin (7.5 mg/kg) or amikacin (15–20 mg/kg IM or IV) should be given. If the child does not improve in 48 h, intravenous ceftriaxone 50–75 mg/kg/day 12 hourly may be prescribed instead. The antibiotic may be changed according to the culture sensitivity report. For preventing infection, hand hygiene is very important. Measles vaccination should be given if the child is above 6 months and not

immunized. Mother should be taught about hand hygiene, to maintain a growth chart and vaccination schedule.

6. **Micronutrients:** Double dose of vitamins and minerals should be given except vitamin A. On day 1, vitamin A is prescribed as per age: for 0<6 months of age 50,000 IU, 6–12 months of age 100,000 IU and for more than 1 year 200,000 IU. On day 1, folic acid 5 mg should be given and thereafter 1 mg/day. The daily doses of trace elements are as follows: zinc 2 mg/kg/day, copper 0.2–0.3 mg/kg/day and iron 3 mg/kg/day. Iron is started after 1 week because its impaired absorption and gastrointestinal irritation during first week. All the supplementations should be continued till the child gains weight after the initial stabilization.

7. **Feeding:** Small and frequent feeds should be started as soon as possible. There should be a gradual increase to prevent refeeding syndrome. The total fluid intake is 130 ml/kg/day, and it is 100 ml/kg/day when edema reduces. Encourage breastfeeding, and start with F75 starter feed 2 hourly. If the child has diarrhea, low-lactose F75 formula should be advised, and if diarrhea persists, lactose-free F75 formula should be used. Children with malnutrition when fed may develop refeeding syndrome. Attention should be paid to diagnose and manage these complications.

8. **Catch-up growth:** The child catches growth after 2 weeks of stabilization. After 2–3 days when appetite returns, the intake may be increased by increasing the volume and decreasing the frequency of feed, gradually to six feeds a day. The children on breastfeeding should be continued till 2 years of age. There should be a gradual transition from F75 to F100 formula. The calorie should be calculated as 150–250 kcal/kg/day in which protein should be 4–6 g/kg/day. The parents should be encouraged to give a supplementary food.

9. **Sensory stimulation:** The children should be in a good cheerful environment with facilities for playing for 15–30 min/day. Age-appropriate physical activity should be encouraged as soon as possible. Both child and parent need emotional support.

10. **Prepare for follow-up:** If the child is stabilized with the above-mentioned treatment, they may be prepared for rehabilitation and home care after 2–6 weeks. The primary treatment failure is suspected by the following indicators:

a. Appetite that is not regained by 4th day
b. Edema that is not decreased by 4th day
c. Persistence of edema by 10th day
d. Failure to gain weight of 5 g/kg/day till 10 days
e. Secondary treatment failure is suspected if child is not gaining 5 g/kg/day during rehabilitation.

PREVENTION OF MALNUTRITION

Prevention of malnutrition is possible if there is political will and commitment of the government. Improved food production, supply and attention to distribution are important for the elimination of malnutrition. Food fortification, salt iodization and supplementation of food as mid-day meal are organized by many governments as national program. Nationwide surveillance of the vulnerable population may help in better planning. At the community level, health and nutritional education are important regarding the quality and quantity of food. Community education is also important for the removal of prejudice and false beliefs. It is important to encourage those dietary items that are locally available, culturally acceptable, have nutritive value and are affordable. Improvement in literacy and education with empowerment to the females of the reproductive age may reduce the incidence of malnutrition. Mothers should be encouraged to maintain a growth and vaccination card of the child. Primary health care facilities, including universal free immunization, hydration, periodic deworming and early diagnosis and treatment of infections, can help in preventing malnutrition. Mothers should be encouraged to breastfeed their children till 2 years of age. Supplementation of food after 6 months of age and maternal education about child health and common infection are important. In India, integrated child development scheme, national mid-day school meal and national anemia prophylaxis program have been undertaken to overcome malnutrition. Health care system has to be revamped to take care of common acute infections (Table 2.4). UNESCO and WHO have several child welfare programs. The prevention of malnutrition in elderly isolated people needs special attention, including family and social levels.

Table 2.4 Interventions to prevent malnutrition

A. Nutrition for specific intervention:
   1. Promoting breastfeeding 6–24 months
   2. Complementary feeding after 6 months of age
   3. Diversity in diet to increase micronutrient
   4. Supplementing micronutrient (iron, folate) to pregnant women and to young children (vitamin A, iron, zinc in deficient areas)
   5. Children with diarrhea: zinc 10–20 m daily for 2 weeks. Improve water sanitation, hygiene
   6. Fortification of food

B. Nutrition-sensitive intervention:
   1. Credit and microfinance to needy persons
   2. Postharvesting food processing and preservation
   3. Vaccination
   4. Accessibility to health care
   5. Improve water sanitation, hygiene
   6. Preventing and treating acute viral infection
   7. Gender equality with empowerment in economy and education
   8. Social protection, cash transfer
   9. Control of vector-borne and water-borne diseases
   10. Birth spacing and pregnancy after 18 years of age
   11. Reduce heavy physical activity during pregnancy

CONCLUSIONS

Malnutrition is still prevalent, and the burden of stunting, wasted and underweight is highest in Asia followed by Africa. Asia is facing both undernutrition and overweight problems. It is important to eliminate malnutrition to avoid undernutrition-related death, infection and poor immunity on one hand, and overnutrition, hypertension, metabolic syndrome, coronary artery disease and diabetes mellitus on the other. In the recent era, undernutrition in chronic diseases and in intensive care setting is quite common; attention to these issues is important for survival and better functional recovery.

REFERENCES

Bembenek, J. P., Karlinski, M., Niewada, M., Kurkowska-Jastrzębska, I., Członkowska, A. 2018. Measurement of nutritional status using body mass index, waist-to-hip ratio, and waist circumference to predict treatment outcome in females and males with acute first-ever ischemic stroke. *Journal of Stroke and Cerebrovascular Diseases: The Official Journal of National Stroke Association* 27(1):132–139.

Bhutta, Z. A., Das, J. K., Rizvi, A., et al. 2013. Evidence-based interventions for improvement of maternal and child nutrition: What can be done and at what cost? *Lancet (London, England)* 382(9890):452–477.

Black, R. E., Allen, L. H., Bhutta, Z. A., Caulfield, L. E., de Onis, M., Ezzati, M., Mathers, C., Rivera, J., Maternal and Child Undernutrition Study Group. 2008. Maternal and child undernutrition: Global and regional exposures and health consequences. *Lancet (London, England)* 371(9608):243–260.

Brock, J. F., Autret, M., World Health Organization. 1952. *Kwashiorkor in Africa*. World Health Organization.

Caulfield, L. E., de Onis, M., Blössner, M., Black, R. E. 2004. Undernutrition as an underlying cause of child deaths associated with diarrhea, pneumonia, malaria, and measles. *The American Journal of Clinical Nutrition* 80(1):193–198.

Coats, D., Shelton-Dodge, K., Ou, K., et al. 2012. Thiamine deficiency in Cambodian infants with and without beriberi. *The Journal of Pediatrics* 161(5):843–847.

Flier J. S., & Maratos-Flier E. 2018. Pathobiology of obesity. Jameson J, & Fauci A. S., & Kasper D. L., & Hauser S. L., & Longo D. L., & Loscalzo J. (Eds.), *Harrison's Principles of Internal Medicine*, 20e. McGraw-Hill. https://accessmedicine.mhmedical.com/content.aspx?bookid=2129&sectionid=192288213.

Ghai, O. P., Paul, V. K., Bagga, A. 2013. *Nutrition, Ghai Essential Pediatrics*. 8th Edition. New Delhi, India: CBS.

Hailemariam, B., Landman, J. P., Jackson, A. A. 1985. Thiamin status in normal and malnourished children in Jamaica. *The British Journal of Nutrition* 53(3):477–483.

India State-Level Disease Burden Initiative CGF Collaborators. 2020. Mapping of variations in child stunting, wasting and underweight within the states of India: The Global Burden of Disease Study 2000–2017. *EClinicalMedicine 22*:100317. DOI: 10.1016/j.eclinm.2020.100317.

India State-Level Disease Burden Initiative Malnutrition Collaborators. 2019. The burden of child and maternal malnutrition and trends in its indicators in the states of India: The Global Burden of Disease Study 1990–2017. *The Lancet. Child & Adolescent Health* 3(12):855–870.

Jameson, L. J., Fauci, A. S., Kasper, D. L., Hauser, S. L., Longo, D. L., Loscalzo, J. 2018. *Malnutrition and Nutritional Assessment*. 20th Edition. Harrison's Principles of Internal Medicine. New York: Jensen, G.L. McGraw Hill Education.

Kauffman, G., Coats, D., Seab, S., Topazian, M. D., Fischer, P. R. 2011. Thiamine deficiency in ill children. *The American Journal of Clinical Nutrition* 94(2), 616–617.

Khounnorath, S., Chamberlain, K., Taylor, A. M., et al. 2011. Clinically unapparent infantile thiamin deficiency in Vientiane, Laos. *PLoS Neglected Tropical Diseases* 5(2): e969.

Kliegman, R. M., Stanton, B. M. D., Geme, J. S., Schor, N. F., 2019. *Nelsons Text book of Pediatrics*. Elsevier Health Sciences, Philadelphia, PA.

Lönnroth, K., Williams, B. G., Cegielski, P., Dye, C. 2010. A consistent log-linear relationship between tuberculosis incidence and body mass index. *International Journal of Epidemiology 39*(1): 149–155.

Müller, O., Krawinkel, M. 2005. Malnutrition and health in developing countries. *CMAJ: Canadian Medical Association Journal* 173(3), 279–286.

Nobelstiftelsen: Les Prix Nobel en 1964. Stockholm: Imprimerie Royale, P.A. Norstedt & Söner, 1965.

Pandian, J. D., Jyotsna, R., Singh, R., et al. 2011. Premorbid nutrition and short term outcome of stroke: A multicentre study from India. *Journal of Neurology, Neurosurgery, and Psychiatry 82*(10): 1087–1092.

Pulcini, C. D., Zettle, S., Srinath, A. 2016. Refeeding syndrome. *Pediatrics in Review* 37(12):516–523.

Seligman, H. K., Laraia, B. A., Kushel, M. B. 2010. Food insecurity is associated with chronic disease among low-income NHANES participants. *The Journal of Nutrition* 140(2):304–310.

Sinha, P., Davis, J., Saag, L., et al. 2019. Undernutrition and tuberculosis: Public health implications. *The Journal of Infectious Diseases 219*(9):1356–1363.

Tang, C. M., Rolfe, M., Wells, J. C., Cham, K. 1989. Outbreak of beri-beri in The Gambia. *Lancet (London, England) 2*(8656):206–207.

UNICEF-WHO-World Bank: Joint Child Malnutrition Estimates. 2020 edition – interactive dashboard, https://data.unicef.org/resources/joint-child-malnutrition-estimates-interactive-dashboard-2020/.

Van Rie, A., Westreich, D., Sanne, I. 2011. Tuberculosis in patients receiving antiretroviral treatment: Incidence, risk factors, and prevention strategies. *Journal of Acquired Immune Deficiency Syndromes (1999) 56*(4): 349–355.

Walton, E., Allen, S. 2011. Malnutrition in developing countries. *Paediatrics and Child Health 21*(9):418–424.

Waterlow, J. C., Payne, P. R. 1975. The protein gap. *Nature 258*:113–117.

Waterlow, J. C., Stephen, J. M. L. (eds). 1957. Human protein requirements and their fulfillment in practice. *Proceedings of a Conference in Princeton, United States (1955) Sponsored Jointly by the Food and Agricultural Organization of the United Nations (F.A.O.), World Health Organization (W.H.O.), and Josiah Macy Jr. Foundation*, New York. Bristol, John Wright and Sons.

Williams, C. D. 1935. Kwashiorkor: A nutritional disease of children associated with a maize diet. *The Lancet 226*(5855):1151–1152.

WHO. 1999. *Management of Severe Malnutrition: A Manual for Physicians and Other Senior Health Workers*. Geneva: The Organization.

WHO. 2020a. Malnutrition, https://www.who.int/news-room/fact-sheets/detail/malnutrition.

WHO. 2020b. Nutrition, https://www.who.int/nutrition/topics/2_background/en/.

3

Thiamine deficiency neurological disorders

INTRODUCTION

Thiamine (vitamin B1) is an essential water-soluble sulfur-containing vitamin belonging to vitamin B complex group. Since there is no endogenous synthesis, body store is limited to 30 mg, which is sufficient only for 9–18 days. A constant supply of thiamine is therefore essential. The clinical picture of thiamine deficiency is quite variable, and there are no easily available laboratory tests; therefore, thiamine deficiency is often unrecognized or diagnosed late. Thiamine deficiency is more common in low-income countries because of dietary deficiency and lack of food fortification. About 90% of world's rice is consumed in Asian countries, and polished rice with high-carbohydrate diet renders the population in this region vulnerable to thiamine deficiency. In the developed countries, thiamine deficiency also occurs because of food faddism, depression, isolation, alcoholism and critical illness. Thiamine deficiency, if untreated, results in high mortality especially in children, and if treated late, it results in sequelae. Early clinical suspicion and prompt management is the key for good outcome of thiamine deficiency.

HISTORY

Beriberi-like illness has been reported as early as 2600 BC in Chinese literature. The term "beriberi" means *weak* or *I cannot* in Sinhalese language. In the third century, there is a reference to beriberi-like illness characterized by leg weakness, numbness and swelling of feet. In 1580, a Portuguese priest reported beriberi from East

Indies Portuguese colony; the patient was unaware of sandals coming out from his feet. Even before the establishment of etiology, the disease was subtyped as affecting the nervous system manifesting with dropsy, and in the final stage with pounding heart and death. In 1880, beriberi-like illness was reported in Dutch troops in Indonesia. Eijkman, a Dutch physician, was investigating beriberi in chicks to explore the microbiological basis. He noted paralysis in control chicks. These chicks surprisingly improved when their diet was changed from polished rice to ordinary brown rice due to logistic reasons. Eijkman believed that the disease was due to a nutrient in rice which was lost while polishing (Eijkman, 1898). It is a pity that Eijkman's hypothesis was drowned in Industrial Revolution in Europe especially due to rice industry. The work of Eijkman was carried on by Grijns who confirmed the nutritional basis of beriberi (Grijns, 1935). Pure crystals of nutrient were isolated in 1926 by Jansen and Donath (1926). The chemical structure was confirmed by Robert Williams and was named thiamine in 1935, and its chemical production started in 1936 (Williams and Cline, 1936). In 1929, Eijkman and Hopkins were awarded the Nobel Prize (Carpenter, 2012; Figure 3.1).

The contribution of Japanese naval doctor Takaki Kanehiro in 1884 was unique. He studied 376 Japanese sailors: 169 of whom developed beriberi and 25 died. He sent another mission to the same destination (Hawaii) with changed diet, including meat, fish, rice and beans in contrast to diet of rice only in the earlier expedition. This time, there were only 14 patients with mild beriberi

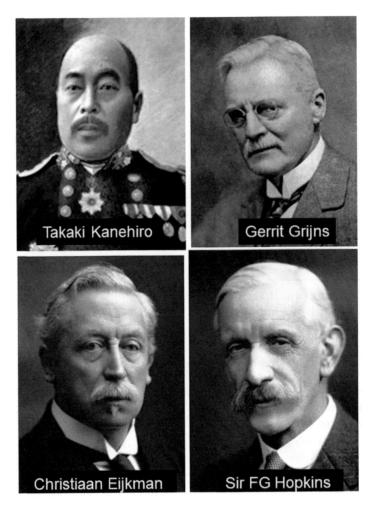

Figure 3.1 Photograph of some scientists who have worked in the discovery of thiamine. In 1929, Christiaan Eijkman and Sir FG Hopkins were awarded the Nobel Prize in physiology or medicine.

and there was no death (Sugiyama and Seita, 2012). These findings were ignored till 1905 when Takaki became the Baron. As a reward for eliminating beriberi from Japanese Navy, he was named as *Barley Baron*. Following his suggestion, sailors were advised to eat barley to prevent beriberi. He was honored after his death by naming the Takaki promontory in Antarctica on his name, the only such peninsula named after a Japanese.

Thiamine is a colorless organosulfur compound, and it consists of an aminopyrimidine and a thiazolium ring linked by a methylene bridge. The thiazole is substituted with methyl and hydroxyethyl side chains. Thiamine is soluble in water, glycerol and methanol, and is stable at acidic pH and frozen storage, but unstable in alkaline pH, UV light, gamma radiation and heat. There are five known

natural thiamine phosphate derivatives: thiamine monophosphate (TMP), thiamine diphosphate (TDP), thiamine triphosphate (TTP), adenosine thiamine triphosphate (ATTP) and adenosine thiamine diphosphate (ATDP) (Figure 3.2). The role of TDP as a coenzyme in various intracellular reactions is well characterized. The non-coenzyme action of thiamine and its derivatives has been recently recognized in which thiamine and its derivatives bind to a number of recently identified proteins that do not involve the catalytic action.

PATHOPHYSIOLOGY

Daily requirement of thiamine is 1.2 mg in adult males and 1.1 mg in females. The requirement of thiamine increases during pregnancy

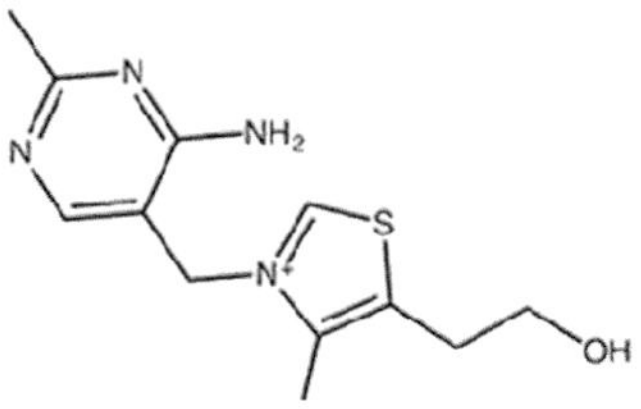

Thiamine (T)

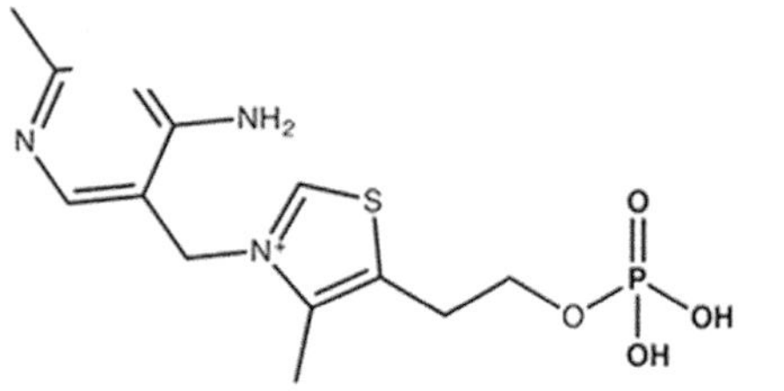

Thiamine monophosphate (TMP)

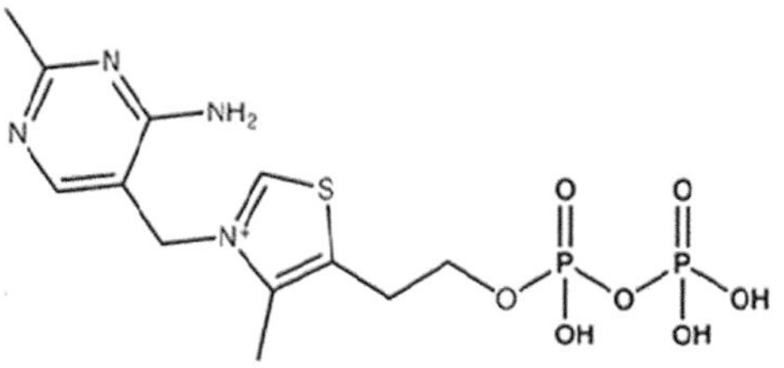

Thiamine diphosphate (TDP)

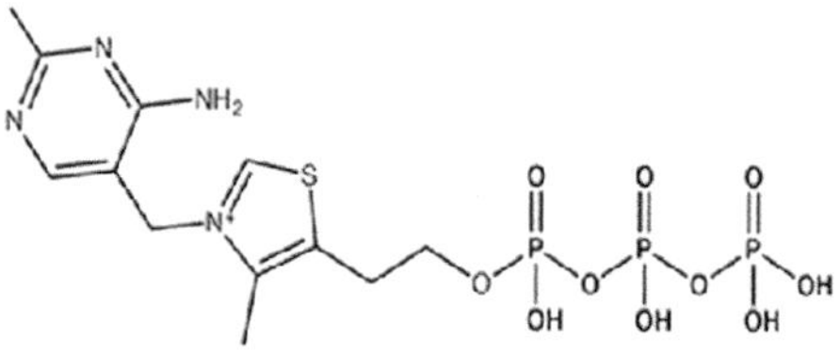

Thiamine triphosphate (TTP)

Figure 3.2 Structures of thiamine and its derivative.

(1.4 mg/day) and lactation (1.5 mg/day). Thiamine requirement depends on the carbohydrate intake of 0.5 mg/1000 calories. Age-wise requirement of thiamine is presented in Table 3.1. There is no upper limit of thiamine, and there is no adverse effect of high dose. Thiamine is found in whole grains, yeast, legumes, nuts and meat (Table 3.2). Thiamine is absorbed from the jejunum. Following hydrolysis of thiamine pyrophosphate, it dissociates to free thiamine. If the concentration of free thiamine is more than 1 µM in the intestinal lumen, it enters the enterocyte through diffusion. In the lower gastrointestinal tract, thiamine is

Table 3.1 Daily requirement of thiamine

Age group	Thiamine requirement (mg/day)
0–6 Months	0.2
7–12 Months	0.3
1–3 Years	0.5
4–6 Years	0.6
7–9 Years	0.9
Adult male	1.2
Adult female	1.1
Pregnancy	1.4
Lactation	1.5

Table 3.2 Dietary sources of thiamine

Source	Thiamine mg/100 gm
A. Cereals	
Wheat – whole grain	0.41
Whole flour	0.13
Rice-brown	0.33
Polished	0.08
Parboiled	0.22
Maize	0.18
Oatmeal	0.63
Sorghum	0.15
Pasta	0.13
B. Pulses, seeds, nuts	
Chickpeas	0.40
Soybeans	
Dry whole seed	1.03
Flour	0.77
Raw ground nut	0.84
Peas	0.77
Lentils	0.50
C. Tubers	
Potato	0.10
Raw sugar	0.09

(Continued)

Table 3.2 (*Continued*) Dietary sources of thiamine

Source	Thiamine mg/100 gm
D. Nonvegetarian diet	
Pork	0.42
Poultry	0.10
Liver-pork	0.40
Beef	0.07
Egg	0.12
E. Milk, milk product	
Milk	0.01
Cheese	0.02–0.06
F. Vegetables	
Cassava leaves	0.16
Cauliflower	0.11
Spinach	0.11
Carrot/cabbage/tomato	0.06
G. Fruits	
Breadfruit	0.09
Orange/pineapple	0.08
Banana	0.05
Apple/apricot/lemon	0.04
H. Others	
Brown yeast	15.6

absorbed through thiamine transporter 1, which is an ATP-dependent active process. After absorption, thiamine is converted to TMP by thiamine phosphokinase 1, and then crosses the basal lamina to enter the bloodstream. About 90% of thiamine is present in the red blood cell and white blood cell. Free thymine in the cell is phosphorylated (monophosphate, diphosphate or triphosphate). TDP is metabolically active and is used as a cofactor for many enzyme processes such as pyruvate dehydrogenase, α-ketoglutarate dehydrogenase complex, branched-chain α-ketoacid dehydrogenase complex and α-transketolase. α-Ketoglutarate dehydrogenase is the most sensitive to thiamine deficiency; therefore in its absence, there is reduced energy metabolism, and increased glutamate and free radical formation in mitochondria. Thiamine mainly circulates in the body through the red blood cell and is delivered to the metabolically active organs such as heart, brain, liver, pancreas and muscles.

The cellular uptake of thymine is mediated by two high-affinity carriers: (a) thiamine transporter 1 (THTR1) encoded by SLC19A2 and (b) thiamine transporter 2 (THTR2) encoded by SLC19A3. These transporters are expressed maximally in the intestine and also in the liver, leukocytes, breast, pancreas and kidney. Inside the cell, thiamine is rapidly phosphorylated to thiamine pyrophosphate through thiamine pyrophosphokinase. Thiamine pyrophosphate may be converted to TMP, TDP and TTP. These phosphorylated thiamines may as well be dephosphorylated. TDP is the most active metabolically, and about 90% of thiamine is in TDP form. In the brain, 10% of thiamine is in the form of TTP, which helps in membrane excitability and nerve conduction by modulating sodium channels. Inside the cell, thiamine acts at the cytosol, mitochondria and peroxisome in various enzymatic reactions.

Cytosol: In the cytosol, thiamine pyrophosphate acts as a cofactor in transketolase enzyme pathway. Transketolase is the key enzyme for nonoxidative pentose phosphate pathway. Pentose monophosphate pathway generates (a) nicotinamide adenosine dinucleotide phosphate (NADPH), which is a cosubstrate for fatty acid biosynthesis as well as antioxidant, and (b) ribose, which is needed for nucleic acid synthesis especially in high proliferating tissues. Impairment of cytosolic functions of thiamine therefore may result in oxidative stress and cell damage, reduced cell proliferation and reduced fatty acid synthesis.

Mitochondria: About 90% of cytosolic TPP is transferred to the mitochondria by mitochondrial TPP transporter, which is regulated by SLC25A19 gene. In the mitochondria, TPP acts in three important enzymatic processes as a cofactor: (a) pyruvate dehydrogenase, (b) α-ketoglutarate dehydrogenase and (c) branched-chain α-ketoacid dehydrogenase. Pyruvate dehydrogenase converts pyruvate to acetyl CoA with the help of TPP. Acetyl CoA enters into the Krebs cycle for energy production. Pyruvate dehydrogenase is the key enzyme and helps in choosing between glycolytic and fatty acid pathways for energy production. In the absence of thiamine, glucose is converted to pyruvate but pyruvate is not converted to acetyl CoA, resulting in the accumulation of pyruvate leading to lactic acidosis and energy depletion. In severe thiamine deficiency, neonates and children may develop fatal lactic acidosis and milder deficiency may result in spasticity, seizure and cognitive decline. α-Ketoglutarate dehydrogenase complex is another TPP-dependent enzyme, which converts α-ketoglutarate to succinyl CoA in Krebs cycle. During this reaction, NADPH is formed. Impairment in this reaction results in a reduction in energy and NADPH production and an increase in glutamate, resulting in oxidative stress and excitotoxicity. Branched-chain α-ketoglutarate dehydrogenase complex is another TPP-dependent enzyme, which converts the branched-chain α-ketoacids to branched-chain acetyl CoA. These amino acids are needed for protein synthesis and energy production in citric acid cycle. Impaired function of this enzyme results in reduced protein synthesis and energy production.

Peroxisomes: Peroxisomes help in the catabolism of hydrogen peroxide and shortening of long-chain fatty acids. In the peroxisomes, TPP-dependent enzyme 2-hydroxy acetyl CoA lyase 1 (HACL1) catalyzes very long-chain fatty acids. An inability to cleave very long-chain fatty acid and phytanic acid results in increased triglyceride levels. Accumulation of these substances leads to cerebellar ataxia, peripheral neuropathy, hearing loss, anosmia, cardiac dysfunction and epiphyseal dysplasia. In humans, the mammillary body, thalamus and hypothalamus are vulnerable to thiamine deficiency in adults, whereas in children, mammillary bodies and basal ganglia are especially vulnerable (Dhir et al., 2019). The functions of thiamine are shown in Figure 3.3.

Thiamine deficiency

Thiamine deficiency is rare in healthy individuals with normal food intake. Thiamine deficiency occurs in the regions where diet mainly comprises starchy carbohydrate-rich food, polished rice and cassava, consuming thiamine antagonist (betel nut, raw fish, African raw silk worm larvae), and with *Clostridium botulinum* infection (Table 3.3). Critically ill patients, prolonged intravenous dextrose infusion, infant and

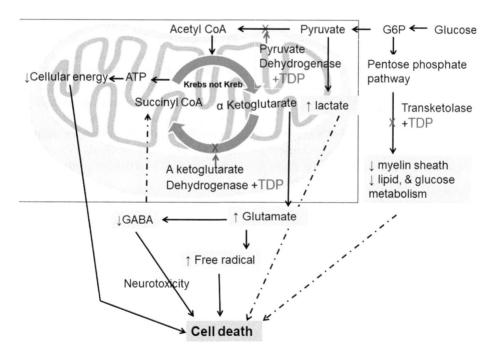

Figure 3.3 Schematic diagram shows the functions of thiamine. (1) Thiamine diphosphate (TDP) works as a cofactor with pyruvate dehydrogenase enzyme to convert pyruvate to acetyl CoA. Lack of this reaction will result in an increased lactate and a reduced supply of acetyl CoA to Krebs cycle. (2) In the Krebs cycle, TDP acts as a cofactor with α-ketoglutarate dehydrogenase, which converts α-ketoglutarate to succinyl CoA. Impairment of this function will lead to increased glutamate and oxidative stress. (3) In the pentose phosphate pathway, TDP acts as a cofactor with transketolase.

Table 3.3 Causes of thiamine deficiency

A. Increased demand
  Carbohydrate-rich diet
  Pregnancy
  Lactation
  Hyperthyroidism
  Fever
  Cancer
  Intensive care unit
  Exercise
B. Increased depletion
  Diarrhea
  Diuretics
  Dialysis
  Hyperemesis gravidarum
  Hyperthyroidism
C. Reduced absorption
  Chronic intestinal diseases
  Alcoholism
  Malnutrition
  Gastrointestinal bypass surgery
  Malabsorption due to celiac disease, Crohn's
    disease, sprue
D. Dietary deficiency and intake thiamine
  antagonist
E. Genetic
  Inactivation of thiamine transporter

children on formula feed, and severe malnutrition may also be associated with thiamine deficiency. Prolonged starvation, alcoholism, bariatric surgery, dialysis, food faddism, anorexia nervosa, depression and isolation may also result in thiamine deficiency (Table 3.4).

CLINICAL MANIFESTATIONS OF THIAMINE DEFICIENCY

Thiamine deficiency primarily results in neurological, cardiac and gastrointestinal manifestations (Table 3.5; Figure 3.4).

NEUROLOGICAL MANIFESTATIONS OF THIAMINE DEFICIENCY

The neurological manifestations of thiamine deficiency are mainly:

1. Wernicke encephalopathy (WE) or Wernicke–Korsakoff syndrome
2. Beriberi.

Wernicke encephalopathy

WE is a common neuropsychiatric manifestation of thiamine deficiency. In 1881, Wernicke described three patients characterized by confusion, stumbling gait and bilateral VIth cranial nerve palsy with normal pupillary reflex (Kulkarni et al., 2005). Subsequently, Korsakoff described alcoholic patients with memory impairment. Murawieff in 1897 described the relationship of WE with Korsakoff psychosis (Victor, 1976). WE is characterized by a triad of ocular, cerebellar and

Table 3.4 Antithiamine factors

	Source	Mechanism
A. Thiamine antagonist		
Hemin	Animal tissue	Absorption or digestion
Flavonoids	Tea, fruits, vegetables, buck wheat plants	
Polyphenols	Tea, coffee, betel nuts, red cabbage, blueberries, red currant, red beets, oils seeds	
B. Thiaminase		
Type I	Raw or fermented fish, shell fish, ferns, some bacteria	Alters thiamine structure
Type II	Certain bacteria	↓Biological activity of thiamine

Table 3.5 Involvement of different organs in thiamine deficiency and its clinical manifestations

Organ involved	Clinical manifestation
A. Nervous system	
Central	Encephalopathy, ataxia, ophthalmoplegia, amblyopia, dementia, autonomic dysfunction
Peripheral	Peripheral neuropathy – symmetrical sensory, motor and autonomic
B. Cardiovascular	Cardiomegaly, congestive heart failure
C. Gastrointestinal	Constipation, abdominal distension, anorexia, nausea, vomiting

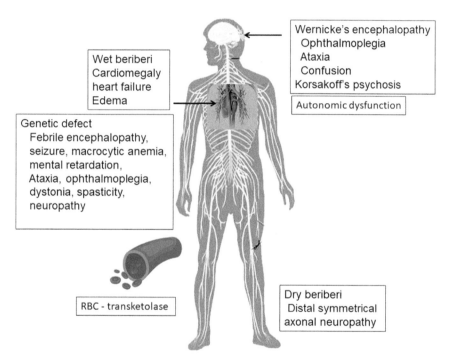

Wet beriberi
Cardiomegaly
heart failure
Edema

Wernicke's encephalopathy
Ophthalmoplegia
Ataxia
Confusion
Korsakoff's psychosis

Autonomic dysfunction

Genetic defect
Febrile encephalopathy,
seizure, macrocytic anemia,
mental retardation,
Ataxia, ophthalmoplegia,
dystonia, spasticity,
neuropathy

RBC - transketolase

Dry beriberi
Distal symmetrical
axonal neuropathy

Figure 3.4 Schematic diagram shows clinical manifestations of thiamine deficiency.

mental changes. The ocular symptoms in order of frequency are nystagmus, bilateral VIth nerve palsy and conjugate gaze palsy. The pupillary reflex is normal, and involvement of IIIrd and IVth cranial nerves is uncommon. There may be retinal hemorrhage. Ataxia is due to vestibular, cerebellar and peripheral nerve involvement. Vestibular dysfunction is evidenced by a universal impaired caloric response. The patient has global confusional state characterized by apathy, insomnia, hallucination, disorientation, lethargy and drowsiness. Stupor and coma occur in less than 4% of patients. The patients have tachycardia, glossitis, angular cheilitis and skin changes. Two-thirds of patients have fatty liver, and 17% may have cirrhosis of liver. The complete triad of WE is found in 16% of patients only (Torvik, 1991). Therefore, it is frequently underdiagnosed. Only one-third of alcoholic and 6% of nonalcoholic WE are diagnosed during life (Day and del Campo, 2014; Galvin et al., 2010). The clinical features of WE are presented in Table 3.6. In a study on 17 patients with nonalcoholic WE, the delay in diagnosis ranged between 0 and 273 days (Yin et al., 2019). In the medical literature, among 600 patients on nonalcoholic WE, the following clinical settings were observed: malignancy,

Table 3.6 Clinical features of Wernicke encephalopathy

A. Acute stage
Classical features:
Mental changes, ophthalmoplegia, ataxia
Uncommon features:
Hallucination, behavioral abnormality, seizure, stupor or coma, tachycardia, hypotension, visual disturbance, hearing loss, papilledema, hypothermia.
B. Late features
Spasticity, hyperthermia, movement disorder – chorea, coma

chemotherapy especially erbulozole, gastrointestinal disease or surgery, hyperemesis gravidarum, fasting, starvation, malnutrition, unbalanced diet and bariatric surgery (Galvin et al., 2010). Psychiatric diseases and food faddism are also important causes of thiamine deficiency (Yin et al., 2019). In these situations, therefore, there should be a high index of suspicion. In a systematic review of autopsy studies on 256 WE, a complete triad was present in 8.2%, altered sensorium in 53%, memory impairment in 23.4%, cerebellar sign in 25.4%, eye sign in 24.2% and seizure in 3.1% (Galvin et al., 2010). In another autopsy study on 106 alcoholic WE, the sensitivity was highest (85%) if two out of four components (dietary deficiency, eye sign, cerebellar signs and memory/altered sensorium) were present. Therefore, it is recommended to consider WE if two out of four above-mentioned symptoms or signs are present (Galvin et al., 2010). The clinical features are similar in alcoholic and nonalcoholic WE; however, the alcoholic WE has slower onset and more frequently has neurological symptoms and signs (Table 3.7).

Neuropathology

There are three stages of WE: acute, subacute and chronic. Sometime there may be acute or chronic in the patients with repeated episodes of WE (Harper and Butterworth, 2002). The autopsy findings in WE depend on the stage of the disease. In the early stage, there are symmetrical grayish congested areas with punctate hemorrhages, which are seen in medial thalamus and dorsolateral thalamus in nearly all the patients with WE. About 50% patients have these changes in periaqueductal gray matter, mammillary bodies and medial thalamus (Figure 3.5). About 30% of patients may have these changes in cerebellar vermis. Other areas involved are cranial nerve nuclei, red nuclei, dentate nucleus, reticular formation and cerebral cortex. There is no capillary proliferation or macrophage infiltration. In the late stage, there is swelling of astrocytes, reduced myelin, minimal neuronal loss gliosis and astrocytosis. The acute on chronic WE shows both the above mentioned pathological changes (Harper and Butterworth, 2002; Olds et al., 2014). The kinetics of neuropathological changes following thiamine deficiency are shown in Figure 3.6.

Clinicopathological correlation: The mammillary body and medial thalamic involvement result in memory impairment, psychosis and behavioral abnormality. Optic nerve edema results in visual loss, and cerebellar involvement results in ataxia. In the late stage of WE, cortical involvement may result in spastic weakness, hypothalamic involvement in refractory hypothermia and basal ganglia involvement in choreiform movement and rigidity.

Computerized tomography and magnetic resonance imaging: CT is usually normal in the acute stage of WE, but may show hypodensity in periaqueductal gray (PAG) and medial part of the

Table 3.7 Comparison of clinical features between alcoholic and nonalcoholic Wernicke encephalopathy

	Alcoholic (N=102)	Nonalcoholic (N=116)
Triad of WE	55 (53.9%)	39 (33.6%)
Altered sensorium	77 (75.5%)	78 (68.2%)
Memory impairment	9 (8.8%)	13 (11.2%)
Cerebellar signs	82 (80.4%)	58 (50%)
Eye signs	92 (98.2%)	82 (70.7%)
Mechanical ventilation	7 (6.9%)	36 (31%)
Deficient diet	4 (3.9%)	96 (82.8%)

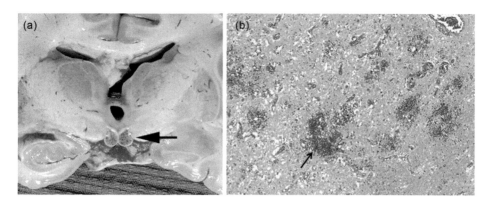

Figure 3.5 Pathological changes of a patient with Wernicke encephalopathy. (a) Macroscopic picture of brain shows hemorrhagic changes in the mammillary bodies (arrow) and periventricular area. (b) Microscopic section of the mammillary bodies showing microhemorrhage (arrow), prominent microvascular proliferation and endothelial swelling (Hematoxylin and Eosin×100). With permission from rOlds, K., Langlois, N. E., Blumbergs, P., Byard, R. W. 2014. The pathological features of Wernicke encephalopathy. *Forensic Science, Medicine, and Pathology 10*(3):466–468.

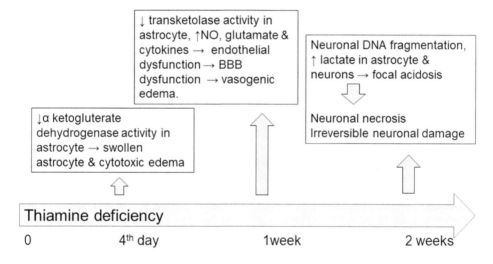

Figure 3.6 The pathophysiological changes of brain at different time points of thiamine deficiency.

thalamus. MRI has a sensitivity of 53% and a specificity of 93% in the diagnosis of WE; therefore, it has been considered as a diagnostic test (Sechi and Serra, 2007; Ota et al., 2020). MRI shows more frequently abnormal results in nonalcoholics (97.6%) than in alcoholics (63.4%) on conventional MRI sequences. Diffusion weighted image (DWI) and fluid attenuation inversion recovery (FLAIR) sequences are more sensitive. Classically, there is an involvement of thalamus (symmetrical, bilateral), hypothalamus, mammillary body, PAG matter and floor of the fourth ventricle (Figures 3.7 and 3.8). In a study, the frequency of involvement of these areas is as follows: around the third ventricle in 80%, PAG matter in 59%, mammillary body in 45%, tectal plate in 36%, cranial nerve nuclei in 18%, floor of the 4th ventricle in 7%, cerebellum in 5%, vermis in 4%, dentate nuclei in 1.8%, and pre- and post-central cortex in 1.8% patients. Contrast enhancement of mammillary body, tectal plate, PAG matter and cranial nerve nuclei is seen in 63% (Zuccoli et al., 2009). Cranial nerve nuclei involvement is a feature of nonalcoholic WE. In children, putaminal involvement is typical and is attributed to high thiamine-dependent metabolism (Zuccoli et al., 2010). FLAIR sequence is more sensitive and accurate than T2 sequence in detecting the abnormalities in WE because

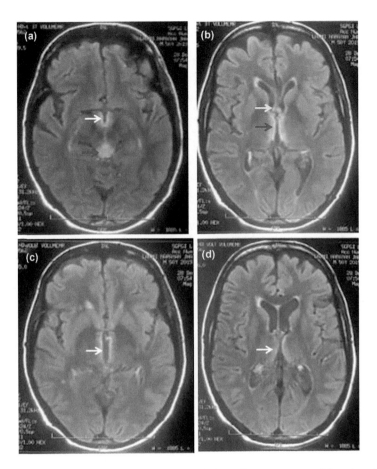

Figure 3.7 MRI in FLAIR sequence of Wernicke encephalopathy. A 61-year-old male addicted to alcohol presented with ataxia and confusion, and improved on the third day following IV thiamine treatment of 300 mg 8 hourly. His MRI shows (a) hyperintensities in mammillary bodies bilaterally (white arrow) and periaqueductal gray matters (red arrow), (b) Fornix (yellow arrow) and medial thalamus (red arrow), (c) periventricular (third ventricle) region (white arrow) and (d) medial thalamus (white arrow).

CSF appears black in FLAIR sequence and periventricular hyperintensity is clearly seen. DWI is also sensitive for detecting cytotoxic edema and differentiating from vasogenic edema. On DWI sequence, cytotoxic edema appears hyperintense but apparent diffusion coefficient (ADC) values are low; however in vasogenic edema, DWI is hyperintense with high ADC value. In acute WE, DWI may reveal the underlying pathological changes of brain. In 50% of patients with WE, there may be contrast enhancement and sometimes enhancement of mammillary body may be the only finding (Mascalchi et al., 1999). Magnetic spectroscopy reveals a reduced NAA/creatine ratio, suggesting an impairment of neuronal metabolism, and an increased lactate peak, suggesting glycolysis (Figure 3.9). Improvement in NAA/creatine ratio

parallels a clinical improvement (Murata et al., 2001). The classical MRI lesions in WE should be differentiated from Japanese encephalitis (JE), atypical Creutzfeldt–Jakob disease, deep cerebral venous thrombosis, paramedian thalamic syndrome and top of basilar syndrome. The distinguishing features of WE are mammillary body, and symmetric tectal and PAG involvement. The MRI lesion in metronidazole encephalopathy may simulate WE and is attributed to a reduced conversion of thiamine to its active analogue (Zuccoli et al., 2009).

In a study on six infants with thiamine deficiency, MRI revealed a bilateral symmetrical hyperintensity in periaqueductal area, basal ganglia and thalami in T2-, FLAIR- and proton-attenuated sequences. Five patients had mammillary

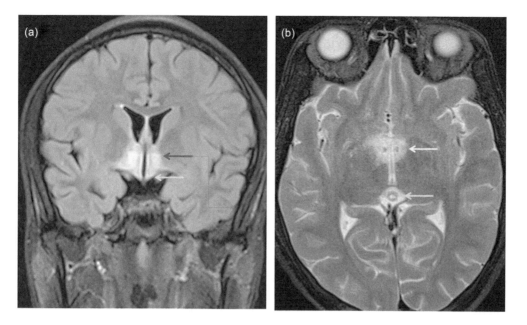

Figure 3.8 A 56-year-old alcoholic male with Wernicke encephalopathy. (a) Coronal FLAIR image shows hyperintensities in mammillary bilaterally bodies (yellow arrow) and periaqueductal gray matters (red arrow). (b) Axial T2FS showed the T2 hyperintensities in periaqueductal gray matters and minimal affection of antero-medial thalami. (Courtesy Dr D Baruah, Associate Professor, Tezpur Medical College, Assam.)

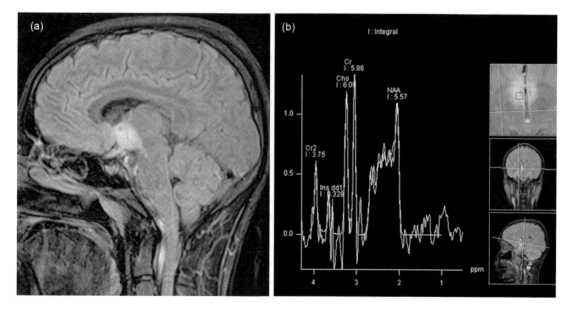

Figure 3.9 A 17-year-old boy, chronic alcoholic with Wernicke encephalopathy. (a) Sagittal FLAIR image showed the hyperintensity of hypothalamus. (b) Low TE (30) MR spectroscopy showed minimally raised choline peak with a reduction of NAA. (Courtesy Dr D Baruah, Associate Professor, Tezpur Medical College, Assam.)

Table 3.8 Thiamine biomarkers and thiamine status

Biomarkers	Thiamine	TMP	TDP	ETK activity
Specimen	Plasma	Plasma	Blood/RBC	Washed RBC
Indicator of thiamine status	Recent intake	Recent intake	Bioactive thiamine	Functional activity
Limitation	Do not indicate thiamine status	Do not indicate thiamine status	Unstable, needs expertise	Not widely available

body, three had brainstem involvement, and all had frontal, cortical and subcortical involvement. MR spectroscopy revealed the lactate doublet in periaqueductal area. After 2–5 months, only one child had normal MRI and others had residual damage. Clinically, only one child improved completely, and the remaining children had developmental delay, dysphagia and ataxia (Kornreich et al., 2005).

Laboratory tests: Whole-blood TDP measurement using HPLC is the most practical method. Measurement of ETK is sensitive, but is not widely available. Blood in EDTA, amber-colored vial is collected and frozen till analyzed. The normal TDP level in adults is 70–180 nM/l, but a normal value does not exclude WE (Table 3.8).

Treatment

The patient with suspected WE should be treated with thiamine of 200 mg IV 8 hourly before starting IV glucose. Thiamine is dissolved in 100 ml saline and infused in 30 min. Half-life of thymine is 96 min; hence, 2–3 dosages daily are recommended. In alcoholic patients, the dose of thiamine is 500 mg 8 hourly. This treatment is continued for 2–3 days or till improvement ceases. Those resistant to thiamine, a magnesium deficiency should be checked and corrected. After the initial improvement, the patient should be treated with 200 mg thiamine daily for 3–5 days to replenish the body store depending on the severity of thiamine deficiency. Intravenous regimen is followed by oral supplementation indefinitely (Thomson et al., 2012; NICE, 2011; Sechi and Serra, 2007).

Outcome and recovery pattern of WE

Death in WE per se occurs in 15%–20% of patients. In the remaining patients, the death may be due to alcohol and alcohol-withdrawal cardiac complications. Alcohol is associated with prolonged QT interval, cardiac failure and sudden cardiac death (George et al., 2010). WE patients recover in a predictable manner following the treatment. The ocular symptoms improve within hours; VIth cranial nerve palsy improves completely within a week followed by ptosis and gaze paralysis. Vertical nystagmus improves by 2–3 months. Ataxia and vestibular dysfunction improve slowly over weeks to months. Ataxia clears in 40% of patients only. Global confusion starts improving in 1–2 weeks, and a complete recovery occurs in 15% of patients only. Once global confusion subsides, the memory impairment becomes apparent and persists in 85% of patients as Korsakoff psychosis (Sechi and Serra, 2007). In a study on 11 patients, 73% had, however, had a complete resolution of symptoms following 500 mg of thiamin daily for 3 days after a median duration of 92 h (Nishimoto et al., 2017).

Korsakoff syndrome

Korsakoff syndrome (KS) is defined as a disproportionate memory impairment in comparison with other cognitive functions due to thiamine deficiency as a sequel of WE (Kopelman, 1995). Korsakoff psychosis has two major components: (a) retrograde amnesia and (b) impaired ability to acquire new information due to anterograde amnesia. Confabulation is regarded as a typical symptom but not an essential prerequisite for the diagnosis of KS (Kopelman, 1995). These patients are conscious, alert, oriented and co-operative, but apathetic. These features help the patients with KS to differentiate from other psychiatric disorders. Anterograde amnesia is of varying severity in which registration is intact but retention is impaired; hence, the learning of new information and skill are grossly affected. The patient is therefore able to perform the habitual tasks only. Retrograde amnesia is relatively severe and may antedate the onset of illness by several years. Recent memory is impaired more than the remote. The other cognitive and behavioral abnormalities include impaired digital symbol task, calculation, block design, shifting task and concept formation. The patient may also have a lack of spontaneity and initiation. Two-third patients with KS may have lower limb weakness. Cranial nerve involvement is rare except vagus nerve resulting in dysphagia or dysphonia.

Neuropathology: The neuropathological findings are similar to WE but reveal chronic pathological changes. There may be a dilatation of the third and lateral ventricles. Petechiae seen in WE are replaced by brown- or tan-colored areas of gliosis and necrosis. In KS, mammillary bodies are invariably involved. The involvement of mammillary bodies, mammillothalamic tract and anterior thalamus is responsible for anterograde amnesia. Frontal lobe involvement is responsible for retrograde amnesia, apathy and emotional blunting (Kril et al., 1997; Brokate et al., 2003).

Treatment: Treatment of KS is similar to that of WE. Timely and adequate treatment of WE with thiamine may prevent the development of KS.

Prognosis: The prognosis of KS is not good; only 20% recover completely, 40% partially and another 40% have minimal or no improvement. The improvement starts after weeks of treatment and may continue for months to years.

BERIBERI

Beriberi refers to edema of legs and unsteadiness in walking. Beriberi is common in East Africa, East Asia and South America where rice is a staple diet. Low-protein, low-fat and high-carbohydrate meals result in beriberi. The causes of thiamine deficiency have been mentioned above. Beriberi has diverse presentations, and can be broadly categorized into wet beriberi, dry beriberi and mixed types. These disorders are also grouped as thiamine deficiency disorders (TDDs). The presentation of beriberi varies in different age groups.

Infantile beriberi: Infantile beriberi occurs in low-income countries in the infants who are on exclusive breastfeeding of thiamine-deficient mother (Whitfield et al., 2017; Allen, 2012). Infantile beriberi manifests with diverse clinical features, including heart failure, and central and peripheral nervous system involvement; therefore, it is also referred as "thiamine deficiency disorder" (TDD).

Infantile beriberi manifests before 4 months of age but not during the neonatal period. It manifests with varied clinical features such as irritability, refusal to feed, vomiting and tachypnea. Initially, the infant has a shrill cry, which is replaced by aphonia in later stage. The child may be dyspneic because of heart failure and may even be cyanosed. At times, infantile beriberi may be triggered by an infection, rendering the differentiation difficult. These infants have a rapid downhill course unless thiamine is corrected (Luxemburger et al., 2003). Beriberi may be misdiagnosed as malaria, typhoid or pneumonia, and the patient may die undiagnosed due to cardiogenic shock, lactic acidosis and multiorgan failure.

Beriberi in older infants and children: Beriberi in older infants and children may manifest with nystagmus, anorexia, ophthalmoplegia, bulging of fontanelle and altered sensorium (Wani et al., 2016; Harel et al., 2017). These patients are confused with meningoencephalitis. In older children and adolescences, beriberi manifests with neuropathic symptoms and signs such as tingling, numbness, paresthesia, pain, weakness and loss of reflexes.

Beriberi in adults: In the adults and children, dry beriberi refers to neuropathy. The patients may have pins and needles burning sensations in feet and hands with widespread sensory abnormalities, including legs, thigh, chest, forearm and occasionally lips. If untreated, the patient may develop foot drop and wrist drop, loss of tendon reflexes and muscle tenderness. The severely affected patients may also have deafness, as well as dysphonia and dysphagia due to the vagal nerve involvement (Duce et al., 2003; McCandless, 2009). The other cranial nerves are usually normal unless associated with WE. In beriberi, the neuropathy is usually subacute to chronic, but rarely it may be acute mimicking Guillain–Barre syndrome or acute flaccid paralysis. In a study on 13 patients with beriberi neuropathy, 11 had chronic and 2 had acute presentation. The underlying causes of beriberi were anorexia, recurrent vomiting and alcohol abuse. Twelve patients had weakness, six dysautonomia, four bulbar weakness and three nystagmus. Cerebrospinal fluid analysis was normal, and the nerve conduction study revealed sensory motor axonal neuropathy. Following thiamine treatment, 11 patients improved, 2 had sequelae and 1 died of pulmonary embolism (Saini et al., 2019). In another study, 7 out of 11 patients with dietary thiamine deficiency neuropathy had acute presentation (Koike et al., 2008).

Pathology of beriberi: In the early stage, there is segmental demyelination giving a beaded appearance, and in the late stage, there is evidence of axonal degeneration. Beriberi in alcoholic patients may have both segmental demyelination and primary axonal degeneration. The diverse pathology in alcoholic patients may be due to multiple etiologies of neuropathy. Nerve conduction studies reveal the features of axonal degeneration evidenced by marginal slowing of nerve conduction velocity, with reduced sensory nerve action potentials. Electromyography may reveal evidence of denervation and reinnervation in the distal muscles. Beriberi should be differentiated from other causes of neuropathy such as diabetes mellitus, toxic neuropathy and porphyria.

The patient with beriberi should be given a vitamin-rich high-calorie diet and thiamine of 5–25 mg orally thrice daily. A higher dose of thiamine (>50 mg/day) has no advantage (Whitfield et al., 2018). About 50% of patients with beriberi neuropathy improvement. The neuropathic symptoms in mildly affected patients improve within weeks, whereas it takes months to years in severely affected patients.

THE OTHER SYNDROMES POSSIBLY RELATED TO THIAMINE DEFICIENCY

The other syndromes possibly related to thiamine deficiency are as follows:

a. **Tropical ataxic neuropathy:** Tropical ataxic neuropathy is characterized by gait ataxia, bilateral optic atrophy and sensory polyneuropathy. This condition is primarily reported from Nigeria, Ghana and other West African countries. Tropical ataxic neuropathy is attributed to cassava consumption, which contains cyanogenic glycoside. These patients show an improvement with thiamine supplementation highlighting an etiological link (Monekosso et al., 1964; Adamolekun, 2011).
b. **Epidemic spastic paraparesis (Konzo):** Konzo is the leading cause of disability in African

children especially in Democratic Republic of Congo, Mozambique, Tanzania, Cameroon, Central African Republic and Angola. Konzo is associated with food shortage, famine or drought, and is also attributed to the consumption of cyanogenic glycoside from partially processed cassava. Konzo patients have spastic paraparesis with some overlapping features with beriberi. Thiamine deficiency is attributed to the etiology of this disease (Nzwalo and Cliff, 2011).
c. **Seasonal ataxia in Nigeria:** During rainy season, the consumption of roasted African silk worms (*Anaphe venata*), which contain thiaminase, results in WE-like symptoms. The patient has nausea, vomiting, dizziness progressing to nystagmus, tremor, ataxia, dysarthria, confusion and coma. The patient recovers fully within 72 h of thiamine treatment (Adamolekun and Ndububa, 1994).

Case definition of thiamine deficiency disorders

There should be a high index of suspicion for the diagnosis of TDD in view of nonspecific presentation, high mortality in untreated patients and good response to early treatment without any side effects. The laboratory confirmation of thiamine deficiency is difficult and not widely available. Therefore, a case definition based on clinical and therapeutic responses to 50–100 mg of thiamine is available (Table 3.9). In an appropriate clinical setting if the patient responds to thiamine treatment with in 24 h, it is regarded as "most likely thiamine deficiency disorder", and if the response occurs within 72 h, it is regarded as "probable thiamine deficiency disorder".

Genetic defect resulting in thiamine deficiency disorders

Thiamine is essential for various cytosolic, mitochondrial and peroxisomal functions. Genetic mutations in these steps may lead to thiamine metabolism disorders with diverse clinical manifestations. They may manifest in infancy to adolescence and respond to high-dose thiamine (Table 3.10).

Table 3.9 Case definition of thiamine deficiency disorders in adults and children

	Major manifestations	Minor manifestations
Children and adult	Ataxia Abnormal eye movement Behavioral change, confusion Impaired consciousness, coma	Pins and needle in limbs Lethargy, apathy Tachycardia with warm extremities Signs of vitamin B deficiency – angular stomatitis

Infant	Sudden heart failure
	Increased cry, hoarseness
	Breathing difficulty, cyanosis
	Hepatomegaly
	Nystagmus
	Bulging fontanelle
	Muscle twitching
	Seizures (without fever)
		Refusal to feed, reduced sucking
		    for >48h
		Vomiting
		Constipation
		Tachycardia with warm extremities
		    without fever

Table 3.10 Diseases related to genetic defect of thiamine metabolism

Disease	Age onset	Clinical feature	Mutation/ protein	Treatment
Rogers syndrome/ TRAM	Neonate to adolescence	Diabetes, deafness, optic atrophy, short stature, macrocytic anemia, congenital heart disease	SLC 19A2/ THTR1	Thiamine (50–100 mg)/ day
Biotin-thiamine- responsive basal ganglia disease	Birth to adolescence	Episodic encephalopathy with seizure, fever, external ophthalmoplegia, ataxia, basal ganglia lesion	SLC19A3/ THTR 2	Biotin (5–10 mg)+ Thiamine (100–300 mg)/ day
Amish lethal microcephaly/ THMD3	Birth	Episodic encephalopathy with lactic acidosis, α-ketoglutaric aciduria, microcephaly, seizure, mental retardation, lactate in urine	SLC25A19/ Mitochondrial TTP carrier.	Thiamine 100–200+ high-fat diet
THMD4 (thiamine metabolism dysfunction)	Adolescence	Episodic febrile encephalopathy, neurologic deficit (transient), progressive polyneuropathy, bilateral striatal degeneration	SLC25A29/ MTPC	High-dose thiamine
THMD5	Early childhood	Episodic encephalopathy, high lactate, ataxia, dystonia, spasticity	TPK I/thiamine phosphokinase I	High dose of thiamine

THMD, thiamine metabolism dysfunction syndrome; TRAM, thiamine-responsive megaloblastic anemia syndrome.

PREVENTION

Thiamine is a water-soluble vitamin; therefore, a regular supply is essential. In intensive care setting, there is high incidence of thiamine deficiency, which may remain undiagnosed or be attributed to primary disease. After one week, critically ill patients should be supplemented with thiamine. Community awareness about the source of thiamine is important for its prevention. Thiamine is degraded in food processing. The following methods are recommended to minimize the thiamine degradation (WHO, 1999):

1. Use minimum water in vegetable preparation, and do not discard the water.
2. Avoid high-flame cooking.
3. Cover by a lid while cooking.
4. Avoid storing for long time.
5. Wash vegetable just before cooking.
6. Use parboiled rice.
7. Alkali, and oxidizing and reducing agents enhance the thiamine degradation.

CONCLUSION

TDDs are common in infants and children in low-income countries, leading to high infant mortality. It is also common in alcoholics, elderly, undernourished, psychiatric diseases, in isolation, in chronic illness and in hospitalized patients. TDDs are characterized by the central and peripheral nervous system involvement with some overlapping features. Associated cardiac involvement and autonomic dysfunction may result in higher mortality. High index of suspicion and prompt treatment is life-saving, and an improvement occurs without sequelae.

REFERENCES

Adamolekun, B. 2011. Neurological disorders associated with cassava diet: A review of putative etiological mechanisms. *Metabolic Brain Disease* 26(1):79–85.

Adamolekun, B., Ndububa, D. A. 1994. Epidemiology and clinical presentation of a seasonal ataxia in western Nigeria. *Journal of the Neurological Sciences* 124(1):95–98.

Allen, L. H. 2012. B vitamins in breast milk: Relative importance of maternal status and intake, and effects on infant status and function. *Advances in Nutrition (Bethesda, MD)* 3(3):362–369.

Brokate, B., Hildebrandt, H., Eling, P., Fichtner, H., Runge, K., Timm, C. 2003. Frontal lobe dysfunctions in Korsakoff's syndrome and chronic alcoholism: Continuity or discontinuity? *Neuropsychology* 17(3):420–428.

Carpenter, K.J. 2012. The discovery of thiamin. *Annals of Nutrition and Metabolism* 61(3):219–223.

Day, G. S., del Campo, C. M. 2014. Wernicke encephalopathy: a medical emergency. *CMAJ: Canadian Medical Association Journal = journal de l'Association medicale canadienne* 186(8):E295.

Dhir, S., Tarasenko, M., Napoli, E., Giulivi, C. 2019. Neurological, psychiatric, and biochemical aspects of thiamine deficiency in children and adults. *Frontiers in Psychiatry* 10:207.

Duce, M., Escriba, J. M., Masuet, C., Farias, P., Fernandez, E., de la Rosa, O. 2003. Suspected thiamine deficiency in Angola. *Field Exchange* 20:25.

Eijkman, C. 1898. Beri-beri: Zur Abwehr. *Arch Schiffs Tropen Hyg* 2:103.

Galvin, R., Bråthen, G., Ivashynka, A., Hillbom, M., Tanasescu, R., Leone, M. A., EFNS. 2010. EFNS guidelines for diagnosis, therapy and prevention of Wernicke encephalopathy. *European Journal of Neurology* 17(12):1408–1418.

George, A., Figueredo, V. M. 2010. Alcohol and arrhythmias: A comprehensive review. *Journal of Cardiovascular Medicine (Hagerstown, MD)* 11(4):221–228.

Grijns, G. 1935. *Researches on Vitamins. 1901–1911.* Holland: Gorinchen.

Harel, Y., Zuk, L., Guindy, M., Nakar, O., Lotan, D., Fattal-Valevski, A. 2017. The effect of subclinical infantile thiamine deficiency on motor function in preschool children. *Maternal & Child Nutrition* 13(4):e12397.

Harper, C., Butterworth, R. 2002. Nutritional and metabolic disorders. In *Greenfield's Neuropathology*. 7th ed. Graham, D. I., Lantos, P. L., Eds. Arnold Publishing: London. pp. 607–651

Jansen, B.C.P., Donath, W.F. 1926. On the isolation of the anti-beri-beri vitamin. *Proc Konink Akad van Wetensch Amsterdam* 107:1390–1400.

Koike, H., Ito, S., Morozumi, S., Kawagashira, Y., Iijima, M., Hattori, N., et al. 2008. Rapidly developing weakness mimicking Guillain-Barré syndrome in beriberi neuropathy: Two case reports. *Nutrition (Burbank, Los Angeles County, CA)* 24(7–8):776–780.

Kopelman, M. D. 1995. The Korsakoff syndrome. *The British Journal of Psychiatry: The Journal of Mental Science, 166(2):154–173.*

Kornreich, L., Bron-Harlev, E., Hoffmann, C., Schwarz, M., Konen, O., Schoenfeld, T., et al. 2005. Thiamine deficiency in infants: MR findings in the brain. *AJNR. American Journal of Neuroradiology* 26(7):1668–1674.

Kril, J. J., Halliday, G. M., Svoboda, M. D., Cartwright, H. 1997. The cerebral cortex is damaged in chronic alcoholics. *Neuroscience* 79(4):983–998.

Kulkarni, S., Lee, A. G., Holstein, S. A., Warner, J. E. 2005. You are what you eat. *Survey of Ophthalmology* 50(4):389–393.

Luxemburger, C., White, N. J., ter Kuile, F., Singh, H. M., Allier-Frachon, I., Ohn, M., et al. 2003. Beriberi: the major cause of infant mortality in Karen refugees. *Transactions of the Royal Society of Tropical Medicine and Hygiene* 97(2): 251–255.

Mascalchi, M., Simonelli, P., Tessa, C., Giangaspero, F., Petruzzi, P., Bosincu, L., et al. 1999. Do acute lesions of Wernicke's encephalopathy show contrast enhancement? Report of three cases and review of the literature. *Neuroradiology* 41(4): 249–254.

McCandless, D.W. 2009. *Thiamine Deficiency and Associated Clinical Disorders in Contemporary Clinical Neuroscience Series*, pp. 31–46. New York: Humana Press.

Monekosso, G. L., Annan, W. G., Ashby, P. H. 1964. Therapeutic effect of vitamin b complex on an ataxic syndrome in western Nigeria. *Transactions of the Royal Society of Tropical Medicine and Hygiene* 58:432–436.

Murata, T., Fujito, T., Kimura, H., Omori, M., Itoh, H., Wada, Y. 2001. Serial MRI and (1)H-MRS of Wernicke's encephalopathy: report of a case with remarkable cerebellar lesions on MRI. *Psychiatry Research* 108(1):49–55.

National Collaborating Centre for Mental Health (UK). 2011. *Alcohol-Use Disorders: Diagnosis, Assessment and Management of Harmful Drinking and Alcohol Dependence*. Leicester: British Psychological Society.

Nishimoto, A., Usery, J., Winton, J. C., Twilla, J. 2017. High-dose parenteral thiamine in treatment of Wernicke's encephalopathy: Case series and review of the literature. *In Vivo (Athens, Greece)* 31(1):121–124.

Nzwalo, H., Cliff, J. 2011. Konzo: from poverty, cassava, and cyanogen intake to toxico-nutritional neurological disease. *PLoS Neglected Tropical Diseases* 5(6):e1051.

Olds, K., Langlois, N. E., Blumbergs, P., Byard, R. W. 2014. The pathological features of Wernicke encephalopathy. *Forensic Science, Medicine, and Pathology* 10(3):466–468.

Ota, Y., Capizzano, A. A., Moritani, T., Naganawa, S., Kurokawa, R., Srinivasan, A. 2020. Comprehensive review of Wernicke encephalopathy: Pathophysiology, clinical symptoms and imaging findings. *Japanese Journal of Radiology* DOI: 10.1007/s11604-020-00989-3. Advance online publication.

Saini, M., Lin, W., Kang, C., Umapathi, T. 2019. Acute flaccid paralysis: Do not forget beriberi neuropathy. *Journal of the Peripheral Nervous System: JPNS* 24(1):145–149.

Sechi, G., Serra, A. 2007. Wernicke's encephalopathy: New clinical settings and recent advances in diagnosis and management. *The Lancet. Neurology* 6(5):442–455.

Sugiyama, Y., Seita, A. 2013. Kanehiro Takaki and the control of beriberi in the Japanese Navy. *Journal of the Royal Society of Medicine* 106(8):332–334.

Thomson, A. D., Guerrini, I., Marshall, E. J. 2012. The evolution and treatment of Korsakoff's syndrome: Out of sight, out of mind? *Neuropsychology Review* 22(2):81–92.

Torvik, A. 1991. Wernicke's encephalopathy: prevalence and clinical spectrum. *Alcohol and alcoholism (Oxford, Oxfordshire)*. Supplement 1:381–384.

Victor, M. 1976. The Wernicke-Korsakoff syndrome. In *Handbook of Clinical Neurology*. Part II. Vol. 28; Vinken, P. J., Bruyn, G. W., Eds.; Amsterdam: North-Holland Publishing Company, pp. 243–270.

Wani, N. A., Qureshi, U. A., Ahmad, K., Choh, N. A. 2016. Cranial ultrasonography in infantile encephalitic beriberi: A useful first-line imaging tool for screening and diagnosis in suspected cases. *AJNR: American Journal of Neuroradiology* 37(8):1535–1540.

Whitfield, K. C., Smith, G., Chamnan, C., Karakochuk, C. D., Sophonneary, P., Kuong, K., et al. 2017. High prevalence of thiamine (vitamin B1) deficiency in early childhood among a nationally representative sample of Cambodian women of childbearing age and their children. *PLoS Neglected Tropical Diseases* 11(9):e0005814.

Whitfield, K. C., Bourassa, M. W., Adamolekun, B., Bergeron, G., Bettendorff, L., Brown, K. 2018. Thiamine deficiency disorders: Diagnosis, prevalence, and a roadmap for global control programs. *Annals of the New York Academy of Sciences* 1430(1):3–43.

Williams, R.R., Cline, J.K. 1936. Synthesis of vitamin B1. *Journal of the American Chemical Society* 58:1504–1505.

World Health Organization, United Nations High Commissioner for Refugees. 1999. Thiamine deficiency and its prevention and control in major emergencies. https://www.who.int/nutrition/publications/emergencies/WHO_NHD_99.13/en/.

Yin, H., Xu, Q., Cao, Y., Qi, Y., Yu, T., Lu, W. 2019. Nonalcoholic Wernicke's encephalopathy: A retrospective study of 17 cases. *The Journal of International Medical Research, 47*(10):4886–4894.

Zuccoli, G., Santa Cruz, D., Bertolini, M., Rovira, A., Gallucci, M., Carollo, C., Pipitone, N. 2009. MR imaging findings in 56 patients with Wernicke encephalopathy: nonalcoholics may differ from alcoholics. *AJNR: American Journal of Neuroradiology 30*(1):171–176.

Zuccoli, G., Siddiqui, N., Bailey, A., Bartoletti, S. C. 2010. Neuroimaging findings in pediatric Wernicke encephalopathy: a review. *Neuroradiology 52*(6):523–529.

4

Niacin deficiency: Pellagra

INTRODUCTION

Pellagra is a complex metabolic disorder presenting with dermatitis, dementia and diarrhea, which is attributed to the deficiency of niacin or tryptophan. In the past, pellagra occurred in large epidemics in Europe, Africa and Asia. Pellagra epidemics have declined significantly after the 1970s; however, sporadic cases and outbreaks are reported from refugee camps and drought-affected areas.

HISTORICAL BACKGROUND

The spread of pellagra throughout the world is linked to the expedition of Christopher Columbus. He introduced maize to Europe. Columbus considered maize to be the tastiest food in any form – boiled, roasted or ground to flour. Portuguese traders brought maize to India and Africa. In 1555, there were reports of maize cultivation in China and Tibet. In the last voyage in 1521, Columbus introduced maize in the Philippines. In this way, maize became available globally and led to a widespread occurrence of pellagra. Pellagra was first described in Spanish farmers as *mel de la rosa* by Casal in 1735. Casal observed dermatitis, diarrhea and dementia in the farmers. He also observed that corn was the staple diet of laborers and may be responsible for this disease. He, however, regarded *mel de la rosa* a form of leprosy. Casal noted the therapeutic benefit of diets containing milk, eggs and fresh meat. In 1771, Frapoli, an Italian physician to Ospedale Maggiore of Milan, termed this disease as "pellagra" (rough skin). He reported three stages of pellagra: initially dry itchy skin followed by infiltrated fissured skin with neuropsychological abnormalities, stupor, fever, diarrhea, failure of mental power and emaciation and finally death (Still, 1977). Goldberger disproved the infective theory of pellagra that pellagra (infection) cannot be transmitted to monkeys. He, his wife and colleagues consumed blood, nasal secretion, urine and feces of the pellagra patients, but did not develop pellagra. He also confirmed that pellagra can be prevented by consuming proteins (Barrett-Connor, 1967). In 1937, Conrad Arnold Elvehjem and his colleagues from Wisconsin, USA, isolated the pellagra-preventing factor from the liver extract and demonstrated that nicotinic acid could cure black tongue in dogs, other animals and humans (Elvehjem et al., 1937; Fouts et al., 1937). This treatment resulted in a dramatic improvement of patients within 48–72 h (Pies et al., 1939). These studies confirmed the therapeutic efficacy of niacin in pellagra (Lanska, 2010). In the 1950s, it was noted that pellagra could not be accounted by niacin only. The diet in some area where pellagra was rare used lower niacin compared to pellagra-endemic areas. The difference was milk consumption in low pellagra-endemic area, which has resulted in the concept of niacin–tryptophan link. The amino acid tryptophan is converted to niacin by the intestinal bacteria (Lanska, 2012).

Till the 1970s, there were several epidemics of pellagra in Europe, Asia, Africa and America. In South Africa, more than 100,000 patients were reported every year during the 1970s. Currently, large-scale outbreaks are not reported because of education and availability of alternative sources of niacin. Pellagra has declined substantially in 1900 and disappeared since 1916. Pellagra, however, has been reported as a major problem in Romania and Central Europe. In Romania, more than 55,000 patients were reported in 1932, with 1654 deaths (WHO, 2000). In Moldavia, about

10% of population suffered from pellagra in spring season because most of the villagers took maize as a staple diet comprising 70% of calorie intake (WHO, 2000).

Dogs fed on the diet of pellagra patients developed black tongue. Low tryptophan in maize may be compensated by animal protein and other cereals. Maize is also deficient in riboflavin and thiamine, which are deficient in pellagra patients. The generic name of niacin is pyridine 3-carboxylic acid, which is biologically active form of nicotinamide. Nicotinic acid and nicotinamide are white crystals – the latter is more stable. 60 mg of tryptophan is converted into 1 mg of niacin. Riboflavin, pyridoxine and iron are needed for the conversion of tryptophan to niacin.

SOURCES OF NIACIN

Niacin is composed of two vitamers: nictotinic acid and nicotinamide (Figure 4.1). Niacin has exogenous and endogenous sources. The endogenous niacin is formed from the conversion of tryptophan. The exogenous sources are meat, fish, egg, milk, cheese, cereals, legumes and seeds. Vegetables, coffee and tea also contain niacin. In animal tissues, niacin is present as nicotinamide and in plants as nicotinic acid. Niacin in mature grain, especially in corn, is present as niacin-glycoside and the minor proportion as peptide-bound niacin – these are collectively known as "niacinogen". Niacin in grain is therefore poorly available because intestinal enzyme cannot free niacin from niacinogen. The availability of niacin may be improved by soaking maize in lime water, heating

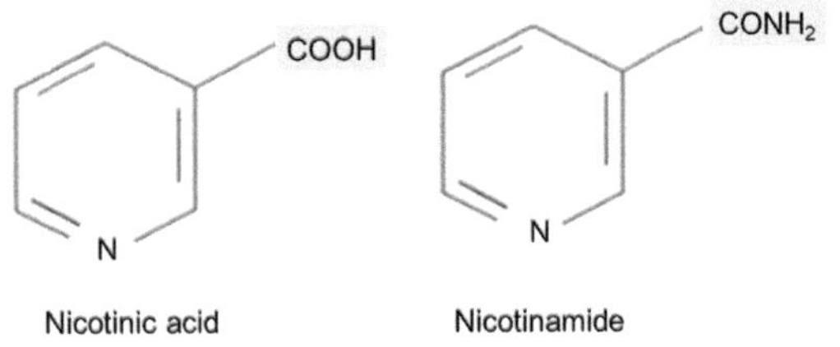

Figure 4.1 Schematic diagram showing the structures of nicotinic acid and nicotinamide.

or roasting. Protein deficiency results in the metabolism of tryptophan to maintain nitrogen balance, but in the presence of adequate protein, it is converted to niacin. It is interesting to note that milk prevents pellagra. Rice eaters do not have pellagra in spite of lower niacin content in rice. Both rice and milk have higher protein and tryptophan contents than maize. Cooking methods also influence niacin levels: boiling and blanching reduce the niacin levels (40%) compared to boiling alone. Hence if cooking water is not discarded, then niacin loss is minimal. Similar to thiamine, milling reduces the niacin levels in cereals. The fermented food using yeast has a higher niacin content. Sprouted grains have higher riboflavin, ascorbic acid and niacin levels. In certain countries, cereals like rice, pasta and breakfast cereals are fortified with riboflavin, niacin and folic acid, as these fortified cereals cannot be differentiated by the consumer from nonfortified foods because of similar taste, smell and flavor (Table 4.1).

Endogenous niacin is produced by the conversion of tryptophan by kynurenine pathway mainly in the liver. Several nutritional, hormonal and physiopathological factors influence the

Table 4.1 Dietary sources of niacin

Nonvegetarian source	mg/100 g	Vegetarian source	mg/100 g
Tuna	10–22.1	Yeast	56.0
Bacon	10.4	Peanuts	14.3
Salmon	10.0	Almond	3.6
Turkey	7–12	Mushroom	3.6
Chicken	7–12	Avocado	1.7
Beef	4–8	Potato	1.4
Pork	4.8	Corn	1.0
Cod fish	2.5	Rice	0.5
Egg	0.1	Kale	0.4
		Milk, cheese	0.1
		Tofu	0.1

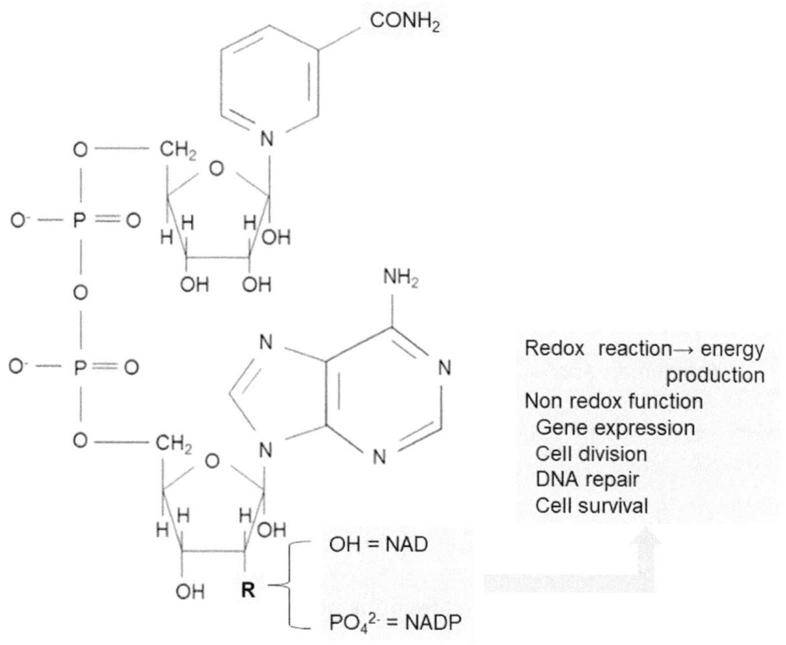

Figure 4.2 Schematic diagram showing coenzymatic form of niacin and its action. NAD=nicotinamide adenine dinucleotide. NADP=nicotinamide adenine dinucleotide phosphate.

kynurenine pathway. Deficiency of thiamine, pyridoxine, heme, iron, copper and zinc, and low-protein diet impair the conversion of tryptophan to niacin. Leucine-containing foods such as maize and sorghum also reduce the biosynthesis of niacin. The endogenous synthesis is increased with estrogen, glucocorticoid, unsaturated fatty acid and sucrose (Gasperi et al., 2019).

ABSORPTION AND METABOLISM

Niacin is a water-soluble vitamin and is almost completely absorbed from the small intestine. There are two active forms of nicotinamide in blood and tissues of various organs: nicotinamide adenine dinucleotide (NAD) and nicotinamide adenine dinucleotide phosphate (NADP) (Figure 4.2). There is little storage of niacin in the liver; hence, it has to be replenished daily. Absorption of niacin is not affected by food but can be inhibited by drugs like isoniazid, 6-mercaptopurine, 5-flurouracil, chloramphenicol and alcohol, and in malabsorption syndrome. In Hartnup disease, pellagra occurs due to the tryptophan metabolism abnormality. Tryptophan, nicotinamide and nicotinic acid can be converted to NAD and NADP. Niacin is important for oxidation in the cells, and it helps

in the release of energy from fat, protein and carbohydrate. Nicotinamide biosynthesis can occur in the brain via kynurenine reaction (Figure 4.3). Nicotinamide can cross blood–brain barrier freely. Nicotinamide helps in neuronal differentiation, growth and development (Williams and Ramsden, 2005; Fricker et al., 2018). It inhibits cytochrome c oxidase and caspase 3 and 9 activities, thereby reducing oxidative stress and cell death. Niacin and niacin metabolites are excreted in urine. Pellagra is the first disorder of electron transport chain affecting humans (Chong et al., 2004).

EPIDEMIOLOGY

Endemic pellagra was prevalent in maize-eating zone from 58° North to 40° South latitude. In the first half of 20th century, pellagra declined globally except in Africa and India. In the Upper Egypt, the incidence of pellagra in 1958–1963 was 45/100,000 population, which declined to 10.3/100,000 population during 1964–1966. At the same time, the incidence of pellagra in Lower Egypt was 83.2/100,000 population (Barrett-Connor, 1967; Patwardhan and Darby, 1972). In Italy, the new cases of pellagra in 1906 were 6783 with 437 deaths, which declined to 91 new cases and 0.2/100,000 deaths in

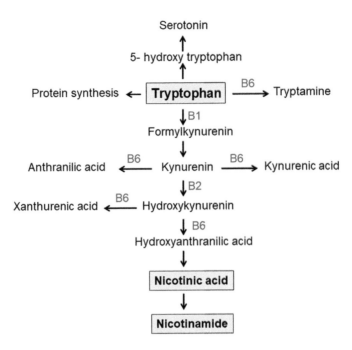

Figure 4.3 Schematic diagram showing the synthesis of niacin from tryptophan and the role of B1 (thiamine), B2 (riboflavin) and B6 (pyridoxine) as cofactors in this pathway.

1928 (Lavinder and Babcock, 1910; Aykroyd, 1933). In 1932, new cases of pellagra in Romania were 55,013 with 1654 deaths (Aykroyd, 1935; Roe, 1973). Replacement of maize by wheat eradicated pellagra from Romania in 1966. In South Carolina, death due to pellagra was 44.8/100,000 population in 1916, which dropped to 8.5/100,000 in 1940 (Davis, 1964). The incidence of pellagra rapidly declined in the USA due to a universal fortification of bread, corn meal and flour with niacin which was legally enforced. In the 1960s, during Green Revolution, opaque 2 mutant gene of maize was introduced. This variety of maize had 86% increase in protein and 38% reduction in leucine (Mertz, 1964). In the 1930s, the incidence of pellagra in most of the countries declined but it remained a public health problem in 1960 and 1970 in some countries of Asia, Egypt and South Africa. Pellagra has been reported from Hyderabad in Sorghum (Jowar)-eating population but has not been found in Sorghum eaters in Africa and Europe (Gopalan and Srikantia, 1960). In Malawi, 690 patients with pellagra from a local Kasese Catchment area of 30,000 people were identified during July 2015 and April 2016. About 96% patients were above 15 years of age. They had typical skin disease, which was considered as eczema in 60%. The skin lesions responded to multivitamin tablet containing 20 mg of niacin daily or twice daily for 30 days (Matapandeu et al., 2017). In recent years, the pellagra outbreaks have been reported in the refugee camps and in the areas with food sanctions and war (Table 4.2).

Table 4.2 Outbreaks of pellagra in the past few decades

Year	Location	Underlying situation	Prevalence
1988	Zimbabwe	Refugee camp	1.5%
1989	Malawi	Refugee camp	0.5%
1990	Malawi	Mozambican refugees	2.0%
1994	Nepal	Bhutanese refugees	0.5/10,000/day
1995	Mozambique	Population survey	1.4%
1999	Angola	Population survey	2.6/1000/week

Table 4.3 Clinical features of pellagra

Organ	Symptoms and signs
Nervous system	Neuropsychiatric abnormality: insomnia, irritability, depression, apathy Cognitive: dementia Peripheral neuropathy
Skin	Symmetrical erythema of skin in the sun-exposed area (face, neck, hand and feet), hyperpigmentation, hyperkeratosis, swelling and thickening of skin, dark red or purple skin rash followed by exfoliation with demarcated line between normal and abnormal skin
Gastrointestinal tract	Stomatitis, glossitis, anorexia, dysphagia, indigestion, diarrhea and constipation
Others	Asthenia, weight loss, cachexia, infection, neck traction and epileptic fit

CLINICAL FEATURES OF NIACIN DEFICIENCY

Niacin deficiency results in a clinical triad of diarrhea, dermatitis and dementia. In the early stage, the patient may have vague clinical symptoms such as anorexia, asthenia, weight loss, dysphagia, indigestion, diarrhea and constipation, which may lead to the aggravation of symptoms and signs in a vicious manner (Table 4.3). The patient may manifest with neuropsychiatric abnormalities, such as insomnia, irritability, nervousness, depression, apathy and mild memory impairment. If the patients remain untreated, they develop dementia. Pellagra is recognized by the typical skin lesions, which are symmetrical, erythematous, in the sun-exposed areas and looking like sunburn. There are symmetrical face involvement, Casal's necklace, and glove and stocking appearance of pigmented lesions. These lesions are scaly and exfoliative, and may have itching or burning sensations. The demarcation from the normal skin is very clear and typical, as opposed to other dermatitides (Figures 4.4 and 4.5). The patient has progressive weight loss, disappearance of subcutaneous fat, muscle atrophy, increased weakness, bulbar palsy, psychotic behavior along with cardiac decompensation, reduced immunity and secondary infection. In the terminal phase, the patient may have fever, neck retraction and epileptiform attack (typhoid pellagra). If the patient is untreated, death ensues in a few months. In recent years, the classical triad of pellagra is rare, and often the patient presents with skin changes. In a retrospective study from a dermatology department, 178 of 47,219 (0.4%) had pellagra-like skin lesions. All the patients

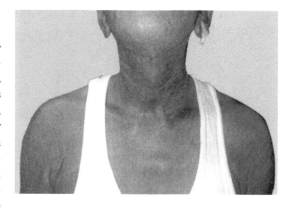

Figure 4.4 Clinical photograph of a patient with pellagra showing a scaly pigmented skin lesion in the neck area (Casal's necklace). (With permission Brahmaiah, U., Parveda, A.R., Hemalatha, R., Laxmaiah, A. 2019. Pellagra: A forgotten entity. *Clinical Dermatology Review* 3:126–129.)

had at least one skin lesion in sun-exposed area. Diarrhea was present in 12.4%, peripheral neuropathy in 8.4% and insomnia in 8.4%. 42.1% patients were alcoholic, and 6.7% patients had dietary deficiency. These patients improved on nicotinamide and multivitamins (Akakpo et al., 2019). Another study from a de-addiction center from India reported 31 out of 2947 (1%) patients with pellagra. 64.5% were from low-income group, all had dermatitis, 58% were delirious and 19% had diarrhea. 61% of these patients had the associated alcohol-withdrawal symptoms. Peripheral neuropathy was present in 32%, Wernicke encephalopathy in 26% and seizure in 16% patients (Narasimha et al., 2019). In a report of 335 patients from Andhra Pradesh, typical skin lesions were seen on the dorsum of hand and extensor surface of forearm

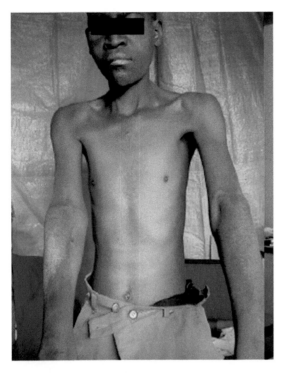

Figure 4.5 Pigmented scaly skin lesion in a male with pellagra from Malawi. (With permission Matapandeu, G., Dunn, S.H., Pagels, P. 2017. An outbreak of pellagra in the Kasese catchment area, Dowa, Malawi. *American Journal of Tropical Medicine and Hygiene* 96(5):1244–1247. DOI:10.4269/ajtmh.16-0423.)

DIAGNOSTIC CRITERIA

The diagnosis of pellagra is easy in a patient with likely deficiency of niacin and tryptophan with a characteristic skin lesion. In a patient without skin lesion, the laboratory tests are required. Urinary metabolites are usually measured for the diagnosis of pellagra. Fasting urine normally has N^1-methyl nicotinamide (mg/g of urinary creatinine) more than 0.6 mg in adults and more than 2.5 mg in the third trimester of pregnancy. A level below those aforementioned levels is associated with niacin deficiency.

PATHOPHYSIOLOGY

Both niacin and nicotinamide are easily absorbed from the small intestine. In the tissue, niacin is converted to NAD with the help of kinase; it is phosphorylated to NADP. Liver can produce niacin from tryptophan. Sixty milligrams of tryptophan is equivalent to 1 mg of niacin. The conversion of nicotinic acid, nicotinamide and tryptophan to NAD and NADP requires Cu, Zn and pyridoxine. Blood, kidney, brain and liver store NAD and NADP for a very short time. NAD and NADP act as coenzymes for many dehydrogenases participating in H^+-transfer processes. NAD is needed for enzyme production from carbohydrate, fat, protein and alcohol, and also helps in cell signaling and DNA repair. NADP helps in the anabolic reaction of fatty acid and cholesterol synthesis, resulting in increased HDL and a reduction in LDL and VLDL, thereby improving the endothelial function and plaque stability. Niacin also upregulates the brain-derived neurotrophic factor and tropomyosin receptor kinase B. The effect of niacin is mediated through G-protein-coupled receptor, including niacin receptors R1 and R2. These receptors are expressed in the adipose tissue, spleen and

followed by neck and face. Skin lesions were less common in feet and legs. Peripheral neuropathy was present in 2% and anemia in 1.8% (Brahmaiah et al., 2019). The dermatitis in niacin deficiency is due to the reduced ADP ribose polymerase activity, which is needed for DNA repair. The dermatitis in pellagra may simulate xeroderma pigmentosum, subacute dermatitis or dermatitis of kwashiorkor; their differentiating points are mentioned in Table 4.4.

Table 4.4 Differential diagnosis of pellagra dermatitis

Subacute dermatitis	Dry hyperkeratotic, fissured, hyperpigmented skin affecting dorsum of hand, feet, leg and forearm especially during winter. Absence of demarcated line separating normal to abnormal and rim scales, and response to moisturizing agent differentiated from pellagra
Dermatitis of kwashiorkor	Extensive pigmented skin desquamation bilaterally in infant especially localized to buttocks and thigh
Xeroderma	Generalized dryness with thin atrophic, bran-like desquamation in leg

immune cells of adipocytes but not in the heart, intestine and kidneys.

Niacin is excreted in urine as N^1-methylnicotinamide and 1-methyl 6-pyridone 3-carboxamide. Daily excretion of niacin by-product is 30 mg. In case of high niacin intake, it may be excreted as such. Interconvertibility of NADH and NADPH has been demonstrated. NADPH has a synergistic effect on the oxidation of NADH through NADH dehydrogenase cytochrome system. NADPH is also directly oxidized by cytochrome P450. Cerebral tissues are rich in NADH glutathione reductase, which catalyzes the reduction of oxidized glutathione at the rate of 250 μmol/h/g of brain tissue. NADH-related enzyme reactivity is mainly present in blood vessels, glia, white matter and other brain tissues, except catecholaminergic neurons and cerebellar molecular layer. This helps in maintaining the myelin integrity (by NADPH-mediated reductase biosynthesis of lipids), phagocytosis (by pentose phosphate pathway for the utilization of oxidative burst activity), and detoxification of drugs and chemicals (by NADPH cytochrome P450 reductase system).

PATHOLOGY

The pathological changes in pellagra have been observed in almost all the structures of the body. Brain is diffusely atrophied in chronic niacin deficiency and moderately edematous in acute stage. Dura matter is opaque, thickened and adherent to the cranium. There are punctate cerebral hemorrhages, sclerosis and softening of the cerebellum and spinal cord. In the gastrointestinal system, there are ulcers in mouth, stomach and intestine. There is a cystic dilatation of the crypts of Lieberkuhn. Ulcers are also seen in the colon, which are covered by fibrinous material. There may be atrophic gastritis and achlorhydria.

Skin ulcers are characterized by the rarefaction of superficial corium, endothelial proliferation and dilatation of blood vessels giving rise to erythematous spongy appearance in the initial stage. Hyperkeratotic epithelium is separated from the corium due to the formation of intraepidermal and subepidermal vesicles containing fluid, RBC, fibrin and melanin. Rupture of vesicles and bullae and proliferating capillaries result in desquamation beginning at the center of the lesion. Tongue may be inflamed and atrophic with fungiform papillae.

TREATMENT

Pellagra is treated with nicotinamide 300 mg in divided doses for 3–4 weeks. Appetite and general health improve rapidly. Stomatitis, glossitis and gastrointestinal symptoms improve within a few days. Dermatitis and dementia improve by weeks. A longer treatment is required for the chronic patients. It is also recommended to administer other B vitamins as there may be multiple deficiencies of thiamine, riboflavin and pyridoxine. In severely affected patients with encephalopathy and vomiting, parenteral administration is needed in the patients with gastrointestinal upset and coma.

HARTNUP DISEASE

In 1956, Hartnup disease was first described in two siblings of Hartnup family. Hartnup disease is an autosomal recessive disorder due to the transporter gene SLC6A19, located on the short arm of chromosome 5 (5p15.33) (Seow et al., 2004). This transporter is found in the kidney and intestine, which helps in the absorption of neutral amino acids, including tryptophan. In Hartnup disease, this defect results in hypoaminoacidemia. Reduced level of tryptophan results in deficiency of niacin, melatonin and serotonin, and these patients clinically manifest with pellagra-like symptoms.

The clinical manifestations of Hartnup disorder vary widely ranging from infancy to adulthood or may remain asymptomatic. Infants may manifest with failure to thrive, delayed development, photosensitivity, dermatitis, episodic ataxia, tremor and nystagmus (Figure 4.6). The underlying defect in Hartnup disorder is in kidney and intestine but its manifestations are in the skin and brain. In children and adults, Hartnup disorder is characterized by short stature, mental retardation, unsteady gait, fainting attacks, headache and psychiatric symptoms, including anxiety, mood changes, hallucination and delusions (Seow et al., 2004). The illness may be triggered by infection, fever, drugs, sunlight, physical and mental stress or underlying gastrointestinal diseases such as coeliac or Crohn's disease (Ciecierega et al., 2014).

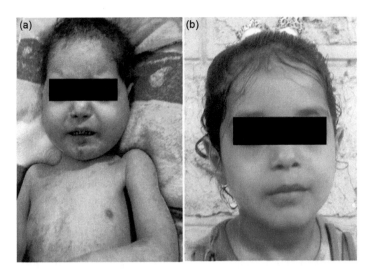

Figure 4.6 A girl with Hartnup disease. (a) Scaly desquamating skin rash with pigmentation involving the whole body. She was irritable. (b) The same girl one month after niacin of 50 mg thrice daily. There was a complete resolution of skin lesion and diarrhea. (With permission from Ciecierega, T., Dweikat, I., Awar, M. et al. 2014. Severe persistent unremitting dermatitis, chronic diarrhea and hypoalbuminemia in a child: Hartnup disease in setting of celiac disease. *BMC Pediatrics* 14:311. DOI:10.1186/s12887-014-0311-6.)

The diagnosis of Hartnup disorder is supported by urinary chromatography, which reveals increased levels of neutral amino acids (glutamine, valine, leucine, isoleucine, phenylalanine, serine, histidine, tyrosine and tryptophan) (Milovanović et al., 2003). The diagnosis is confirmed by SLC6A19 gene defect. The treatment of Hartnup disease includes high-protein diet, which overcomes neutral amino acid deficiency. The patient should be advised to have good nutrition and protect from sunlight using sun screen. Symptomatic patients should be treated with niacin as in pellagra.

PREVENTION

An average intake of 15–20 mg niacin daily prevents pellagra in all age groups. In a stressful condition such as coinfection, a higher daily dose may be needed because of higher metabolic need. Mass administration of niacin as a preventive measure is not recommended, because it is not stored in the body (Table 4.5).

Preventing pellagra in the community: Pellagra can be prevented by health education, changing the cooking process and food fortification. Niacin is widely available in both animal and plant foods. In the plants, niacin is present in the form of niacytin or niacinogen. In maize, niacin is bound to small peptide and carbohydrate; therefore, a substantial amount may not be bioavailable. The method of food processing or cooking may render niacin bioavailable. Though maize is a staple diet in South and Central America, pellagra is rare in these regions because maize is soaked in lime water or consumed after boiling. The water in which maize is boiled contains niacin, hence, it should not be discarded. Similarly, roasting coffee beans increases the bioavailability of niacin from 20 to 500 mg/kg. Niacin is lost during milling of grains. Whole wheat bread contains five times more niacin compared to white bread (WHO, 2000). A number of ethnic cooking methods preserve niacin. In Indonesia, "Tempeh", which is a fermented dehould with partially cooked soybean with molds of genus *Rhizopus*, results in 7-fold increase in niacin (van Veen, 1970). In Nigeria, "Logi" is prepared by fermenting maize with lactobacilli, and yeast also improves the bioavailability of niacin and other vitamins (Uzogara et al., 1990). Germination of cereals and legumes also increases the bioavailability of niacin, riboflavin and other vitamins (Chen et al., 1975; Lay and Fields, 1981).

In a study from Malawi, the risk factors of pellagra in a community were female gender, unemployed head of the family, residence in a close camp rather than living in a village, absence of

Table 4.5 Daily requirement of niacin in healthy subjects

Age	Energy requirement kcal/day	Niacin (mg)
0–6 months	117/kg, breastfed	5
7–12 months	1000	6.6
1–2 years	1300	8.6
3 years	1450	9.6
4–6 years	1700	11.2
7–9 years	2100	13.9
10–12 years	2500	16.5
13–15 years (males/females)	3100/2600	20.4/17.2
16–19 years (males/females)	3600/2400	23.8/15.8
>19 years (males/females)	3200/2300	21.1/15.2
Pregnancy	+300	+2
Lactation	+500	+4

1 mg niacin = 60 mg tryptophan.

groundnut and fish in the diet, lack of kitchen garden and domestic poultry, and absence of home-based milling (Toole, 1992). These results throw a light on the preventing strategies of pellagra in the community. Groundnut and beans are rich in niacin but have relatively low levels of riboflavin and pyridoxine, which are needed for the conversion of tryptophan to niacin.

The other strategies to prevent pellagra are shifting of staple diet from maize to other cereals such as rice, millet or sorghum. Consumption of other cereals, pulses and nuts may be advised to get the desired amount of niacin. Fortification of maize flour with niacin and multivitamin may also be tried.

Preventing pellagra in special groups: In the last decade, there are only a few outbreaks of pellagra in the community, which are mainly in refugee camps or following food sanctions. Food ration containing adequate bioavailable niacin or niacin equivalent may be followed as mentioned below:

1. Maize-based ration should be supplemented with legumes, pulse, meat, nuts and fish.
2. Use staple general rations such as maize and fortified breakfast with cereals or maize with other cereals like rice, millet and sorghum. If the ration is only maize, it should be fortified with niacin.
3. Provide supplementation with vitamin B complex.

TOXICITY OF NIACIN

Niacin in a dose of 50–500 mg may be associated with flushing, abdominal pain, nausea, vomiting, diarrhea, headache, rash, pruritus or rhinitis. These adverse effects may be reduced by starting at low dose and increasing slowly. Very high dose of 1–3 g/day of niacin may result in fatigue, hypotension, insulin resistance, impaired glucose tolerance, hepatic dysfunction, visual blurring and maculopathy. At 2 g/day of niacin, there are reports of ischemic and hemorrhagic stroke, gastric ulcer and hematemesis. Flushing in niacin toxicity is mediated by prostaglandin, and serotonin plays a secondary role (Makri et al., 2013; Alsheikh-Ali and Karas, 2008; Papaliodis et al., 2008).

CONCLUSIONS

Niacin is a water-soluble vitamin, which is widely available in diet, and its deficiency is rarely encountered in contemporary medical practice. In recent years, pellagra is rare except in refugee camps and in alcoholics. The complete triad of pellagra – diarrhea, dermatitis and dementia – may not occur but may have partial manifestations. Pellagra recovers completely following the niacin treatment. Pellagra can be prevented by ensuring high-protein diet containing 15–20 mg of niacin daily.

REFERENCES

Akakpo, A. S., Saka, B., Teclessou, J. N., Mouhari-Toure, A., Moise Elegbede, Y., Kombate, K., Tchangai-Walla, K., & Pitche, P. 2019. Pellagra and pellagra-like erythema in a hospital setting in Lomé, Togo: retrospective study from 1997 to 2017. Pellagre et érythèmes pellagroïdes en milieu hospitalier à Lomé, Togo: étude rétrospective de 1997 à 2017. *Medecine et sante tropicales* 29(1):68–70.

Alsheikh-Ali, A. A., & Karas, R. H. 2008. The safety of niacin in the US Food and Drug Administration adverse event reporting database. *The American Journal of Cardiology* 101(8A):9B–13B.

Aykroyd, W.R., 1933. Pellagra. *Nutrition Abstracts and Reviews* 3:337–344.

Aykroyd, W.R., Lexa, I., 1935. Nitzulescu: Study of the alimentation of peasants in the pellagra area of Moldavia (Romania). *Archives Roumaines de Pathologie Experimentale et de Microbiologie* 8:407–426.

Barrett-Connor, E. 1967. The etiology of pellagra and its significance for modern medicine. *The American Journal of Medicine* 42(6):859–867.

Brahmaiah, U., Parveda, A.R., Hemalatha, R., Laxmaiah, A. 2019. Pellagra: A forgotten entity. *Clinical Dermatology Review* 3:126–129.

Chen, L.H., Wells, C.E., Fordham, J.R. 1975. Germinated seeds for human consumption. *Journal of Food Science* 40:1290–1294.

Chong, Z. Z., Lin, S. H., Maiese, K. 2004. The NAD+ precursor nicotinamide governs neuronal survival during oxidative stress through protein kinase B coupled to FOXO3a and mitochondrial membrane potential. *Journal of Cerebral Blood Flow and Metabolism: Official Journal of the International Society of Cerebral Blood Flow and Metabolism* 24(7):728–743.

Ciecierega, T., Dweikat, I., Awar, M. et al. 2014. Severe persistent unremitting dermatitis, chronic diarrhea and hypoalbuminemia in a child: Hartnup disease in setting of celiac disease. *BMC Pediatrics 14:* 311.

Davis, J. N. P. 1964. The decline of pellagra in the Southern United States. *Lancet* 2:195–196.

Elvehjem C. A., Madden R. J., Strong F. M. Woolley, D. W. 1937. Relation of nicotinic aid and nicotinic acid amide to canine black tongue. *Journal of the American Chemical Society* 59(9):1767–1768.

Fouts, P. J., Helmer, M., Lepkovsky, S., Jukes, T. H. 1937. Treatment of pellagra with nicotinic acid. *Proceedings of the Society for Experimental Biology* 37:405.

Fricker, R. A., Green, E. L., Jenkins, S. I., Griffin, S. M. 2018. The influence of nicotinamide on health and disease in the central nervous system. *International Journal of Tryptophan Research: IJTR* 11: DOI: 10.1177/1178646918776658.

Gasperi, V., Sibilano, M., Savini, I., Catani, M. V. 2019. Niacin in the central nervous system: An update of biological aspects and clinical applications. *International Journal of Molecular Sciences* 20(4): 974.

Gopalan, C., Srikantia, S.G., 1960. Leucine and pellagra. *Lancet* 1(7131):954–957.

Lanska D. J. 2010. Chapter 30: Historical aspects of the major neurological vitamin deficiency disorders: The water-soluble B vitamins. *Handbook of Clinical Neurology* 95:445–476.

Lanska D. J. 2012. The discovery of niacin, biotin, and pantothenic acid. *Annals of Nutrition & Metabolism* 61(3):246–253.

Lavinder, C. H., Babcock, J.W., 1910. *Pellagra by Dr. A Marie.* Columbia, SC: The State Company.

Lay, M.M.-G., Fields, M.L. 1981. Nutritive value of germinated corn and corn fermented after germination. *Journal of Food Science* 46: 1069–1073.

Makri, O. E., Georgalas, I., Georgakopoulos, C. D. 2013. Drug-induced macular edema. *Drugs* 73(8):789–802.

Matapandeu, G., Dunn, S.H., Pagels, P. 2017. An outbreak of pellagra in the Kasese catchment area, Dowa, Malawi. *American Journal of Tropical Medicine and Hygiene* 96(5):1244–1247.

Mertz, E.T., Bates, L.S., Nelson, O.E., 1964. Mutant gene that changes protein composition and increases lysine content of maize endosperm. *Science* 145(3629):279–280.

Milovanović, D.D. 2003. A clinicobiochemical study of tryptophan and other plasma and urinary amino acids in the family with Hartnup disease. *Advances in Experimental Medicine and Biology* 527:325–335.

Narasimha, V. L., Ganesh, S., Reddy, S., Shukla, L., Mukherjee, D., Kandasamy, A., Chand, P. K., Benegal, V., Murthy, P. 2019. Pellagra and alcohol dependence syndrome: Findings from a tertiary care addiction treatment centre in India. *Alcohol and Alcoholism (Oxford, Oxfordshire)* 54(2): 148–151.

Papaliodis, D., Boucher, W., Kempuraj, D., et al. 2008. Niacin-induced "flush" involves release of prostaglandin D2 from mast cells and serotonin from platelets: Evidence from human cells in vitro and an animal model. *The Journal of Pharmacology and Experimental Therapeutics* 327(3): 665–672.

Patwardhan, V. N., Darby, W. J., 1972. *The state of nutrition in the Arab middle east*. Nashville, TN: Vanderbilt University Press.

Pies, T. D., Grant, J. M., Stone, R. E., Mclester, J. B. 1938. Recent observations on the treatment of six-hundred pellagrins with special emphasis on the use of nicotinic acid in prophylaxis. *Southern Medical Journal 31*(12):1231–1237.

Roe, D. A., 1973. *A plague of corn: The social history of pellagra*. Ithaca, NY: Cornell University Press.

Seow, H. F., Bröer, S., Bröer, A., Bailey, C. G., Potter, S. J., Cavanaugh, J. A., Rasko, J. E. (2004). Hartnup disorder is caused by mutations in the gene encoding the neutral amino acid transporter SLC6A19. *Nature Genetics 9*:1003.

Still, C.N. 1977. Nicotinic acid and nicotinamide: Pellagra and related disorders of the nervous system. In: *Handbook of clinical neurology*. Vol. 28. Vinken, P.J., Bruyn, G.W. *Metabolic and deficiency disease of the nervous system, Part-II, in collaboration with H. L. Klawans Amsterdam*. New York: North Holland Publishing Company.

Toole, M. J. 1992. Micronutrient deficiencies in refugees. *Lancet (London, England) 339*(8803):1214–1216.

Uzogara, S.G., Agu L.N., Uzogara E.O. 1990. A review of traditional fermented foods, condiments and beverages in Nigeria: Their benefits and possible problems. *Ecology of Food and Nutrition 24*(4):267–288.

van Veen, A. G., Steinkraus, K. H. 1970. Nutritive value and wholesomeness of fermented foods. *Journal of Agricultural and Food Chemistry 18*(4):576–578.

Williams, A., Ramsden, D. 2005. Nicotinamide: A double edged sword. *Parkinsonism & Related Disorders 11*(7):413–420.

World Health Organization, United Nations High Commissions for Refugees. 2000. Pellagra and its prevention and control in major emergencies. https://www.who.int/nutrition/publications/emergencies/WHO_NHD_00.10/en/.

5

Neurological manifestations of pyridoxine deficiency

INTRODUCTION

Vitamin B6 is a family of compounds, including pyridoxine, pyridoxamine, pyridoxal and their 5′ phosphate derivatives. Chemically, vitamin B6 is a derivative of 2-methyl-3-hydroxy 5-hydroxymethyl pyridine. Substitution at C4 position determines the three components: these are hydroxymethyl ($-CH_2OH$) in pyridoxine, aminomethyl ($-CH_2NH_2$) in pyridoxamine and aldehyde ($-CHO$) in pyridoxal. The 5′ alcohol group can be esterified to phosphate, producing pyridoxine-5′-phosphate (PNP), pyridoxamine-5′-phosphate (PMP) and pyridoxal-5′-phosphate (PLP). When pyridoxine is linked to glucose, it forms pyridoxine-β-glucoside (PNG) (Figure 5.1).

HISTORY

Rudolf Peters in 1932 noted acrodynia in rats exposed to a semisynthetic diet in addition to thiamine and riboflavin. Paul Gyorgy in 1934 treated acrodynia in rats by pyridoxine. Deficiency of pyridoxine has resulted in convulsions and microcytic

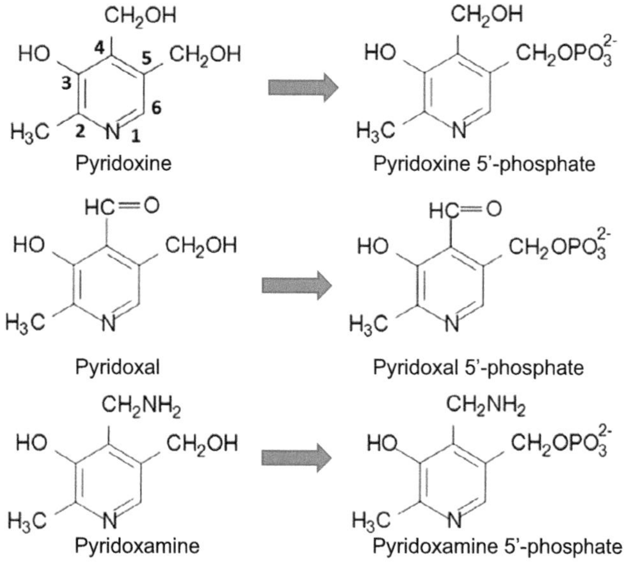

Figure 5.1 Management protocol of pyridoxine-responsive neonatal seizure.

anemia in experimental animals. Vitamin B6 was purified and crystallized by Samuel Lepkovsky in 1938. The chemical structure of vitamin B6 is similar to the pyrimidine derivative, and Gyorgy named it as pyridoxine. In 1942, the derivatives of pyridoxine, pyridoxamine and pyridoxal were described (Rosenberg, 2012).

MECHANISM OF ACTION

Pyridoxal-5′-phosphate acts as a cofactor in more than 140 enzymatic reactions; 70% of these reactions occur in humans. Because of its active aldehyde group, PLP acts in the metabolism of protein, amino acids, carbohydrate, lipid and folate as well as polyamine synthesis. Vitamin B6 also participates in protein and polyamine synthesis, mitochondrial functioning and erythropoiesis. Impairment in PLP functioning in these reactions is evident in its deficiency states, and can be associated with biomarker abnormalities such as elevated plasma threonine and glycine, and reduced cerebrospinal fluid GABA (gamma amino butyric acid).

Vitamin B6 acts in the cell as an antioxidant similar to vitamin C and vitamin E. Pyridoxal-5′-phosphate can also modify the expression and action of steroid hormone receptors, can also modulate the immune functions and has an antiepileptic activity. PLP blocks P2X7 (P2 purinoceptor 7). During neuroinflammation, intracellular ATP release is increased leading to the activation of P2X7, which can produce epilepsy.

UNWANTED EFFECTS OF PLP

Aldehyde component renders PLP highly reactive. With intracellular macromolecules, PLP participates in the production of reactive oxygen species (ROS) and can alter amino acid structure. Intracellular concentration of PLP above $10–100\,\mu M$ can inhibit the enzyme activity, thereby leading to DNA damage and mutagenesis (Garaycoechea et al., 2018). Reactivity of PLP with small molecules leads to the production of thiazolidines. Aldehyde group of PLP also reacts with Knoevenagel condensation with Δ^1 pyrroline 5-carboxylate and Δ^1 piperideine 6-carboxylate. In ALDH7A1 deficiency and hyperprolinemia type II, PLP deficiency occurs due to above-mentioned mechanisms (Mills et al., 2006). Aldehyde group of PLP also reacts with hydralazine, isoniazid, penicillamine and cycloserine. The cell

maintains a PLP level around $1\,\mu M$ concentration to avoid unwanted reactions (di Salvo et al., 2011).

SOURCES OF PYRIDOXINE

Pyridoxine is available in all the vegetarian and nonvegetarian diets. The rich sources of pyridoxine are legumes, nuts, wheat bran, fruits, vegetables, meat, eggs and fish. The plant source of vitamin B6 is pyridoxine, and its animal source is 5′-pyridoxal phosphate. Gut microbiota can also synthesize vitamin B6. The rich sources of vitamin B6 are summarized in Table 5.1.

ABSORPTION AND DISTRIBUTION

For entering in any compartment, the phosphorylated form of vitamin B6 needs to be dephosphorylated, which is again phosphorylated to be biologically active once it enters the compartment. Vitamin B6 is absorbed from the small intestine in nonphosphorylated form. The phosphorylated and glucoside forms of pyridoxine are first hydrolyzed by the intestinal phosphatases and glucosidases, respectively. Once within the enterocytes of the small intestine, pyridoxine or pyridoxamine can be converted prior to transportation to liver. In the liver, pyridoxine, pyridoxal and pyridoxamine are re-phosphorylated by pyridoxal kinase. Pyridoxal-5′-phosphate is exported from the liver and bound to the lysine residue of albumin in the circulation. Excessive amount of PLP is de-phosphorylated to pyridoxal, which is again oxidized to pyridoxic acid before it is excreted in urine. Aldehyde dehydrogenase or aldehyde oxygenase helps in the conversion of pyridoxine to pyridoxic acid. Pyridoxal-5′-phosphate is bound to albumin present in the blood; hence, it cannot cross the blood–brain barrier; therefore, it has to be de-phosphorylated to pyridoxal. De-phosphorylation of PLP to pyridoxal is done by the enzyme alkaline phosphatase. Pyridoxal crosses the blood–brain barrier by diffusion, and in the brain cell or in the choroid plexus, it is converted again to PLP. Next to the liver, the choroid plexus can rapidly release PLP. This explains the high level of pyridoxal in the CSF. In the CSF and extracellular space, PLP has to be de-phosphorylated for entry into the brain cells.

The uptake of vitamin B6 by the cells is regulated by genes or proteins, which are yet to be characterized in humans. Intracellular PLP is maintained at

Table 5.1 Rich sources of vitamin B6

Nuts and seeds	mg/100 g	Fruits	mg/100 g
Pistachio	1.7	Mamey sapote	0.7
Sunflower seed	1.3	Apricot	0.5
Sesame seed	0.8	Banana	0.4
Butter nut, hazelnut, lotus	0.6	Jackfruit, mango, raisins, avocado	0.3
Peanut, walnut	0.5	**Dairy and poultry**	
Cashew nuts	0.4	Cheese	0.6
Vegetables		Milk/yogurt	0.1
Peppers	3.5-4.2	Egg	0.2
Garlic	1.2	Chicken	0.9
Mushroom	1	Meat and fish	
Mustard green	0,2	Beef	0.5
Potato	0.3	Salmon	0.9

$1\,\mu M$ to prevent inappropriate reaction (aldehyde and carbonyl stress). In the muscle, low PLP level is maintained by glycogen phosphorylase, in RBC by hemoglobin and in plasma by albumin. Free PLP is degraded by phosphatases.

CAUSES OF PYRIDOXINE DEFICIENCY

The daily requirement of vitamin B6 varies from 0.1 to 1.7 mg depending upon the age and physiological conditions (Table 5.2). In healthy individuals, pyridoxine deficiency is rare because of its wide availability in food. The risk of pyridoxine deficiency is increased in pregnant and lactating women, and in exogenous estrogen use. Pyridoxine deficiency has been reported in 12.4% of females of child-bearing age in Canada, and 49% of Norwegian nursing home residents (Ho et al., 2016; Kjeldby et al., 2013). Patients with malabsorption and those undergoing bariatric surgery

may develop pyridoxine deficiency due to an impaired absorption. Following bariatric surgery, up to 17.6% of patients may develop pyridoxine deficiency (Clements et al., 2006). In neonates, vitamin B6 deficiency can occur because the gut microbiota in neonates is not well established. Neonate may also suffer from vitamin B6 deficiency if the mother is pyridoxine-deficient. About 24%–56% of patients on hemodialysis may develop vitamin B6 deficiency due to the loss and impaired conversion of PLP in uremic state (Kosmadakis et al., 2014). Drugs like hydralazine, isoniazid, phenelzine, cycloserine and penicillamine may also be responsible for pyridoxine deficiency due to the activation of phosphokinase, leading to an increased metabolism of pyridoxine. Levodopa utilizes pyridoxine, folate and vitamin B12 in its metabolism; therefore, patients treated with levodopa for a long time are prone to develop pyridoxine deficiency. Nearly all the patients treated with levodopa at a dose of 2000 mg/day develop neuropathy (Table 5.3).

CLINICAL SYNDROMES OF PYRIDOXINE DEFICIENCY

Pyridoxine deficiency results in three major clinical manifestations:

1. Seizures and encephalopathy
2. Peripheral neuropathy
3. Systemic manifestations such as seborrheic dermatitis, angular stomatitis, glossitis, microcytic anemia, lactic acidosis and hypoglycemia.

Table 5.2 Daily requirement of pyridoxine

Age	Daily dose (mg/day)
0–6 months	0.1
7–12 months	0.3
1–3 years	0.5
4–8 years	0.6
9–13 years	1.0.
14–50 years	1.3
>50 years	1.7 male, 1.5 female
Pregnancy	1.9
Lactation	2.0

Table 5.3 Causes of pyridoxine deficiency

A. Population at risk:

Pregnancy, lactation, nursing home residents, neonate of vitamin B6-deficient mother

B. Malabsorption:

Inflammatory bowel disease, intestinal resection, surgery or bariatric surgery

C. Increased loss:

Hemodialysis

D. Drugs:

Hydralazine, isoniazid, penicillamine, cycloserine, phenelzine, levodopa

E. Genetic causes

Pyridoxine-responsive epilepsy (PRE): The basis of pyridoxine-responsive seizures has been attributed to the role of pyridoxine in the formation and degradation of GABA. Pyridoxal 5'-phosphate has lower susceptibility to the decarboxylase system compared to the transaminase system (Frimpter et al., 1969). The differential enzymatic susceptibility of PLP leads to lower GABA concentration in pyridoxine deficiency leading to seizure (Figure 5.2). There are seven well-characterized autosomal recessive diseases associated with PRE, which are as follows:

1. ALDH7A1 deficiency
2. PNPO deficiency
3. PLPBP deficiency
4. Hyperprolinemia type II (ALDH4A1)
5. Hypophosphatasia (ALPL)
6. GP1-anchor defect (PIGO, PIGV/+others)
7. Molybdenum cofactor deficiency (MOCS1, GPHN).

Out of these PRE, ALDH7A1 deficiency is the commonest. PRE is a rare genetic disease, and its prevalence in the UK is 1/100,000 (Baxter et al., 1996), in Ireland 1/700,000 (Baxter, 1999) and in the Netherlands 1/396,000 (Been et al., 2005). A summary of PRE is presented in Table 5.4.

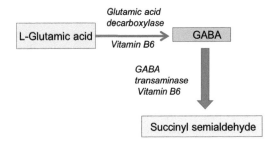

Figure 5.2 Role of pyridoxine in gamma amino butyric acid (GABA).

ALDH7A1 deficiency: ALDH7A1 deficiency is an autosomal recessive disorder due to mutations in ALDH7A1 gene. More than 165 pathogenic mutations have been reported. The frequency of carrier is 1:127, and that of ALDH7A1 deficiency is 1:64352 (Coughlin et al., 2019). It is characterized by seizures that are resistant to antiepileptic drugs (AEDs). Seizures occur on the first day of life or may occur in the neonatal period. This disease may manifest during childhood with developmental delay, learning disability and attention deficit hyperkinetic disorder. Seizures are resistant to AEDs, but respond to a high dose of pyridoxine. In the third trimester, mother may feel increased fetal movements due to seizures. Pyridoxine-dependent epilepsy should be considered in the following clinical settings:

1. Neonatal or infantile seizures without apparent brain malformation, perinatal or gestational injury or in the absence of hypoxic–ischemic encephalopathy.
2. Seizure may be prolonged focal, myoclonic, tonic–clonic, atonic, infantile spasm or status epilepticus. The neonate may manifest with facial grimacing and abnormal eye movements.
3. Inadequate response to AEDs.
4. In children with epilepsy having mental retardation and developmental delay, and epilepsy is not responding to AEDs.
5. Seizures respond to pyridoxine or folinic acid.
6. Seizures are preceded by vomiting, irritability and crying.
7. Consanguinity, family history of seizures or status epilepticus in the first week of life leading to death of sibling.

Besides seizure, the patient may have encephalopathy, low Apgar score and hypoxia in the cord blood mimicking hypoxic–ischemic encephalopathy.

Table 5.4 Clinical, MRI and biochemical changes in pyridoxine-responsive seizures

	Genetic locus	Age of onset	Skeletal abnormalities	Cranial CT/MRI	Biochemical findings
ALDH7A1 deficiency	ALDH7A1	PRE seizures – prenatal, 0–6 months, developmental delay	Macrocephaly, facial dysmorphism	Corpusstriatal, callosal, cerebellar atrophy, ventricular dilation	↑ α-AASA in urine/plasma
PNPO deficiency	PNPO	PRE seizures – day 1–3 years, dyskinesia, dystonia	Microcephaly	WM hypomyelination, brain atrophy	↑ Pyridoxamine/pyridoxic acid ratio, ↓ PNPO enzyme activity
PLPBP deficiency	PLPBP	PRE seizures day 1–30, days pneumonia, colitis, electrolyte abnormality	Developmental delay, microcephaly	Broad gyri, shallow sulci, WM abnormality	–
Hyperprolinemia type II	ALDH4A1	PRE seizure (infancy-childhood), may be asymptomatic	–	–	↑ Plasma proline & P5C, ↑ Urine P5C & N-(pyrole-2 carboxyl) glycine
Hypophosphatasia	ALPL	Seizure late, 50% PRE	Predominant teeth & bone abnormality (Rickets-like)	–	↓ Plasma alkaline phosphate & ↑ plasma phosphate, & ↑ urine phosphoserine & phosphoethanolamine
GPI-anchor deficiency	PIGO PIGV (+others)	Variable, PRE	–	Hypomyelination, BG & brain stem lesion	↑ plasma alkaline phosphate
Molybdenum cofactor deficiency	MOCS1, MOCS2, GPHN	PRE, Survival rare beyond early childhood	Microcephaly	Cerebral, cerebellar & callosal atrophy, hypomyelination	↑ Plasma & urine α-AASA

−, not present; α-AASA: α-aminoadipic semialdehyde; CC: corpus callosum; GPI: glycosylphosphatidylinositol; P5C: Δ¹-pyrroline-5-carboxylate; PLPBP: PLP-binding protein; PNPO: pyridoxamine phosphate oxidase; MRI: magnetic resonance imaging; PRE: pyridoxine-responsive epilepsy.

There may be atypical manifestations of ALDH7A1, such as expressive language defect in the later stage or rarely normal intellect with seizures up to 3 years of life. Mental retardation may also occur along with macrocephaly. Electroencephalogram may reveal multifocal seizure discharges, burst suppression, hypsarrhythmia or may be normal (Bok et al., 2010). Magnetic resonance imaging may show callosal hypoplasia, large cisterna magna, ventriculomegaly, cortical atrophy, and rarely white matter abnormality or focal cortical dysplasia (Bennett et al., 2009).

Laboratory diagnosis: Pyridoxine deficiency may be associated with (a) elevated plasma and urinary α-aminoadipic semialdehyde (α-AASA), (b) elevated CSF and plasma pipecolic acid, and (c) monoamine metabolite abnormality in plasma and urine measured by HPLC. Neonatal screening can be done by demonstrating α-AASA level in the dried blood spot test (Wempe et al., 2019; Coughlin et al., 2019). The diagnosis is confirmed by genetic studies by demonstrating allelic pathogenic variants of ALDH7A1. The commonest mutation (> 30%) is P. glu 399Gln (Bennett et al., 2005). There is no genotype and phenotype correlation.

Treatment: Seizure responds to pyridoxine treatment in 90% of children, and 75% of them have intellectual and developmental delay irrespective of treatment (Coughlin et al., 2019). Additional treatment such as low lysine and high arginine has been evaluated. Lysine-restricted diet reduces the toxic α-AASA, and arginine competes with lysine at the intestinal absorption site. The beneficial effect of triple therapy (pyridoxine, arginine and restricted lysine) in ALDH7A1 deficiency has been reported (Coughlin et al., 2015).

Pyridoxine phosphate oxidase (PNPO) deficiency: PNPO deficiency is an autosomal recessive disease due to mutation in PNPO gene, which results in PNPO deficiency. This enzyme is needed for the conversion of pyridoxine to PNP. PNPO deficiency manifests with seizures similar to ALDH7A1, but the onset of seizure may occur after 1 week (1 day–3 years), typically within 2 weeks of life. The seizures are refractory to AED. Three groups of patients with PNPO mutations have been described in relation to their seizure response:

(a) Those with neonatal-onset seizures responding to PLP, (b) infantile spasms responding to PLP and (c) seizures occurring below 3 months of age responding to pyridoxine. Seizures in R225H/C and D33V genotypes are responsive to pyridoxine (Mills et al., 2014). These neonates may have fetal distress, prematurity, developmental delay, seizure, and brain damage if treatment is delayed. These children may be flaccid or spastic, have orofacial dyskinesia, dystonia, irritability, lethargy and encephalopathy. The systemic manifestations include abdominal distension, anemia, cardiac abnormality, renal dysfunction, hepatomegaly and microcephaly. The children may also have hypoglycemia, metabolic acidosis, elevated lactate and coagulopathy. Plasma threonine and glycine and urinary vanillactate are elevated. Cerebrospinal fluid analysis reveals the reduced levels of HVA and HIAA, and elevated 3-methoxytyrosine. PNPO is necessary in many enzymatic processes of monoamine synthesis (Clayton et al., 2003).

EEG may show epileptiform discharges, burst suppression or hypsarrhythmia. MRI reveals white matter abnormalities, basal ganglia and hippocampal atrophy, hypomyelination, diffuse cortical atrophy, encephalomalacia and cortical laminar necrosis. Plasma and CSF pyridoxine is elevated on the dried blood spot but PNPO enzyme activity is reduced. The diagnosis is confirmed by PNPO mutation analysis. R116Q genotype has a milder phenotype with later clinical manifestation and better developmental outcome (Wilson et al., 2019).

Congenital hypophosphatasia (CHP): The clinical manifestations of CHP are widely variable. Due to low alkaline phosphatase enzyme level, the children with CHP manifest with bone and teeth abnormality. There are hypomineralization of bone, rickets like changes on radiograph, restrictive lung disease due to thoracic deformity, and premature fall of deciduous teeth and poor dentition. In severely affected patients, there may be neonatal seizures before the bone changes. Seizures are resistant to AEDs but respond to pyridoxine in 50% of patients only. There are isolated reports of subacute brainstem degeneration, which are attributed to high level of extracellular PLP-related toxicity (de Roo et al., 2014). There are low serum ALP level, high urinary phosphoethanolamine, high plasma PLP and PLP-to-pyridoxine ratio (Akiyama et al., 2018). The diagnosis is confirmed by ALPL gene mutation. Recently, enzyme replacement therapy especially in the early stage has been reported to be beneficial (Whyte et al., 2017)

Hyperprolinemia type II: Hyperprolinemia type II (HP II) is due to mutation in the gene ALDH4A1, which results in the deficiency of pyrroline-5 carboxylate dehydrogenase. This enzyme is necessary in the second stage of proline catabolism. Absence of this enzyme results in hyperprolinemia as high as 1000 μM. Neonatal seizures are rare. About 50% of patients develop seizures during infancy and childhood, which are usually triggered by fever. Unlike other pyridoxine-dependent epilepsy, the seizures in HP II respond to AED. During seizures, there is elevated urinary xanthurenic acid, suggesting PLP deficiency. In one study, all the patients had seizures, behavioral abnormality and hallucinations with low plasma PLP level. The diagnosis is confirmed by the demonstration of ALDH4A1 gene mutation. The disease course is nonprogressive and is independent of pyridoxine treatment (van de Ven et al., 2014).

Pyridoxal phosphate-binding protein (PLPBP) deficiency: PLPBP deficiency is a rare disease and is due to mutation of PLPBP gene. PLPBP deficiency results in seizures either in intrauterine or in neonatal period (1–30 days). The neonate may have pneumonia, enterocolitis, electrolyte imbalance and microcephaly. Electroencephalography may be normal or may show a burst suppression. MRI shows broad gyri, shallow sulci and white matter abnormalities (Wilson et al., 2019).

Treatment: New enzymopathies related to pyridoxine are being reported. The common pyridoxine-responsive epileptic encephalopathies are ALDH7A1, PNPO or PLPBP deficiency. The neonatal/infantile seizures or status epilepticus not responding to AED should be treated with iv pyridoxine. If pyridoxine fails to respond, iv folinic acid followed by PLP should be tried. The recommended treatment protocol is shown in Figure 5.3.

PERIPHERAL NEUROPATHY

After infancy, the brain is protected from PLP deficiency due to the maturation of protective mechanism. The major neurological deficit of PLP deficiency after infancy therefore manifests with peripheral neuropathy. Peripheral neuropathy in acquired vitamin B6 deficiency is not well characterized, except in relation to isoniazid treatment. Pyridoxine neuropathy is a length-dependent distal symmetrical predominantly sensory neuropathy manifesting with painful paresthesia. Neuropathy also occurs in penicillamine, hydralazine, isoniazid and cycloserine therapy, if these drugs are not

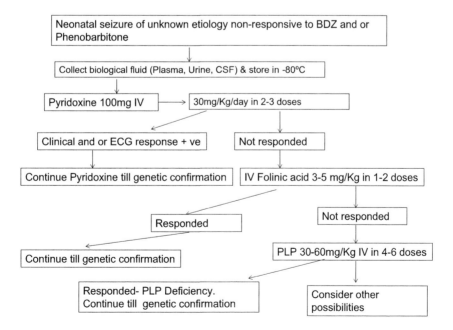

Figure 5.3 Schematic diagram shows the structures of pyridoxine, pyridoxal, pyridoxamine and its phosphorylated forms.

supplemented with pyridoxine. Isoniazid-induced neuropathy may be prevented with as low as 6 mg/day pyridoxine supplementation.

SYSTEMIC MANIFESTATIONS OF PYRIDOXINE DEFICIENCY

Angular stomatitis, glossitis, stomatitis and seborrheic dermatitis may occur. Pyridoxine is also required in heme synthesis, and its deficiency results in microcytic anemia. Pyridoxine also acts as a cofactor in various enzymatic reactions in carbohydrate metabolism; therefore, congenital deficiency of pyridoxine is associated with hypoglycemia.

PYRIDOXINE HYPERVITAMINOSIS

Pyridoxine toxicity is rare and occurs following supratherapeutic dosage or as an iatrogenic complication. Pyridoxine has been used in high dose by food faddists, alcoholics and patients on treatment with isoniazid, cycloserine or penicillamine. Some health food and drinks also contain a high amount of pyridoxine.

The clinical picture of pyridoxine toxicity is similar to that of pyridoxine deficiency. High-dose pyridoxine inhibits PLP formation, which is the active form of vitamin B6. Neuropathy, encephalopathy and fetal malformation have been reported following pyridoxine toxicity. Maternal abuse of pyridoxine may result in fetal phocomelia. High dose of pyridoxine may also result in encephalopathy.

Peripheral neuropathy: Pyridoxine toxicity is a rare cause of peripheral neuropathy. In a study on 284 patients with peripheral neuropathy, only 7 (2.5%) were attributed to pyridoxine toxicity (Farhad et al., 2016). In an experimental study, neuropathic and neurotoxic effects have been demonstrated. Pyridoxine toxicity is dependent on dose and duration of exposure; neuropathy develops at a dose of 5 g/day in 3 months, and below 500 mg/day by 2 years. Pyridoxine intake below 50 mg is safe. The clinical features depend on the pattern of neuropathy. Four patterns of neuropathy have been described in pyridoxine toxicity:

1. Sensory neuronopathy due to dorsal root ganglia involvement
2. Sensory and autonomic neuropathy
3. Painful axonal sensory motor neuropathy
4. Demyelinating sensory motor neuropathy.

The patients manifest with the features of large fiber involvement predominantly sensory neuropathy. These patients manifest with tingling paresthesia in glove and stocking distribution. There may be sensory ataxia, numbness in hand and feet, and rarely Lhermitte's sign and autonomic dysfunction. In normal volunteers, increased vibration threshold precedes the onset of symptoms. There are two reports of acute sensory neuronopathy following intravenous doses of 132 and 189 mg of pyridoxine for 3 days for the treatment of mushroom poisoning (Albin et al., 1987).

Nerve conduction studies in pyridoxine toxicity neuropathy are consistent with sensory axonopathy with absent or reduced sensory nerve action potentials, and relatively normal motor conductions. Biopsy of sural nerve reveals the nonspecific axonal degeneration.

DIAGNOSIS AND TREATMENT

Serum PLP assay may help in the diagnosis of pyridoxine toxicity. Treatment is withdrawal of pyridoxine source or to reduce it to a safe dose if pyridoxine supplementation is essential. There may be deterioration initially after withdrawal due to the coasting effect, but eventually most of the patients improve.

CONCLUSION

Pyridoxine is widely available in vegetarian and nonvegetarian foods; hence, pyridoxine deficiency is rare. Pyridoxine deficiency manifests with encephalopathy and seizure during neonatal period and neuropathy in adults. Pyridoxine-responsive seizures due to the genetic defect are important to recognize because these patients respond to a high-dose pyridoxine and not to antiepileptic drugs.

REFERENCES

Akiyama, T., Kubota, T., Ozono, K., et al. 2018. Pyridoxal 5'-phosphate and related metabolites in hypophosphatasia: Effects of enzyme replacement therapy. *Molecular Genetics and Metabolism* 125(1–2):174–180.

Albin, R. L., Albers, J. W., Greenberg, H. S., et al. 1987. Acute sensory neuropathy-neuronopathy from pyridoxine overdose. *Neurology* 37(11): 1729–1732. DOI: 10.1212/wnl.37.11.1729.

Baxter, P. 1999. Epidemiology of pyridoxine dependent and pyridoxine responsive seizures in the UK. *Archives of Disease in Childhood* 81(5):431–433.

Baxter, P., Griffiths, P., Kelly, T., Gardner-Medwin, D. 1996. Pyridoxine-dependent seizures: Demographic, clinical, MRI and psychometric features, and effect of dose on intelligence quotient. *Developmental Medicine and Child Neurology* 38(11):998–1006.

Been, J. V., Bok, L. A., Andriessen, P., Renier, W. O. 2005. Epidemiology of pyridoxine dependent seizures in the Netherlands. *Archives of Disease in Childhood* 90(12):1293–1296.

Bennett, C. L., Chen, Y., Hahn, S., et al. 2009. Prevalence of ALDH7A1 mutations in 18 North American pyridoxine-dependent seizure (PDS) patients. *Epilepsia* 50(5):1167–1175. DOI: 10.1111/j.1528–1167.2008.01816.x.

Bennett, C. L., Huynh, H. M., Chance, P. F., Glass, I. A., Gospe, S. M., Jr, 2005. Genetic heterogeneity for autosomal recessive pyridoxine-dependent seizures. *Neurogenetics* 6(3):143–149.

Bok, L. A., Maurits, N. M., Willemsen, M. A., et al. 2010. The EEG response to pyridoxine-IV neither identifies nor excludes pyridoxine-dependent epilepsy. *Epilepsia* 51(12):2406–2411.

Clayton, P. T., Surtees, R. A., DeVile, C., Hyland, K., Heales, S. J. 2003. Neonatal epileptic encephalopathy. *Lancet (London, England)* 361(9369):1614.

Clements, R. H., Katasani, V. G., Palepu, R. 2006. Incidence of vitamin deficiency after laparoscopic Roux-en-Y gastric bypass in a university hospital setting. *The American Surgeon* 72(12):1196–1204.

Coughlin, C. R., 2nd, Swanson, M. A., Spector, E., et al. 2019. The genotypic spectrum of ALDH7A1 mutations resulting in pyridoxine dependent epilepsy: A common epileptic encephalopathy. *Journal of Inherited Metabolic Disease* 42(2):353–361.

Coughlin, C. R., 2nd, van Karnebeek, C. D., Al-Hertani, W., 2015. Triple therapy with pyridoxine, arginine supplementation and dietary lysine restriction in pyridoxine-dependent epilepsy: Neurodevelopmental outcome. *Molecular Genetics and Metabolism* 116(1–2):35–43. DOI: 10.1016/j.ymgme.2015.05.011.

de Roo, M., Abeling, N., Majoie, C. B. 2014. Infantile hypophosphatasia without bone deformities presenting with severe pyridoxine-resistant seizures. *Molecular Genetics and Metabolism* 111(3): 404–407.

di Salvo, M. L., Contestabile, R., Safo, M. K. 2011. Vitamin B(6) salvage enzymes: Mechanism, structure and regulation. *Biochimica et Biophysica Icta* 1814(11):1597–1608.

Farhad, K., Traub, R., Ruzhansky, K. M., Brannagan, T. H., 3rd 2016. Causes of neuropathy in patients referred as "idiopathic neuropathy". *Muscle & Nerve* 53(6):856–861.

Frimpter, G. W., Andelman, R. J., George, W. F. 1969. Vitamin B6-dependency syndromes. New horizons in nutrition. *The American Journal of Clinical Nutrition* 22(6):794–805.

Garaycoechea, J. I, Crossan, G. P., Langevin, F., et al. 2018. Alcohol and endogenous aldehydes damage chromosomes and mutate stem cells. *Nature* 553(7687):171–177.

Ho, C. L., Quay, T. A., Devlin, A. M., Lamers, Y. 2016. Prevalence and predictors of low vitamin B6 status in healthy young adult women in metro Vancouver. *Nutrients* 8(9):538.

Kjeldby, I. K., Fosnes, G. S., Ligaarden, S. C., Farup, P. G. 2013. Vitamin B6 deficiency and diseases in elderly people: A study in nursing homes. *BMC Geriatrics* 13:13.

Kosmadakis, G., Da Costa Correia, E., Carceles, O., Somda, F., Aguilera, D. 2014. Vitamins in dialysis: Who, when and how much? *Renal Failure* 36(4):638–650.

Mills, P. B., Camuzeaux, S. S., Footitt, E. J., 2014. Epilepsy due to PNPO mutations: Genotype, environment and treatment affect presentation and outcome. *Brain: A Journal of Neurology* 137(Pt 5):1350–1360.

Mills, P. B., Struys, E., Jakobs, C. 2006. Mutations in antiquitin in individuals with pyridoxine-dependent seizures. *Nature Medicine* 12(3):307–309.

Rosenberg, I. H. 2012. A history of the isolation and identification of vitamin B(6). *Annals of Nutrition & Metabolism* 61(3):236–238. DOI: 10.1159/000343113.

van de Ven, S., Gardeitchik, T., Kouwenberg, D., Kluijtmans, L., Wevers, R., Morava, E. 2014. Long-term clinical outcome, therapy and mild mitochondrial dysfunction in hyperprolinemia. *Journal of Inherited Metabolic Disease* 37(3):383–390.

Wempe, M. F., Kumar, A., Kumar, V., Choi, Y. J., Swanson, M. A., Friederich, M. W., Hyland, K., Yue, W. W., Van Hove, J., Coughlin, C. R., 2nd. 2019. Identification of a novel biomarker for pyridoxine-dependent epilepsy: Implications for newborn screening. *Journal of Inherited Metabolic Disease* 42(3):565–574.

Whyte M. P. 2017. Hypophosphatasia: Enzyme replacement therapy brings new opportunities and new challenges. *Journal of Bone and Mineral Research: The Official Journal of the American Society for Bone and Mineral Research* 32(4):667–675.

Wilson, M. P., Plecko, B., Mills, P. B., Clayton, P. T. 2019. Disorders affecting vitamin B6 metabolism. *Journal of Inherited Metabolic Disease* 42(4):629–646.

6

Neurological effects of Vitamin B12 deficiency

INTRODUCTION

Vitamin B12 is also known as cobalamin, a water-soluble vitamin, and is essential for cell metabolism and cell functioning. Vitamin B12 is a group of compounds formed by a porphyrin-like corrin nucleus that contains a cobalt atom, which is bound to benzimidazolyl nucleotide. Vitamin B12 acts as a cofactor in DNA synthesis and helps in metabolism of fatty acids and amino acids. Vitamin B12 deficiency though can occur because of vegetarianism and dietary deficiency, it can occur as well due to autoimmune, genetic and a variety of other causes. Since vitamin B12 deficiency has diverse clinical manifestations including hematological, psychiatric and neurological, it may be clinically overlooked. A high index of suspicion therefore is required to diagnose it especially at an early stage. Vitamin B12 deficiency is the most misdiagnosed and most cost-effective treatable condition.

HISTORICAL BACKGROUND

Pernicious anemia (PA) was first reported by Thomas Addison and associated neuropathy by William Gardner and William Osler. Hayem reported "giant blood corpuscle", and Paul Ehrlich reported megaloblast in the bone marrow. Ludwig Lichthein reported myelopathy, which was named as subacute combined degeneration in 1900. In 1920, George Whipple reported liver as antianemia therapy in dogs that were anemic because of blood loss. Taking this analogy to PA, Edwin Cohn prepared liver extract which was 50–100 times more potent than liver. William Castle noted

an intrinsic factor in gastric juice; when this was mixed with liver extract, it helped in treating PA. In 1934, George Whipple, William P Murphy and George Minot were awarded Nobel Prize for treatment of PA. Marry Shaw Shorb, who was working on *Lactobacillus lactis* Dorner culture, used liver extract in this process. Incidentally, her father-in-law had PA and was being treated with liver extract. This observation paved the way for discovery of vitamin B12. In Cambridge, Shorb, Folker and Todd extracted a PA factor from the extract of *Lactobacillus lactis* Dorner, and they named it vitamin B12. Todd in 1957 was awarded Nobel Prize in chemistry. In 1964, Dorothy Hodgkin reported the structure of vitamin B12 using crystallography for which she was awarded the Nobel Prize (Scott and Molloy, 2012) (Figure 6.1).

STRUCTURE AND FUNCTION OF VITAMIN B12

Vitamin B12 is chemically the most complex of all the vitamins. It is based on a corrin ring similar to porphyrin ring in the heme. It has central metal ion cobalt, and four out of six coordination sites are occupied by nitrogen atom and fifth by dimethyl-benzimidazolyl group, which is linked to a ribose-3-phosphate. The ribose-3-phosphate binds to aminoisopropanolyl group. Cobalt atom may be in 1+, 2+ or 3+ oxidation state (Figure 6.2). In the β position, different ligands such as methyl, cyanide, adenosyl and hydroxyl groups are attached, and depending on their attachment, the vitamers are named methylcobalamin, adenosylcobalamin, cyanocobalamin and hydroxycobalamin. Cobalt is

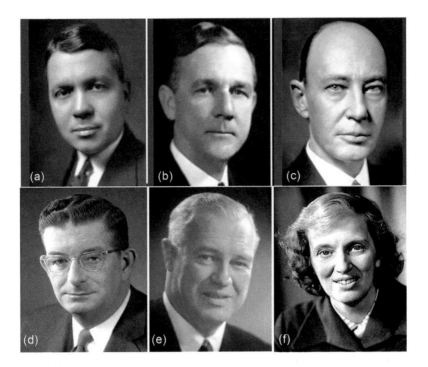

Figure 6.1 Six Nobel Prizes have been awarded to the scientists who worked on vitamin B-12: **(a)** William Parry Murphy, **(b)** George Hoyt Whipple and **(c)** George Richards Minot in 1934 for the discovery of vitamin B-12; **(d)** Robert B Woodward received it in 1965 for synthesis of vitamin B-12 and **(e)** Lord Todd and **(f)** Dorothy Crowfoot Hodgkin were awarded in 1957 and 1964, respectively, for discovering the structure of vitamin B-12.

naturally in trivalent state and is known as cob(III) alamin, and when cobalt is in monovalent state, it is known as Cob(1)alamin. This monovalent state can be attached either to methyl group producing methylcobalamin or to a 5′-adenosyl group giving rise to adenosylcobalamin. Methyl and adenosylcobalamin are found in mammalian cells. The industrial forms of hydroxycobalamin and cyanocobalamin have to be converted to methyl or adenosylcobalamin for its cellular functions.

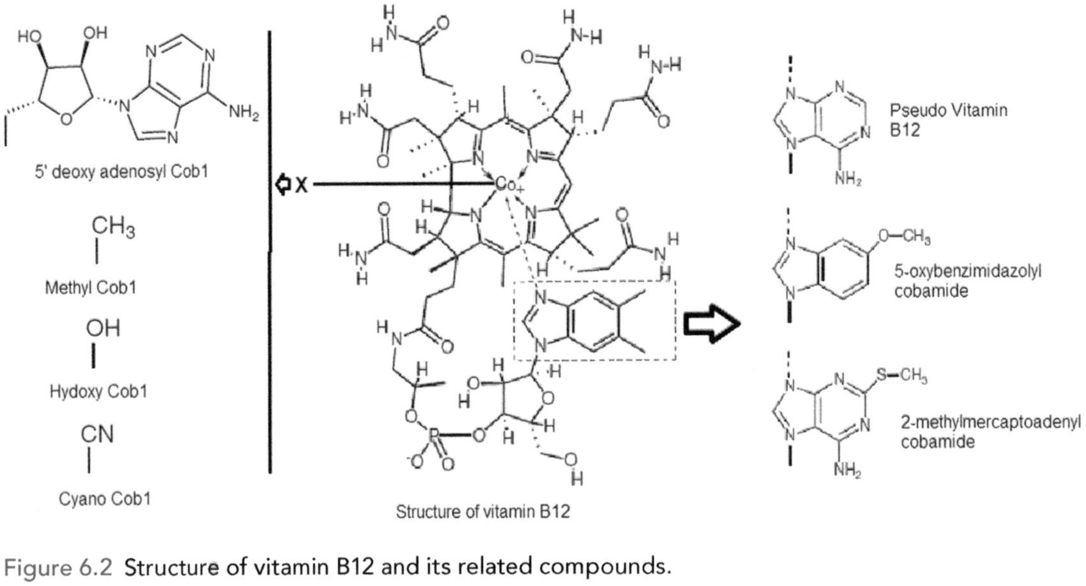

Figure 6.2 Structure of vitamin B12 and its related compounds.

DIETARY SOURCES OF VITAMIN B12

Vitamin B12 is synthesized by certain anaerobic bacteria and by archaeon and not by animals or plants. Vitamin B12 synthesized by bacteria and archaea is accumulated in animal tissues especially in organs and muscles. Meat and milk of ruminant herbivorous animals are good sources of vitamin B12. Bovine milk mainly binds to transcobalamin (TC); therefore vitamin B12 is more bioavailable. In human milk, vitamin B12 is bound to haptocorin (HC), which needs processing for its absorption. The rich dietary sources of vitamin B12 are organ meat (mainly liver and kidney). Beef, pork, lamb, mutton and chicken are also good sources of vitamin B12. Bovine milk is a better source of vitamin B12 than cow milk. The vitamin B12 content of nonruminant animals depends on the livestock. Fish, egg and mushroom also contain vitamin B12. Sea weeds (red and green algae) are a rich source, whereas cereals and fruits are a poor source. The details of dietary vitamin B12 content are presented in Table 6.1. Cooking though reduces vitamin B12, it improves its bioavailability due to loss of moisture and lipids. Fermentation of dairy products by bacteria increases vitamin B12 because fermenting bacteria not only consumes vitamin B12 but also produces B12. In healthy adults, the bioavailability of vitamin B12 is about 50%, and remaining unabsorbed vitamin B12 maintains the microbial ecology in human intestine and may impact human health through gut microbiota. The vegetarians and vegans should consume fortified food to meet their daily requirement.

DAILY REQUIREMENT OF VITAMIN B12

The daily requirement of vitamin B12 in adults is about 2–3 μ. The dietary intake of vitamin B12 in Americans is higher, about 4 μ/day. The requirement is higher in pregnancy, lactation and elderly. The recommended daily dose is mentioned in Table 6.2.

ABSORPTION

Absorption of cobalamin is a well organzied activity of gastric, duodenum, ilium, liver and pancreatic functions. About 50%–60% of ingested vitamin B12 is absorbed (Carmel, 2008). In the food, cobalamin is bound to R-proteins or R-binders. The

Table 6.1 Vitamin B12 content of different food items

Food item	Vitamin B12 (μg/100 g)
Liver	
Beef	52.8
Pork	25.2
Chicken	24.4
Meat	
Beef	0.7–6.2
Lamb, mutton	1.2–2.9
Pork	0.4–2.0
Chicken	0.2–0.6
Kidney beef	27.0–31.0
Fish	2.1–13.3
Snail	20.0
Egg (yolk)	6.9
Dairy milk	
Sheep	0.71
Cow	0.35
Goat	0.06
Human	0.04
Cheese	2.8–4.2
Mushroom	0.1–2.65
Algae	
Red	2.8–66.8
Green	0.1–415

R-proteins are digested by pepsin in the stomach at low pH and the released cobalamin binds to haptocorin (HC), a protein ligand secreted in the saliva and to transcobalamin (Cob1-TC). In the next phase, when cobalamin (Cob1)–HC reaches the duodenum, biliary and pancreatic proteases digest TC and HC and liberate Cob1 which binds to intrinsic factor (Cob1-IF). In distal ilium Cob1-IF is attached to cubulin and megalin receptors which are present in the brush border of ileal enterocyte. Cubulin and megalin receptors both are involved in the absorption of Cob1 but have some differences. Megalin is a single spanning transmembrane glycoprotein, whereas cubulin is a glycoprotein attached to plasma membrane. Megalin is more widely available and belongs to low density lipoprotein. Megalin also mediates endocytosis of cubulin and helps in uptake of Cob1-TC complexes from the proximal

Table 6.2 Recommended daily dose of vitamin B12

Age group	Recommended dose µg/day	
	USA (Institute of Medicine, 1998)	Europe (German Society Nutrition, 2013)
0–<12 months	0.4–0.5	0.4–0.8
1–<13 years	0.9–1.8	1.0–2.0
>13 years	2.4	3.0
Pregnancy	2.6	3.5
Lactation	2.8	4.0

renal tubule. Both CobI and cubulin have epidermal growth factor type repeats. Human astrocytes also secrete TC II. Once inside the enterocyte, the intrinsic factor is degraded in the lysosome. The released cobalamin binds to TC or HC, and these are released in the plasma. About 80% of Cob1 in plasma is bound to HC and is not available for cellular functioning. The Cob1-TCII is available for cellular functions in different organs (Figure 6.3). Unused cobalamin is stored in the liver, kidney and muscles. The total body store of cobalamin is 2–3 mg (Institute of Medicine, 1998). The half-life of cobalamin is 1–4 years (Stahl and Heseker, 2007).

CELLULAR FUNCTION OF COBALAMIN

Vitamin B12 acts as a cofactor in two most important reactions in the mammalian cells. In the cytoplasm, conversion of homocysteine (Hcy) to methionine (Me) occurs with the help of methionine synthase (MeS) in which methyl cobalamin acts as a cofactor. Methionine and its subsequent products are involved in the formation of neurotransmitters, phospholipids, DNA and RNA. In the mitochondria, methyl-malonyl CoA is converted to succinyl-CoA with the help of L-methylmalonyl CoA mutase in which adenosyl Cob1 acts as a cofactor. Succinyl CoA is involved in the catabolism of cholesterol, fatty acids and amino acids (Scalabrino, 2005) (Figure 6.4).

CAUSES OF VITAMIN B12 DEFICIENCY

Vitamin B12 deficiency is closely linked to pernicious anemia and is an autoimmune gastropathy targeting the parietal cells that produce gastric acid and intrinsic factor. Dietary deficiency of cobalamin may occur in vegetarians and vegans.

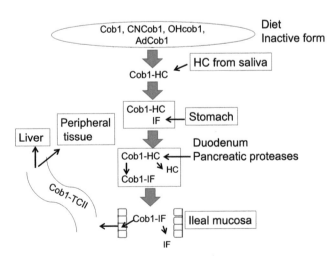

Figure 6.3 Schematic diagram shows the process of absorption of dietary vitamin B12. Ado = adenosyl, Cob1 = Cobalamin, CN = Cyano, HC = Haptocorin, IF = Intrinsic factor, OH = Hydroxyl, TC II = Transcobalamin II.

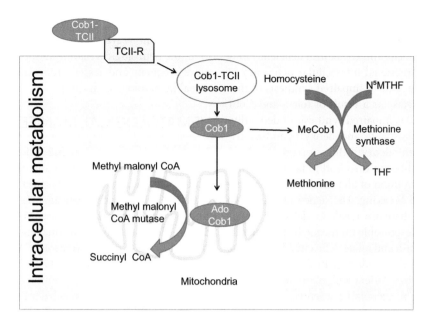

Figure 6.4 Intracellular metabolism of cobalamin, THF = tetrahydrofolate, MTHF = methyl tetrahydrofolate, MeCob = methyl cobalamin, Ado = adenosyl, TC = transcobalamin, TCII-R = transcobalamin receptor (cubulin and megalin).

Various infective and inflammatory diseases of small intestine, pancreas and liver, atrophic gastritis, infestations and infections of small bowel, gastrectomy, small bowel resection and bariatric surgery may result in absorptive defect. A number of drugs such as metformin, H2 receptor blocker, proton pump inhibitors, nitrous oxide, colchicine and neomycin may also reduce the bioavailability of vitamin B12. A number of genetic diseases linked to cobalamin transport and intracellular functioning of cobalamin have been reported. The important causes of vitamin B12 deficiency are presented in Table 6.3.

COBALAMIN AND FOLATE RELATIONSHIP

Cob1 is necessary for synthesis of methionine from Hcy. Tetrahydrofolate is generated from 5 methyl THF, which acts as a coenzyme with thymidylate

Table 6.3 Causes of vitamin B12 deficiency

1. **Autoimmune:**
   Pernicious anemia, inflammatory bowel disease of small intestine
2. **Dietary insufficiency:**
   Vegetarian, vegans
3. **Gastrointestinal disease:**
   Gastrectomy, atrophic gastritis, small intestinal resection, bariatric surgery, infection and infestations, pancreatic or liver disease
4. **Drugs:**
   H-2 receptor blocker, proton pump inhibitors, metformin, nitrous oxide, colchicine, neomycin
5. **Genetic:**
   a. Defective absorption/transport: inherited intrinsic factor deficiency, TC II deficiency, Cubulin/Megalin receptor mutation
   b. Defective intracellular metabolism: Mutation of methionine synthase, methyl malonyl Co-A synthase, MTHFR mutation

synthetase and in DNA synthesis. Thymidylate activity and DNA synthesis are dependent on tetrahydrofolate. Folate and cobalamin deficiency may contribute to functional intracellular deficiency of tetrahydrofolate. Due to impaired synthesis of thymidylate synthetase as a result of folate and Cobl deficiency, there is impaired synthesis of deoxythymidine monophosphate and deoxythymidine triphosphate from deoxyuridine monophosphate. These abnormalities in turn lead to faulty incorporation and recognition of abnormal DNA resulting in DNA strand breaking. Deficiency of these two vitamins may therefore result in defective repair which may be responsible for megaloblastic anemia in both cobalamin and folate deficiency. Since folate deficiency does not produce neurological dysfunction, therefore, in a patient with neurological manifestations with megaloblastic anemia, one should search for cobalamin deficiency (Briani et al., 2013).

CLINICAL FEATURES OF COBALAMIN DEFICIENCY

Cobalamin deficiency has a wide range of clinical features including hematological, gastrointestinal and neurological manifestations (Figure 6.5). Megaloblastic anemia although is common and manifests early, the neurological manifestations may occur without hematological manifestations. In the recent years due to folate fortification of food, the neurological manifestations have become more frequent and lesser proportion of patients reveal hematological findings.

HEMATOLOGICAL MANIFESTATIONS

The patients with vitamin B12 deficiency present with clinical manifestations of anemia such as irritability, fatigue, exertional dyspnea or nocturnal diuresis. Patients with severe anemia may have dizziness, postural hypotension or painful swallowing due to glossitis. Gastrointestinal motility may be affected because of involvement of Meissner's and Auerbach's plexus (Briani et al., 2013). Sometimes, macrocytic anemia may be found in an asymptomatic patient. Anemia in cobalamin deficiency is characterized by macrocytosis, polysegmented (>5 lobes) neutrophils and elevated lactate dehydrogenase. Sometimes raised mean corpuscular volume may be attributed to liver disease, chronic alcoholism and myelodysplastic syndrome. In cobalamin deficiency, DNA synthesis is defective which results in nuclear cytoplasmic asynchrony, slow cell division and arrest at various stages of cell cycle. All three cell lines are affected. In bone marrow, erythroid cells are more affected resulting in altered

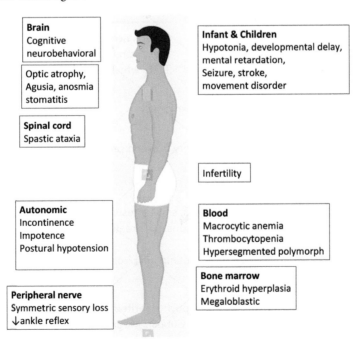

Brain
Cognitive
neurobehavioral

Optic atrophy,
Agusia, anosmia
stomatitis

Spinal cord
Spastic ataxia

Autonomic
Incontinence
Impotence
Postural hypotension

Peripheral nerve
Symmetric sensory loss
↓ankle reflex

Infant & Children
Hypotonia, developmental delay,
mental retardation,
Seizure, stroke,
movement disorder

Infertility

Blood
Macrocytic anemia
Thrombocytopenia
Hypersegmented polymorph

Bone marrow
Erythroid hyperplasia
Megaloblastic

Figure 6.5 Schematic diagram shows the effect of vitamin B12 deficiency in humans.

myeloid erythroid ratio from 3:1 to 1:1. The megalo-blastic changes which are most prominent in bone marrow may spill over to the peripheral blood. The peripheral blood smear reveals large RBC, poi-kilocytosis, anisocytosis, Howell Jolly body (DNA traces) or Cabot ring (nonhemoglobin iron). These changes result in early destruction of RBC, which is responsible for elevated LDH, elevated haptoglo-bin, and low reticulocyte count. The involvement of myeloid series is responsible for hypersegmented polymorphs, which is present in more than 5% of peripheral neutrophils (Figure 6.6). Megakaryocytes may also be hyper-segmented resulting in giant platelets in the peripheral blood. Megaloblastosis is not only restricted to the blood cells but also is seen in rapidly proliferating cells of gastrointestinal epithelium and female genital tract. These changes result in luminal cell atrophy leading to reduce secretion of intrinsic factor thereby reducing cobal-amin absorption in a vicious cycle.

NEUROLOGICAL MANIFESTATIONS

The neurological manifestations of cobalamin deficiency are classically described as subacute combined degeneration (SACD). The neurological manifestations can be grouped as neuropsychiat-ric, cognitive, myelopathy, neuropathy and optic neuropathy. In a study of vitamin B12 deficiency neurological syndromes, myelopathy was present in 93%, encephalopathy in 48% and neuropathy

in 44% of patients, in various combinations and permutations. Combined syndromes occurred in nearly all patients, and pure syndromes occurred as an exception (2%) (Misra and Kalita, 2007). Similar results have been reported in an earlier study including 143 patients with 153 episodes of cobalamin deficiency in which myelopathy was reported in 88% and encephalopathy in 15%; 14% of patients had symptoms only without corre-sponding neurological signs (Healton et al., 1991).

Neuropsychiatric manifestations: Subtle neu-ropsychiatric symptoms are common and often go unnoticed. The frequency of neurobehavioral changes is quite variable ranging from 3% to 42% (Healton et al., 1991; Kalita et al., 2013). This varia-tion in the frequency of neuropsychiatric symptoms may be due to selection of subjects and method of evaluation. The neuropsychiatric symptoms include slow cerebration, confusion, delirium with or without hallucination, delusion, depression and acute psychosis (megaloblastic madness) and rarely it may mimic manic or schizophreniform psychosis (Kalita and Misra, 2008; Hector and Burton, 1988; Dangour et al., 2015). In a study using neuropsy-chiatric inventory on 33 patients with vitamin B12 deficiency, neurologic syndrome revealed abnor-mality in 14 subjects; irritability, aggression and apathy in 7 each, hallucination in 4, delusion in 2 and disinhibition and depression in 1 each. The most of these patients recovered completely follow-ing cobalamin treatment (Kalita et al., 2013).

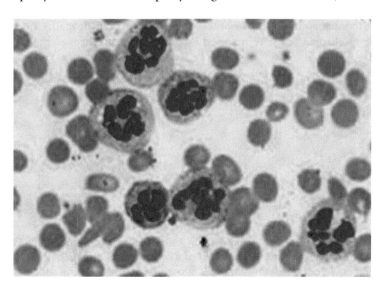

Figure 6.6 Macrocytic anemic with polysegmented polymorph in a patient with subacute combined degeneration.

Cognitive impairment: About 30%–50% patients with SACD have mild to moderate cognitive dysfunction as assessed by Mini Mental Scale Examination (MMSE). In a study on 33 patients, MMSE score was below 18 in 3 patients, and the remaining had milder reduction. The domains involved were recall, calculation, orientation to time, copying and clock drawing. The detailed neuropsychological testing of patients with vitamin B12 deficiency neurological syndrome has revealed impaired category naming, motor speed and precision test, trail making and clock drawing. These findings were consistent with involvement of fronto-subcortical circuit. The cognitive impairment is supported by abnormal cognitive evoked potential. P300 latency was prolonged or unrecordable in the 15 out of 26 patients, which correlated with MMSE score. Following vitamin B12 supplementation, both neuropsychological abnormalities and P300 improved at 3 and 6 months follow up (Kalita et al., 2013). Trail making test and clock drawing test involve executive function and require visuospatial functions and task switching, which depend on fronto-subcortical circuit including frontal cortex, basal ganglia and thalamus (Figure 6.7; Mendez and Cummings, 2003).

Spinal cord: Subacute combined degeneration of spinal cord is typical of cobalamin deficiency. It is characterized by symmetrical dysesthesia of hands and feet, sensory ataxia and spasticity, more marked in the lower limbs. These manifestations are due to the involvement of posterior and lateral columns of cervico-thoracic spinal cord. The onset is usually subacute to chronic but may manifest acutely if there is a high metabolic demand. On examination, the patient has impaired or loss of joint position sensation mainly in the lower limbs. Pinprick and touch impairment may be present in the distal lower limbs, which may be due to associated peripheral neuropathy in SACD (Misra et al., 2008). Severely affected patients with SACD may have micturition disturbance. Urodynamic study in eight patients with SACD having bladder dysfunction revealed voiding and storage abnormality in all, detrusor areflexia in two, neurogenic detrusor over activity with high pressure voiding in three and normal detrusor activity in two patients. These bladder symptoms and urodynamic abnormalities improved following intramuscular hydroxycobalamin treatment in majority (Misra et al., 2008).

Peripheral nerves: Peripheral neuropathy occurs in about 25% patients with cobalamin deficiency (Healton et al., 1991). The onset of peripheral neuropathy is usually subacute to chronic but may be acute especially following nitrous oxide poisoning or in those patients with high demand (Zhao et al., 2020). The neuropathy may be distal axonal in 76% and demyelinating in 24% (Leishear et al., 2012a,b). Some patients may have subclinical neuropathy which may be evident on nerve conduction study. The elderly patents or those on metformin treatment, the possibility of vitamin B12 deficiency should be considered if neuropathic symptoms are present (Leishear et al., 2012a,b). Early diagnosis of neuropathy is important for good outcome. There is a controversy about the coexistence of neuropathy in SACD because of common occurrence of myelopathy. Coexisting

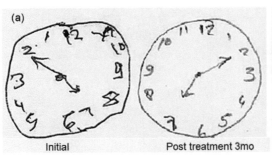
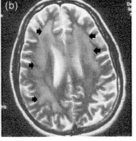

Initial   Post treatment 3mo

Figure 6.7 **(a)** Clock drawing test of a patient with myeloneuropathy due to vitamin B12 deficiency shows improvement from baseline. **(b)** Cranial MRI of a patient with vitamin B12 deficiency who presented with encephalomyeloneuropathy shows T2 hyperintense lesion in the subcortical white matter (arrow). (With permission from Kalita, J., Agarwal, R., Chandra, S., Misra, U. K. 2013. A study of neurobehavioral, clinical psychometric, and P3 changes in vitamin B12 deficiency neurological syndrome. *Nutritional Neuroscience* 16(1):39–46.)

myelopathy may overshadow the neuropathic symptoms. Isolated neuropathy in cobalamin deficiency is uncommon and has been reported in 6% patients only; whereas evidence of neuropathy was present in 69.7% patients with myelopathy.

Nerve conduction studies have revealed both axonal and demyelinating findings (Kalita et al., 2014; Puri et al., 2005; Huang et al., 2011). In view of the controversy about the presence and type of neuropathy in cobalamin deficiency, a sequential NCV study has been conducted in 66 patients. The clinical feature of neuropathy (sensory loss with ankle areflexia) was present in 69.7% patients whereas nerve conduction was abnormal in 54.5% patients. The nerve conduction findings were axonal in 12%, demyelinating in 6.1% and mixed in 66.7%. On follow up, majority of the patients improved both in clinical and neurophysiological parameters. All four patients with isolated neuropathy improved completely. On biopsy, chronic axonal changes of varying severity were noted. Patients with less than 2 months illness had acute axonal degeneration with myelin ovoids (Kalita et al., 2014).

Optic neuropathy: Cohen et al. in 1936 reported the association of optic neuropathy with pernicious anemia. Subsequent studies revealed that visual loss in cobalamin deficiency is rare. In a review of 153 patients with cobalamin deficiency, visual impairment with bilateral centrocecal scotoma was present in one patient only (Fine and Hallett 1980). Visual evoked potential, however, revealed abnormal P100 latency and amplitude without any visual impairment (Misra et al., 2003; Pandey et al., 2004). Experimental studies have revealed patchy areas of demyelination in optic nerve and optic tract (Agamanolis et al., 1976). This has also been confirmed in human studies (Kalita et al., 2018). Sometimes, acute visual loss may be due to macular hemorrhage, which has been reported in a patient with thrombocytopenia due to vitamin B12 (Figure 6.8; Dongre et al., 2021).

PATHOLOGY

The typical neuropathological changes in cobalamin deficiency are referred as SACD, which refers to the involvement of posterior and lateral column of spinal cord. The changes include the swelling of myelin sheath, which are followed by demyelination and astrocytic gliosis. The pathological changes start in the posterior column especially fasciculus cuneatus. The small foci of demyelination coalesce to form large plaque, which extend both horizontally and vertically. The lateral corticospinal tracts are more severely affected than the anterior corticospinal tract. Spinothalamic tracts are usually spared. These changes are prominent in lower cervical, upper thoracic and upper lumbar regions. Focal demyelinating plaques in the subcortical white matter of the brain were initially reported (Kunze and Leitenmaier, 1976; Pant et al., 1968) and may also present in cerebellar white

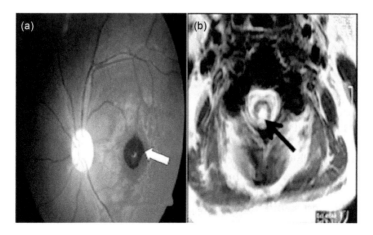

Figure 6.8 **(a)** Macular hemorrhage because of thrombocytopenia in a girl with vitamin B12 deficiency. **(b)** Spinal MRI revealed posterior T2 hyperintensity. (With permission from Dongre, N., Singh, V. K., Kalita, J., Misra, U. K. 2020. Vitamin B12 deficiency presenting as acute febrile encephalopathy and retinopathy. *Postgraduate Medical Journal*, 2021;97:141–142.

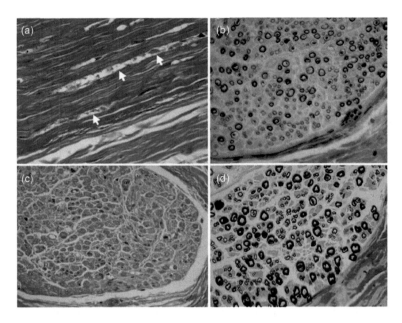

Figure 6.9 Spectrum of findings seen on sural nerve biopsies in B12 deficiency neuropathy.
(a) Acute axonal degeneration and formation of myelin ovoids evident on longitudinal sections
(arrow). The myelin was preserved in these nerve fibers. (b) Focal depletion of large myelinated fibers
with prominent remyelination was seen in cases with short duration of illness (2 months). (c) Increasing
fibrosis of endoneurium accompanied by fiber depletion and (d) prominent axonal regeneration
was seen with increasing duration of disease (24 months). (a) Masson trichrome ×300; (b) Kulchitsky
Pal×280; (c) Masson trichrome ×160; (d): Kulchitsky Pal ×300. (With permission from Kalita, J., Chandra,
S., Bhoi, S. K., Agarwal, R., Misra, U. K., Shankar, S. K., Mahadevan, A. 2014. Clinical, nerve conduction
and nerve biopsy study in vitamin B12 deficiency neurological syndrome with a short-term follow-up.
Nutritional Neuroscience 17(4):156–163.)

matter. Similar changes have also been reported in optic nerve carrying papulomacular bundle. In the peripheral nerve, there is axonal degeneration in the initial stage which is followed by secondary demyelination (Figure 6.9).

LABORATORY DIAGNOSIS

The diagnosis of cobalamin deficiency neurological syndrome is based on the demonstration of low serum vitamin B12 with high serum MMA and Hcy, hematological changes and characteristic spinal MRI findings.

Radiological findings: Following the discovery of MRI, the pathological changes in vitamin B12 deficiency can be visualized in the early and late stage of the disease. The most significant changes are T2 hyperintensity in the posterior column in the cervicodorsal region giving rise to inverted "V" sign (Figure 6.10). There is T2 hyperintensity of lateral column as well. Spinal cord may be swollen in the early stage and atrophic in the late stage.

Patchy gadolinium enhancement may be seen rarely in the patients with acute myelopathy. The spinal cord changes are best seen on T2 sequences as hyperintensity. Using diffusion weighted sequence hyperintensity in posterior and lateral column with restricted diffusion on apparent diffusion coefficient map is consistent with edema in myelin. In experimental studies, myelin edema has been reported (Scalabrino 2005). Cranial MRI reveals subcortical T2 or FLAIR hyperintense lesions in some patients. Subcortical white matter lesions are better seen on FLAIR sequence. The MRI changes in cobalamin deficiency should be differentiated from multiple sclerosis, neuromyelitis optica, post infectious demyelination, copper deficiency and zinc intoxication.

Serum vitamin B12: Serum vitamin B12 level provides a confirmatory evidence of cobalamin deficiency. The radioisotope assay for serum vitamin B12 was done by Schilling test, which is now replaced by chemiluminescence, radio immunoassay or HPLC. About 99% patients with

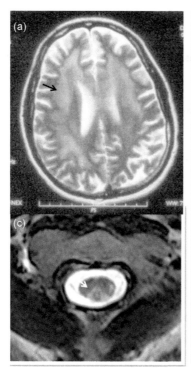
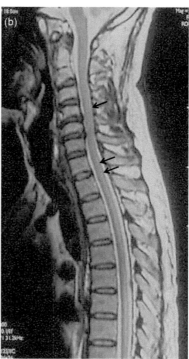

Figure 6.10 MRI changes in subacute combined degeneration manifesting with myelocognitive symptoms. (a) Cranial MRI T2 sequence shows subcortical hyperintensity. (b) Spinal MRI shows posterior T2 hyperintensity in cervicodorsal region and (c) Axial T2 sequence shows inverted "V" sign due to involvement of posterior columns and corticospinal tracts.

hematological or neurological manifestations have serum vitamin level below 300 pg/ml. The level is considered adequate if it is more than 350 pg/ml. In patients suspected of having cobalamin deficiency, but serum vitamin B12 is normal, the measurement of MMA or Hcy is helpful. Methyl malonic acid level of 3SD of controls has a sensitivity of 98.4% and that of Hcy 98.9% for the diagnosis of cobalamin deficiency (Savage et al., 1994). A number of conditions may affect cobalamin, MMA and Hcy levels, which are summarized in Table 6.4.

Electrodiagnostic study: Evoked potential and nerve conduction studies have important role in documenting and prognosticating the patients with cobalamin deficiency. Tibial somatosensory evoked potential is most commonly impaired; the P40 (cortical potential) may be unrecordable or central sensory conduction time may be prolonged. SSEP objectively confirms the proprioceptive sensory loss or may reveal subclinical abnormality. Visual evoked potential is frequently abnormal without impaired visual acuity, color and field of vision. The P100 latency is prolonged

and amplitude may be reduced. Authors find VEP as a useful tool to differentiate SACD from cervical spondylotic myelopathy. If VEP is abnormal, one may investigate for cobalamin deficiency. In electrodiagnostic evaluation of SACD, highest abnormality was noted in tibial SEP 87.3%–100%, VEP in 63.6%–70%, MEP 56.6%, P3 in 58% and NCV in 15%–67% (Figures 6.11 and 6.12; Misra et al., 2007; Pandey et al., 2004; Carmel, 2008; Hemmer et al., 1998; Kalita et al., 2013; Kalita et al., 2018; Kalita and Misra, 2015).

CONUNDRUM OF SUBCLINICAL COBALAMIN DEFICIENCY

There is a group of individuals who do not have clinical manifestations of cobalamin deficiency in spite of low level of serum vitamin B12 (subclinical cobalamin deficiency). These subjects are more in number compared to symptomatic patients. A majority of such patients are due to food bound Cobl malabsorption rather than PA. This may be due to low acid secretion, antacids, proton pump

Table 6.4 Causes of abnormal serum cobalamin, homocysteine and methyl malonic acid level

Biomarkers	Increase	Decrease
Cobalamin	Renal failure	TC1 deficiency
	Liver disease	Folate deficiency
	Myelodysplastic syndrome	HIV
	Hematological malignancy	Myeloma
	Polycythemia rubra vera	Pregnancy
	Carcinoma of breast & colon	Contraceptive pills
		Anticonvulsants
Homocysteine	Renal failure	-
	Hypothyroidism	
	Alcoholism	
	Pyridoxine or folate deficiency	
	Psoriasis	
	Leukemia	
	Renal transplant	
	MTHFR mutation	
	Inborn error of Hcy metabolism	
Methyl malonic acid	Renal failure	-
	Hypovolemia	
	MMA related enzyme defects	
	Methyl malonyl Co mutase deficiency	
	Intestinal bacterial overgrowth	

inhibitors and H2 receptor blockers which may impair dissociation of Cobl from R-protein. It may be a transitory phenomenon, and the offending agents should be withdrawn if possible. Serum vitamin B12 level should be checked after 1–2 months, if low, anti intrinsic factor antibody should be tested to decide about oral or parenteral cobalamin therapy. The patients should be warned about the neurological manifestations which should be immediately reported.

TREATMENT

The patients with vitamin B12 deficiency with clinical manifestations (hematological, neurological, others) require urgent medical treatment. Injection hydroxycobalamin 1000 μg IM on alternate days for 2 weeks followed by 3 monthly is recommended in UK (Shipton and Thachil, 2015). In USA, hydroxycobalamin 1000 μg IM daily is given for 10 days followed by weekly injection for 1 month and then monthly. The hematological improvement occurs earliest; reticulocyte count increases by 1 week, and MCV and hemoglobin normalize by 6–8 weeks. The neurological improvement takes longer time to improve; behavioral, cognitive and bladder dysfunctions improve earlier, and spinal cord manifestations improve later. Sensory ataxia is last to improve and may persist in long standing severely affected patients. The treatment of patients with neurological manifestation should be continued daily till there is no further improvement and then two monthly injection may be continued (Shipton and Thachil, 2015). High dose oral cobalamin tablets are available in Europe and have been reported to be equally effective as parenteral injection (Stabler, 2013). Oral vitamin B12 replacement 1000 μg is adequate to normalize serum vitamin B12 level, cure clinical manifestations related to vitamin B12 deficiency and is safe. High-dose oral vitamin B12 is also safe and effective in absorptive vitamin B12 defect except some neurological syndromes that should be managed with IM injection. Intranasal vitamin B12 as dried powder or nasal gel of cyanocobalamin has been used

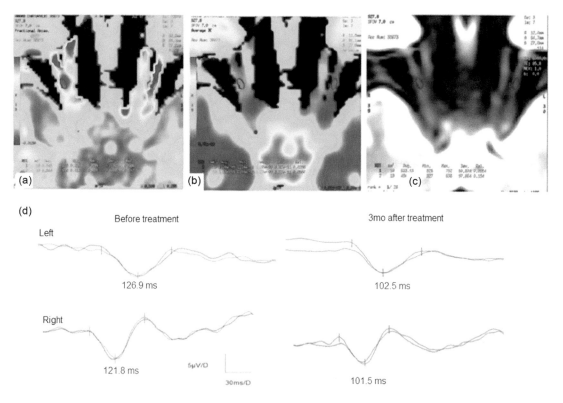

Figure 6.11 (a) FA, (b) ADC, and (c) structural diffusion tensor index maps obtained in a 27-year-old male with subacute combined degeneration. Regions of interest are placed in the middle part of both the optic nerves. (d) VEP of the same patient revealed prolonged P100 latency on both right and left eye (126.9/121.8 ms) which normalized (102.5 /101.5 ms) at 3 months after treatment. ADC, apparent diffusion co-efficient; FA, fractional anisotropy; VEP, visual evoked potential. (With permission from Kalita, J., Soni, N., Dubey, D., Kumar, S., Misra, U. K. 2018. Evaluation of optic nerve functions in subacute combined degeneration using visual evoked potential and diffusion tensor imaging – a pilot study. *The British Journal of Radiology 91*(1091):20180086.)

as an alternative to oral or IM injection. Intra nasal spray 500 μg/0.1 ml has been approved for the treatment of vitamin B12 deficiency and Pernicious anemia (García-Arieta et al., 2001). However, more studies are needed before it can be recommended (Andrès et al., 2018).

COBALAMIN DEFICIENCY IN PEDIATRICS

Cobalamin is essential for the growth and development of CNS both in utero and after birth. During pregnancy, placenta actively concentrates cobalamin, and the fetal cobalamin level may be twice that of maternal level (Fréry et al., 1992). Fetus accumulates cobalamin which fulfills the requirement till 1 year of age (McPhee et al., 1988).

The neurological manifestations of cobalamin deficiency if occurring within 6 months of age are attributed to maternal cobalamin deficiency or fetal cobalamin transporter defect. The newborn depends on the maternal milk for cobalamin supply; therefore, cobalamin deficiency generally manifests after 1 year of age.

Pediatric cobalamin deficiency is commoner in the developing countries. In 3766 children in USA aged 4–19 years, only 1 in 1255 children had serum vitamin B12 less than 100 pg/ml and 1 in 200 had less than 200 pg/ml (Wright et al., 1998). In Mexico, 22% of children had vitamin B12 level below 140 pg/ml and 25% of them were due to intestinal infection or infestation leading to malabsorption (Allen et al., 1995). In Turkey, 41% of newborn have low vitamin B12 levels (Koc et al., 2006).

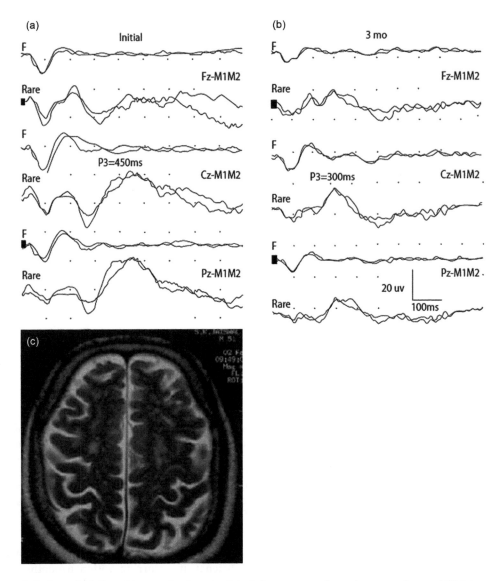

Figure 6.12 (a and b) Cognitive evoked potential of the same patient shows prolonged P3 latency which improved 3-months of B12 therapy. His MMSE score also improved from 23 to 30. F frequent stimuli. (c) Cranial MRI, T2 sequence of the patient revealed multiple white matter T2 hyperintensity. (With permission from Kalita, J., Misra, U. K. 2008. Vitamin B12 deficiency neurological syndromes: Correlation of clinical, MRI and cognitive evoked potential. *Journal of Neurology* 255(3): 353–359.)

Clinical feature: The infants and children with vitamin B12 deficiency have special clinical features which are quite different from adults resulting in delayed diagnosis. The neurological findings may antedate the hematological findings. Low vitamin B12, high Hcy and MMA levels may precede the clinical manifestations. The newborn may have irritability, vomiting, refusal to feed and failure to thrive. The neurological findings include developmental delay, regression of milestone, hypotonia, tremor, chorea focal or generalized seizures. The older children have skin pigmentation of dorsum of hands (knuckles, toes, axilla, arm and medial side of thigh). They may have hypotonia, hyperreflexia, ataxia, paresthesia, chorea and neuropsychiatric changes. Seizures may occur in severely affected children. In a study from Iran, 303 children between 2 and 18 months of age having vitamin B12 deficiency were reported; maternal cobalamin deficiency was present in 163 of them (group I) and not present in 103 (group II). The neurological manifestations were more common in group I compared to group II (29% vs 12.4%). MRI abnormality was also more common in group I. The cranial MRI findings included delayed myelination, demyelination, thin corpus callosum and ventricular dilatation (Tanyildiz et al., 2017). The MRI changes in a girl with mental retardation and spastic hemiplegia due to cobalamin deficiency is shown in Figure 6.13. The clinical presentation in different etiologies of cobalamin deficiency in children and infants is presented in Table 6.5.

The diagnosis of cobalamin deficiency or its enzymatic defect can be evaluated by the following protocol:

1. Vitamin B12 deficiency/transporter defect: Low serum vitamin B12, high MMA and high Hcy
2. Ado Cob1 abnormality: Normal serum vitamin B12, normal Hcy and high MMA
3. Methyl Cob1 defect: Normal serum vitamin B 12 and MMA, and high Hcy.

Treatment: The treatment of cobalamin deficiency in children includes injection hydroxycobalamin 1000 μg IM 2–7 times a week. The duration of treatment is determined by optimal clinical

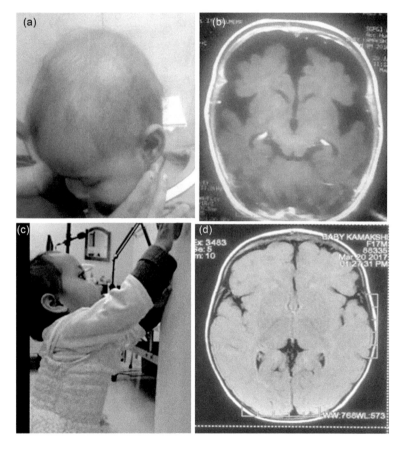

Figure 6.13 (a) A 9-month-old girl with alopecia, failure to thrive and spasticity, and (b) her cranial MRI reveals cortical atrophy and widening of sulci. Her vitamin B12 was low (<150 ng/ml), mean corpuscular volume 104, hemoglobin 6.5 gm/dl. Both parents also had low serum vitamin B12 (<85 ng/ml). Nine months after hydroxycobalamin injection, (c) she could stand and walk with normal black hair and (d) MRI also revealed improvement.

Table 6.5 Clinical and biochemical changes of cobalamin deficiency due to various etiologies in pediatric age group

Defect	Age onset	B12/MMA/Hcy	Hematological	Neurological	Comments
Maternal B12 deficiency	Infancy	L/H/H	Macrocytic anemia	Developmental delay; hypotonia, seizure, movement disorder	Good response to treatment
Pernicious anemia	1–5 years	L/H/H	Macrocytic anemia	Occasional	Good response to IM hydroxycobalamin
TCII deficiency	1–2 months	N/H/H	Megaloblastic anemia, pancytopenia	Development delay	HC level diagnostic
Inborn errors A-G					
Cob1A, B	1 month	N/H/N	?	Same as cobalamin deficiency	MMA normalize after cobalamin treatment
Cob1C,D,F	First few months/late onset	N/H/H	Megaloblastic anemia, hemolysis, pancytopenia	Developmental delay, seizure, hypotonia, hydrocephalous, ocular abnormality	Cardiac disease
Cob1E,G	2 years	N/?/H	Megaloblastic anemia	Hypotonia, seizure, ataxia, developmental delay	Low methionine
MMA (Mut 0, mut-)	Hours to week of life or late onset	N/H/N	Anemia, thrombocytopenia, neutropenia	Encephalopathy, seizure, hypotonia, abnormal posture	Recurrent metabolic acidosis, hyperammonemia

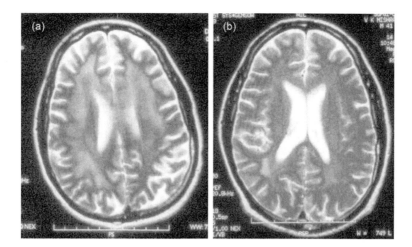

Figure 6.14 Cranial MRI of patient with neurobehavioral and cognitive impairment due to vitamin B12 deficiency. (a) Cranial MRI at presentation revealed severe subcortical white matter T2 hyperintensity, and (b) Follow up MRI after 6 months of injection hydroxycobalamin revealed significant reduction of lesion.

improvement and normalization of hematological and serum vitamin B12, MMA and Hcy level. Dietary deficiency requires additional dietary modification. Intrinsic factor deficiency and absorptive defects require lifelong treatment.

OUTCOME

Adequate vitamin B12 treatment reverses megaloblastosis in 24 h and normalizes marrow hematopoiesis in 48 h. The reticulocyte count increases after 3–4 days and peaks after a week. The polysegmented neutrophils remain in the peripheral blood till 2 weeks. The abnormal hematological parameters start improving by 1 week, and blood picture normalizes by 2 months. Neurological improvement depends on how early the diagnosis is made and treatment is offered. Sleep, taste and smell are earliest to improve usually within a week. Cognitive and neurobehavioral abnormalities improve within 3 months. Posterior column dysfunction and peripheral neuropathy takes several months, and some residual deficit may persist if treated late. The response to treatment in the patients with autoimmune and dietary deficiency of vitamin B12 deficiency is the same because the neurological dysfunction is due to deficiency of vitamin B12 and not due to intrinsic factor deficiency (Misra and Kalita, 2007). Early and adequate treatment improves most of the neurological abnormalities including MRI changes (Figure 6.14).

CONCLUSION

Cobalamin deficiency occurs due to dietary deficiency, pernicious anemia or due to genetic disorders. It occurs more commonly in elderly isolated individuals but is also prevalent among vegetarians and vegans. Majority of vitamin B12 deficiency individuals remain asymptomatic or have subtle neurobehavioral problems. Classically it manifests with megaloblastic anemia, myelopathy, neuropathy and neurobehavioral changes. Genetic cobalamin metabolism disorder may manifest at early age with delayed development, mental retardation, seizure, stroke and movement disorders. The diagnosis of vitamin B12 deficiency is confirmed by low serum vitamin B12, elevated MMA and Hcy levels. Spinal MRI reveals inverted "V" sign. Vitamin B12 deficiency is treated by hydroxycobalamin injection with which patients usually recover.

REFERENCES

Agamanolis, D. P., Chester, E. M., Victor, M., Kark, J. A., Hines, J. D., Harris, J. W. (1976). Neuropathology of experimental vitamin B12 deficiency in monkeys. *Neurology* 26(10):905–914.

Allen, L. H., Rosado, J. L., Casterline, J. E., Martinez, H., Lopez, P., Muñoz, E., Black, A. K. 1995. Vitamin B-12 deficiency and malabsorption are highly prevalent in rural Mexican communities. *The American Journal of Clinical Nutrition* 62(5):1013–1019.

Andrès, E., Zulfiqar, A. A., Serraj, K., Vogel, T., Kaltenbach, G. 2018. Systematic review and pragmatic clinical approach to oral and nasal vitamin B12 (cobalamin) treatment in patients with vitamin B12 deficiency related to gastrointestinal disorders. *Journal of Clinical Medicine* 7(10):304.

Briani, C., Dalla Torre, C., Citton, V., Manara, R., Pompanin, S., Binotto, G., Adami, F. 2013. Cobalamin deficiency: Clinical picture and radiological findings. *Nutrients* 5(11):4521–4539.

Carmel, R. 2008. How I treat cobalamin (vitamin B12) deficiency. *Blood, 112*(6), 2214–2221.

Dangour, A. D., Allen, E., Clarke, R., et al. 2015. Effects of vitamin B-12 supplementation on neurologic and cognitive function in older people: A randomized controlled trial. *The American Journal of Clinical Nutrition* 102(3):639–647.

Dongre, N., Singh, V. K., Kalita, J., Misra, U. K. 2021. Vitamin B12 deficiency presenting as acute febrile encephalopathy and retinopathy. *Postgraduate Medical Journal.* 97(1145): 141–142.

Fine, E. J., Hallett, M. 1980. Neurophysiological study of subacute combined degeneration. *Journal of the Neurological Sciences* 45(2–3):331–336.

Fréry, N., Huel, G., Leroy, M., Moreau, T., Savard, R., Blot, P., Lellouch, J. 1992. Vitamin B12 among parturients and their newborns and its relationship with birthweight. *European Journal of Obstetrics, Gynecology, and Reproductive Biology* 45(3):155–163.

García-Arieta, A., Torrado-Santiago, S., Goya, L., Torrado, J. J. 2001. Spray-dried powders as nasal absorption enhancers of cyanocobalamin. *Biological & Pharmaceutical Bulletin* 24(12), 1411–1416.

Hemmer, B., Glocker, F. X., Schumacher, M., Deuschl, G., Lücking, C. H. 1998. Subacute combined degeneration: Clinical, electrophysiological, and magnetic resonance imaging findings. *Journal of Neurology, Neurosurgery, and Psychiatry* 65(6):822–827.

Healton, E. B., Savage, D. G., Brust, J. C., Garrett, T. J., Lindenbaum, J. 1991. Neurologic aspects of cobalamin deficiency. *Medicine* 70(4):229–245.

Hector, M., Burton, J. R. 1988. What are the psychiatric manifestations of vitamin B12 deficiency? *Journal of the American Geriatrics Society* 36(12):1105–1112.

Huang, C. R., Chang, W. N., Tsai, N. W., Lu, C. H. 2011. Serial nerve conduction studies in vitamin B12 deficiency-associated polyneuropathy. *Neurological Sciences: Official Journal of the Italian Neurological Society and of the Italian Society of Clinical Neurophysiology* 32(1):183–186.

Institute of Medicine. 1998. (US) Standing Committee on the Scientific Evaluation of Dietary Reference Intakes and its Panel on Folate, Other B Vitamins, and Choline. Dietary Reference Intakes for Thiamin, Riboflavin, Niacin, Vitamin B6, Folate, Vitamin B12, Pantothenic Acid, Biotin, and Choline. National Academies Press (US).

Kalita, J., Agarwal, R., Chandra, S., Misra, U. K. 2013. A study of neurobehavioral, clinical psychometric, and P3 changes in vitamin B12 deficiency neurological syndrome. *Nutritional Neuroscience* 16(1):39–46.

Kalita, J., Chandra, S., Bhoi, S. K., Agarwal, R., Misra, U. K., Shankar, S. K., Mahadevan, A. 2014. Clinical, nerve conduction and nerve biopsy study in vitamin B12 deficiency neurological syndrome with a short-term follow-up. *Nutritional Neuroscience* 17(4):156–163.

Kalita, J., Misra, U. K. 2015. Benefit of vitamin B-12 supplementation in asymptomatic elderly: A matter of endpoints. *The American Journal of Clinical Nutrition* 102(3):529–530.

Kalita, J., Misra, U. K. 2008. Vitamin B12 deficiency neurological syndromes: Correlation of clinical, MRI and cognitive evoked potential. *Journal of Neurology* 255(3):353–359.

Kalita, J., Soni, N., Dubey, D., Kumar, S., Misra, U. K. 2018. Evaluation of optic nerve functions in subacute combined degeneration using visual evoked potential and diffusion tensor imaging – a pilot study. *The British Journal of Radiology* 91(1091):20180086.

Koc, A., Kocyigit, A., Soran, M., Demir, N., Sevinc, E., Erel, O., Mil, Z. 2006. High frequency of maternal vitamin B12 deficiency as an important cause of infantile vitamin B12 deficiency in Sanliurfa province of Turkey. *European Journal of Nutrition* 45(5):291–297.

Kunze, K., Leitenmaier, K., 1976. Vitamin B12 deficiency and subacute combined degeneration of the spinal cord (funicular spinal disease). In: Vinken, P.J., Bruyn, G.W., Klawans, H.L. (Eds.), *Metabolic and deficiency diseases of the nervous system (part II)*. Handb. Clin. Neurol. vol. 28. Amsterdam: Elsevier, pp. 141–198.

Leishear, K., Boudreau, R. M., Studenski, S. A., et al. 2012a. Relationship between vitamin B12 and sensory and motor peripheral nerve function in older adults. *Journal of the American Geriatrics Society* 60(6):1057–1063.

Leishear, K., Ferrucci, L., Lauretani, F., Boudreau, R. M., Studenski, S. A., Rosano, C., Abbate, R., Gori, A. M., Corsi, A. M., Di Iorio, A., Guralnik, J. M., Bandinelli, S., Newman, A. B., Strotmeyer, E. S. (2012b). Vitamin B12 and homocysteine levels and 6-year change in peripheral nerve function and neurological signs. *The Journals of Gerontology. Series A, Biological Sciences and Medical Sciences* 67(5):537–543.

McPhee, A. J., Davidson, G. P., Leahy, M., Beare, T. 1988. Vitamin B12 deficiency in a breast fed infant. *Archives of Disease in Childhood 63*(8):921–923.

Mendez, M. F., Cummings, J. L. 2003. *Dementia: A clinical approach.* Oxford, UK: Butterworth-Heinemann.

Misra, U. K., Kalita, J. 2007. Comparison of clinical and electrodiagnostic features in B12 deficiency neurological syndromes with and without antiparietal cell antibodies. *Postgraduate Medical Journal 83*(976):124–127.

Misra, U. K., Kalita, J., Das, A. 2003. Vitamin B12 deficiency neurological syndromes: A clinical, MRI and electrodiagnostic study. *Electromyography and Clinical Neurophysiology 43*(1):57–64.

Misra, U. K., Kalita, J., Kumar, G., Kapoor, R. 2008. Bladder dysfunction in subacute combined degeneration: A clinical, MRI and urodynamic study. *Journal of Neurology 255*(12):1881–1888.

Pandey, S., Kalita, J., Misra, U. K. 2004. A sequential study of visual evoked potential in patients with vitamin B12 deficiency neurological syndrome. *Clinical Neurophysiology: Official Journal of the International Federation of Clinical Neurophysiology 115*(4):914–918.

Pant, S.S., Asbury, A.K., Richardson Jr., E.P., 1968. The myelopathy of pernicious anemia. A neuropathological reappraisal. *Acta Neurologica Scandinavica 44* (Suppl 35):8–36.

Puri, V., Chaudhry, N., Goel, S., Gulati, P., Nehru, R., Chowdhury, D. 2005. Vitamin B12 deficiency: A clinical and electrophysiological profile. *Electromyography and Clinical Neurophysiology 45*(5):273–284.

Savage, D. G., Lindenbaum, J., Stabler, S. P., Allen, R. H. 1994. Sensitivity of serum methylmalonic acid and total homocysteine determinations for diagnosing cobalamin and folate deficiencies. *The American Journal of Medicine 96*(3):239–246.

Scalabrino, G. 2005. Cobalamin (vitamin B(12)) in subacute combined degeneration and beyond: Traditional interpretations and novel theories. *Experimental Neurology 192*(2):463–479.

Scott, J. M., Molloy, A. M. 2012. The discovery of vitamin B(12). *Annals of Nutrition & Metabolism 61*(3):239–245.

Shipton, M. J., Thachil, J. 2015. Vitamin B12 deficiency: A 21st century perspective. *Clinical Medicine (London, England) 15*(2):145–150.

Stabler, S. P. 2013. Clinical practice. Vitamin B12 deficiency. *The New England Journal of Medicine 368*(2):149–160.

Stahl, A., Heseker, H. 2007. Vitamin B-12 (Cobalamine). *Ernahrungs Umschau 54*(10):594–601.

Tanyildiz, H. G., Yesil, S., Okur, I., Yuksel, D., Sahin, G.2017. How does B12 deficiency of mothers affect their infants? *Iranian Journal of Pediatrics 27*(5):e12898.

Wright, J. D., Bialostosky, K., Gunter, E. W., Carroll, M. D., Najjar, M. F., Bowman, B. A., Johnson, C. L. 1998. Blood folate and vitamin B12: United States, 1988–94. *Vital and Health Statistics. Series 11, Data from the National Health Survey 243*:1–78.

Zhao, B., Zhao, L., Li, Z., Zhao, R. 2020. Sub-acute combined degeneration induced by nitrous oxide inhalation: Two case reports. *Medicine 99*(18): e19926.

7

Vitamin D deficiency

INTRODUCTION

Vitamin D is a fat-soluble vitamin, mainly synthesized by the skin when exposed to ultraviolet (UV) light hence known as sunshine vitamin. It is an essential vitamin for calcium regulation and bone health. Vitamin D is also associated with several disorders such as diabetes, heart disease, obesity, depression and many other autoimmune disorders. Vitamin D is traditionally associated with rickets and osteomalacia. About 50% of world population is deficient in vitamin D.

HISTORY

Sir Edward Mellanby was struck by high incidence of rickets in Britain especially in Scotland. Rickets was therefore known as "the English disease". At that time, Mellanby thought that rickets may be a dietary deficiency disease. He produced rickets-like disease in dogs by feeding Scottish diet (oats) and inadvertently kept the dog indoor away from sunlight (Mellanby, 1919; 1976). Mellanby used cod liver oil to treat this disease, and he presumed that rickets may be due to vitamin A deficiency. McCollum at Johns Hopkins University investigated vitamin A and rickets link. He bubbled oxygen through cod liver oil to destroy vitamin A and the remaining product was still able to cure rickets. McCollum concluded that rickets is caused by a new vitamin deficiency and named it vitamin D. Hulshinsky from Vienna and Chick and colleagues from England observed that the children with rickets could be cured by summer sunlight or UV light (Hulshinsky, 1919; Chick et al., 1923). Harry Steenbock exposed goats to sunlight and noted that during summer, they had a positive calcium balance and during winter negative balance (Steenbock and Hart, 1913). These experiments established the link between sunlight and calcium metabolism. He also noted that UV light irradiation to rats and their food also cured rickets. The structure of vitamin D was discovered by Askew et al. (1930). They isolated vitamin D2 from an irradiated mixture of Ergosterol. In 1935, Windaus and colleagues isolated 7-dihydrocholesterol, and in 1937, Windaus and Bock isolated Vitamin D3 which is the natural form of Vitamin D produced following UV irradiation of dihydrocholesterol. The dilemma whether the vitamin D is naturally synthesized product in the skin, or a dietary component was resolved by Esvelt and colleagues in 1978 by identifying vitamin D3 using mass spectroscopy (Esvelt et al., 1978). Discovery of vitamin D resulted in substantial reduction in rickets and research in vitamin D became quiescent. Nicolaysen and colleagues demonstrated that vitamin D increases absorption of calcium from small intestine (Nicolaysen et al., 1953). Carlsson and Bauer demonstrated that Vitamin D mobilizes calcium from bone into the plasma (Carlsson et al., 1952; Bauer et al., 1955). They postulated that vitamin D regulates not only serum and bone calcium but is also important for neuromuscular function.

EPIDEMIOLOGY

Vitamin D deficiency is common, and nearly half of world population is regarded as vitamin D deficient. Vitamin D affects all the age and ethnic groups. In USA, UK and Canada, the prevalence of vitamin D deficiency in elderly ranges between 20% and 100%.

It is also common in Austria, Middle East, Africa, South America and India (Holick, 2007; Marwaha et al., 2005; Thacher et al., 2006). In temperate zone, serum vitamin D level is lower in winter than in summer because of low sun exposure. Pregnant and lactating mothers are at high risk of vitamin D deficiency in spite of vitamin D and calcium supplementation (Hollis and Wagner, 2004). When sun is above or below 30° latitude, vitamin D synthesis is reduced.

The serum vitamin D level above 20 ng/ml is considered sufficient to prevent rickets. Serum vitamin D level of 12–20 ng/ml is considered insufficient and below 12 ng/ml is considered deficient (Table 7.1; European Food Safety Authority, 2016). The data about presence of vitamin D deficiency is related to the cut-off value used for defining vitamin D deficiency. Taking the cut-off value of serum vitamin D below 20 ng/ml, the prevalence of vitamin D deficiency ranges between 25% and 96% is different countries. The highest incidence of osteomalacia and rickets has been reported from Iraq, Pakistan, Afghanistan, Belgium and France, whereas the incidence is lower in Australia and Canada (WHO, 2019).

PATHOPHYSIOLOGY

Vitamin D is a group of secosteroids, which enhances absorption of calcium, potassium and magnesium. It has two important forms: D2 (ergocalciferol) and D3 (cholecalciferol). Vitamin D2 is present in plants and fish, whereas vitamin D3 is produced in skin following sunlight or UV ray exposure (Figure 7.1). The ingested vitamin D is absorbed in small intestine through chylomicrons and reaches venous blood through lymphatics. Vitamin D3 (cholecalciferol) from skin also enters the venous system through chylomicrons and lymphatic. Both vitamin D2 and vitamin D3 need hydroxylation to be in active form. In the liver, vitamin D is hydroxylated to form 25-OH-ergocalciferol or 25-OH-cholecalciferol. These compounds are further hydroxylated in the

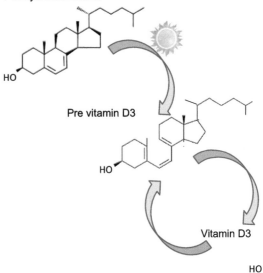

7-dehydrocholesterol

Pre vitamin D3

Vitamin D3

Figure 7.1 Schematic diagram showing how sunlight converts 7-dehydrocholesterol to pre vitamin D3 and vitamin D3.

kidney producing 1–$25(OH)_2$ cholecalciferol which is biologically active vitamin D (calcitriol) (Figure 7.2). Calcitriol circulates in the body like a hormone and acts through vitamin D receptors (VDR).

Vitamin D receptor belongs to nuclear receptor superfamily or steroid hormone receptors. These receptors are present in most of the tissues including skin, brain, heart, prostate, breast, bone and muscles. Vitamin D receptors are located in the nuclei of the target cells and act as a transcription factor leading to gene expression of transport proteins. Vitamin D maintains skeletal calcium balance through enhancing calcium absorption from the intestine. Calcitriol increases intestinal absorption of calcium by 30%–40% and phosphorus by 60%. In the absence of calcitriol, calcium is absorbed by 10%–15% only and phosphorus by 60%. Low calcium diet increases the conversion of 25-OH-D3 to 1–$25(OH)_2D3$, which helps in calcium absorption

Table 7.1 Definition of vitamin D status based on serum 25(OH)D3

Vitamin D status	Serum 25(OH)D3 level	Clinical manifestations	Treatment
Sufficient	• >20 ng/ml	• Healthy	• None
Insufficient	• 12–20 ng/ml	• Disease risk	• Supplementation of vitamin D
Deficient	• <12 ng/ml	• Rickets/osteomalacia	• High dose calciferol

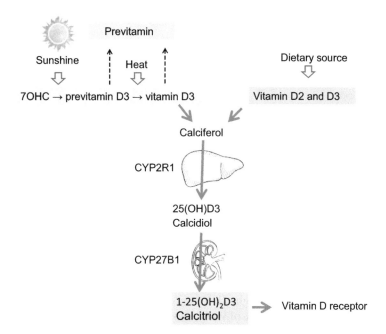

Figure 7.2 Schematic diagram showing conversion of dietary vitamin D and sunshine vitamin D3 to 25(OH)D3 in the liver and 1–25(OH)$_2$D3 in the kidney. The 1–25(OH)$_2$D3 is the active vitamin D and acts through vitamin D receptor.

from small intestine, whereas high calcium content in food suppresses the synthesis of active form of vitamin D (Holick, 2005). Hypocalcaemia is sensed by parathyroid gland which liberates parathormone hormone. Parathyroid hormone acts through G protein to enhance transcription and translation of 1α-hydroxylase enzyme which converts 25-OH-D3 to 1–25-(OH)$_2$-D3 in the proximal renal tubule (Dusso et al., 2006; Holick, 2007). Vitamin D regulates about 200 genes, and their additional action includes inhibition of cellular proliferation, angiogenesis, enhances cell differentiation and apoptosis.

Autophagy and ageing: Autophagy is a process by which healthy cells are maintained by removing damaged protein and malfunctional organelle especially mitochondria. Ageing mitochondria cannot generate ATP resulting in reactive oxygen species (ROS). Calcium at high concentration inhibits autophagy by activating inositol triphosphate receptors, whereas lower level of calcium enhances autophagy. The main driver of ageing is reduction of ATP generation and increased oxidative stress. Increased ROS may also generate inflammatory response. Vitamin D maintains mitochondrial respiratory chain, regulates thermogenesis (Abbas,

2017) and its insufficiency may impair the function of mitochondrial respiratory chain complex. It increases the formation of sirtuin 1, thereby improving mitochondrial biogenesis (Manna et al., 2017). Vitamin D-Clotho-Nrf2 network increases cellular antioxidant (glutathione) which neutralizes ROS.

Vitamin D and Bone: Vitamin D has an important role in bone metabolism because of its action on calcium and phosphorus. Vitamin D deficiency results in reduction in calcium and phosphorus absorption. Reduced calcium increases parathormone, which mobilizes calcium from bone to maintain normal serum calcium. This is due to increased osteoclastic activity, which results in osteopenia and osteoporosis. In children, the deficiency of vitamin D results in bone deformity and muscle weakness.

Vitamin D receptors are also present in brain, but their role is not well understood. Vitamin D receptors are present in most of the body tissue and it has wide range of biological functions. It inhibits cellular proliferation, improves cell differentiation, increases insulin secretion, macrophage and cathelicidin production, and inhibits renin and angiotensin synthesis (Figure 7.3) (Yuk et al., 2009; Berridge, 2017).

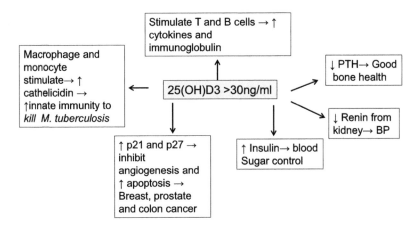

Figure 7.3 Cellular functions and health benefits of vitamin D.

SOURCES OF VITAMIN D

The main source of vitamin D is sunlight (UV 290–315 nm), which is responsible for 90% of vitamin D. Ultraviolet rays penetrate the skin (mainly during 10 am to 3 pm) and convert 7-dihydrocholesterol to previtamin D3, which rapidly converts to vitamin D3. The excess previtamin D3 and vitamin D3 are destroyed by solar UV light, hence, excess sunlight exposure does not result in hypervitaminosis D. Previtamin D3 lasts longer (15 days) than dietary vitamin D (5 days). Exposure to sunlight in a swimming costume till erythema develops produces 10,000–25,000 IU of vitamin D. Face and arm exposure for 20–30 min at mid-May in a fair skin person results in synthesis of 2000 IU vitamin D; two to three such exposures weekly are sufficient to meet vitamin D requirement in a healthy person. Elderly and dark skin person need 2–10 times more exposure than normal (Pearce and Cheetham, 2010). Sunscreen 30 UV application may reduce vitamin D synthesis by 90%. The dietary source of vitamin D is oily fish, cod liver oil, mushrooms, egg yolk and fortified beverages (Table 7.2).

RECOMMENDED DIETARY INTAKE OF VITAMIN D

The daily requirement of vitamin D depends on the age, pregnancy, lactation and associated comorbidities. The daily requirement of vitamin D during infancy is 400 IU/day, 1–18 years of age 600 IU/day, 19–50 years 600 IU/day and after 50 years of age 800 IU/day. During pregnancy and lactation, the vitamin D requirement is higher and may go

Table 7.2 Sources of vitamin D

Sources	Amount of vitamin D
Sunlight/UV	• 20,000 IU per erythema dose of sunbath in swimsuit
	• 3000 IU/ half erythema dose in arms and legs
Dietary source	
Cod liver oil	• 400–1000 IU/10 g
Salmon fish (fresh water)	• 600–1000 IU/100 g
Salmon fish (canned)	• 300–600 IU/100 g
Sardine	• 300 IU/100 g
Tuna	• 236 IU/100 g
Mackerel	• 236 IU/100 g
Mushroom (fresh)	• 100 IU/100 g
Mushroom (sun dried)	• 1600 IU/100 g
Egg yolk	• 20 IU/yolk

Table 7.3 The recommended daily allowance (RDA) of vitamin D in different age groups as per the Institute of Medicine (IOM) and Endocrine Society Clinical Practice Guideline for the patients at risk of Vitamin D deficiency (ESCPG)

Age groups	RDA (IOM)	RDA (ESCPG)
0–1 year	• 400 IU	• 400–1000 IU
2–18 years	• 600 IU	• 600–1000 IU
19–70 years	• 600 IU	• 1500–2000 IU
>70 years	• 800 IU	• 1500–2000 IU
Pregnancy	• 600 IU	• 1500–2000 IU
Lactation	• 600 IU	• 1500–2000 IU

up to 2000 IU/day. The patients receiving antifungal, antiretroviral or corticosteroid therapy require 2–3 times more vitamin D than their counterparts. The details of daily requirement of vitamin D are presented in Table 7.3.

CAUSES OF VITAMIN D DEFICIENCY

The major cause of vitamin D deficiency in both adults and children is inadequate sun exposure. The dietary sources of vitamin D are limited unless fortified. The neonates depend on the mother's milk for vitamin D, hence, mother's vitamin D status is crucial. Human milk contains 25–78 IU/L only, which is inadequate; therefore supplementation is needed if sun exposure is not optimal. Dark skin persons need 3–5 times longer sun exposure than fair skin individuals. Applying sunscreen of 30 UV reduces vitamin D synthesis by 95%. Obesity, malabsorption syndrome, bariatric surgery, nephrotic syndrome, parathyroid disorder, and drugs like corticosteroids, anticonvulsant, antitubercular and antiretroviral drugs result in vitamin D deficiency (Table 7.4).

CLINICAL SYNDROMES OF VITAMIN D DEFICIENCY

Musculoskeletal system

Deficiency of vitamin D and calcium in utero and during childhood reduces bone mineralization. As a result of vitamin D deficiency, parathyroid gland is stimulated resulting in secondary hyperparathyroidism. Parathormone increases conversion of 25-OH-D3 to $1-25(OH)_2D3$; thereby further aggravating the deficiency of 25-OH-D3. Parathormone also increases phosphaturia resulting in hypophosphatemia. Low serum calcium and phosphorus lead to impaired bone mineralization producing rickets in children and osteomalacia in adults. It is important to appreciate

Table 7.4 Causes of vitamin D deficiency

1. Reduced availability
   a. Inadequate sun exposure
2. Reduced synthesis
   a. Dark skin
   b. Short duration sun exposure
   c. Obesity (Body Mass Index > 30)
3. Reduced absorption
   a. Malabsorption syndrome
   b. Bariatric surgery
   c. Intestinal resection
4. Increased excretion
   a. Nephrotic syndrome
5. Increased metabolism
   a. Drugs: anticonvulsant, antitubercular, antiretroviral, antifungal and corticosteroid
6. Impaired 25-hydroxylation: Impaired conversion to 25(OH)D3 due to liver failure and isoniazid
7. Impaired 1α hydroxylation: Hypoparathyroidism, renal failure, ketoconazole, 1α-hydroxylase mutation, oncogenic osteomalacia, X-linked hypophosphatemic rickets
8. Target organ resistance: Vitamin D receptor mutation, phenytoin
9. Granulomatous disease: tuberculosis, lymphoma
10. Primary hyperparathyroidism

that osteomalacia is associated with pain whereas osteoporosis is not unless associated with fracture. The mechanism is that in rickets and osteomalacia, there is hydration of demineralized gelatin matrix just beneath the periosteum. The swelling of matrix pushes the periosteum resulting in throbbing pain. Clinical manifestations of rickets and osteomalacia are attributed to hypocalcaemia in the early stage manifesting with seizure, tetany and cardiomyopathy, and in the later stage poor bone mineralization and muscle weakness.

RICKETS

Vitamin D deficiency in children before the epiphyseal fusion results in rickets, which is characterized by growth retardation and expansion of growth plate. In 1976, rickets was categorized into three stages:

1. Mild rickets in early stage: Early stage of rickets is characterized by osteopenia, low or normal serum calcium and phosphorus, high alkaline phosphate and parathormone, and low vitamin D level. Serum alkaline phosphate is a sensitive marker of vitamin D deficiency.
2. Moderate rickets: Moderate rickets is characterized by radiological changes such as wrist expansion, bowing of legs and periosteal expansion with bone pain. The biochemical changes are similar to early severe stage but more marked.
3. Severe rickets in late stage: In severe rickets, there are skeletal changes, and serum calcium, phosphorus and vitamin D levels are low. Serum alkaline phosphatase and parathormone levels are elevated.

Seizure and tetany are more common during neonatal period. After 6 months of age, vitamin D deficiency manifests with features of rickets. The children have irritability, bone pain, muscle weakness and recurrent infection (Rachitic lung). Rachitic lung is attributed to pliable ribcage and muscle weakness. The common features of rickets include bony deformity such as genu valgum (knock knee), genu varum (bowing of leg), saber tibia (anterior bowing of tibia), anterior bowing of femur, internal rotation of ankle, and costochondral swelling (rickety rosary), Harrison sulcus

widening of wrist, and craniotabes (deformed skull due to softening of bone). Rickets is associated with poor cardiac function, and children with severe rickets may have heart failure. Rickets is due to deficiency of mineralization of growth plate. The underlying pathophysiology in all forms of rickets is low level of serum phosphate leading to reduced apoptosis of hypertrophic chondrocytes in the growth plate. There is reduced mineralization of primary spongiosa in the metaphysis. Hypophosphatemia in rickets is due to secondary hyperparathyroidism. Hypocalcaemia contributed to death in 3 out of 52 children; 2 had cardiomyopathy and 1 had seizure (Scheimberg and Perry, 2014). In another postmortem study in unexpected death in infancy and childhood, 76% children were vitamin D deficient and 69% of them had evidence of rickets (Cohen et al., 2013).

OSTEOMALACIA

Vitamin D deficiency in adults manifests with osteomalacia, which is characterized by bone pain and muscle weakness. Pain occurs in rib, hip, pelvis, joints and back. It simulates fibromyalgia. Generalized aches and pains in osteomalacia differentiate from osteoporosis in which pain is localized. In hospital-based study, vitamin D deficiency was found in 93% in the patients between 10 years and 65 years of age who were referred as fibromyalgia, chronic fatigue, pain or depression (Plotnikoff and Quigley, 2003). In a study on 15 women with nutritional osteomalacic myopathy, all presented with bone pain especially in pelvis. They had pelvic girdle muscle weakness as well as waddling gait. Radiological changes of osteomalacia (demineralization, looser zone, tri-radiate pelvis) were present in 13 patients. Serum alkaline phosphatase was elevated in 12 patients. Electromyography revealed short duration polyphasic potentials in the proximal muscles. Muscle biopsy revealed nonspecific muscle atrophy. These patients improved clinically and electrophysiologically following calcium and vitamin D supplementation for 3 months (Irani, 1976). Osteomalacia in young girls may result in pelvic deformity which may result in obstructed labor subsequently. Elderly patients with osteomalacia may have recurrent falls due to proximal muscle weakness and fractures.

DIAGNOSIS OF VITAMIN D DEFICIENCY, RICKETS AND OSTEOMALACIA

The screening test of vitamin D deficiency is the measurement of serum 25(OH)D3 because 1–25 (OH)$_2$D3 may be elevated due to high parathormone level. Serum calcium is normal but may be low. Serum alkaline phosphatase is elevated even when serum calcium is normal. There is calciuria and phosphaturia resulting in hypophosphatemia.

The characteristic radiological findings of rickets are widened expanded growth plates not only in long bones but also in costochondral junction giving rise to rachitic rosary. There is delayed fusion of sutures of skull bones and radiolucency of long bones. After epiphyseal fusion, the characteristic radiological finding of vitamin D deficiency includes reduced cortical thickness and increased radiolucency of bone. The looser zones or pseudofractures are produced especially in scapula; neck of femur and pelvis due to pulsation of arteries of surrounding bone (Figures 7.4–7.6).

NONSKELETAL FUNCTIONS OF VITAMIN D

Vitamin D receptors are present not only in bone and muscles but also in brain, breast, prostate, colon and immune cells, and these receptors respond to 1–25(OH)$_2$D3. Some tissues also have receptors for 25(OH)D3. Vitamin D regulates a large number of genes which are responsible for cellular proliferation, cell differentiation, apoptosis and angiogenesis.

Osteoporosis and fracture: Chronic vitamin D deficiency is associated with osteoporosis and bone fractures. Above the age of 50 years, about 47% women and 22% men have osteoporosis. Above the age of 80 years, the frequency of osteoporosis rises to 66% (Holick, 2007). A number of studies have shown that supplementation of vitamin D below 700 IU per day or those who have vitamin D less than 26 ng/ml are unlikely to reduce fracture risk (Holick, 2007). In a meta-analysis of seven trials, 700–800 IU vitamin D daily reduced the relative risk of hip fracture by 26% and nonvertebral fracture by 23%. Studies using vitamin D 400 IU daily

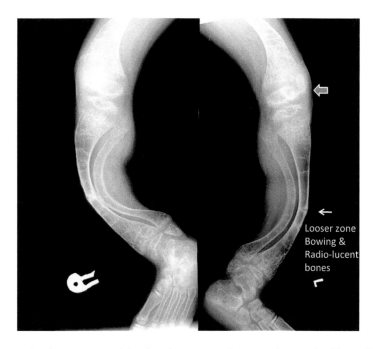

Figure 7.4 Radiograph of an 11-year-old girl with severe rickets. Radiograph of legs shows bowing of leg bones, radiolucency, expansion of epiphyseal growth plate and looser zone. (Courtesy Dr DK Boruah, Associate Professor, Tezpur Medical college, Assam.)

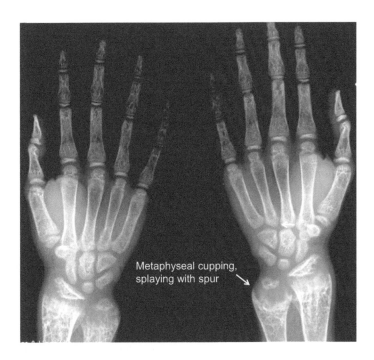

Figure 7.5 Radiograph of hands of an 11-year-old girl showing metaphyseal cupping splaying with spur. (Courtesy Dr DK Boruah, Associate Professor, Tezpur Medical college, Assam.)

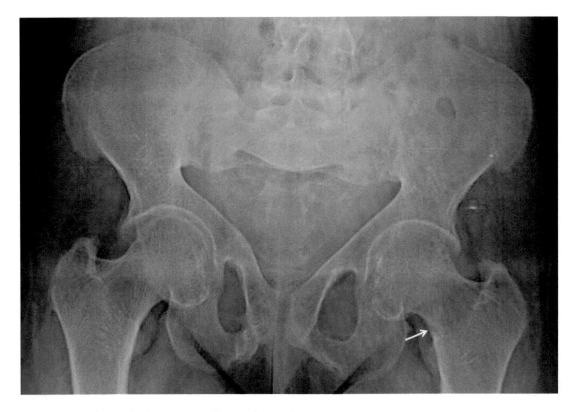

Figure 7.6 Radiograph showing triradiate pelvis and looser zone.

have shown little advantage in reducing fracture compared to placebo (Bischoff-Ferrari et al., 2006).

Muscle strength and falls: Since vitamin D deficiency causes muscle weakness, improving 25-OH vitamin D from 4 to 16 ng/ml improves muscle power and performance speed. A meta-analysis of seven trials including 1237 subjects recorded reduction of falls by 22% compared to placebo and found that vitamin D 400 IU was not effective but 800 IU with calcium was (Bischoff-Ferrari et al., 2006). Vitamin D has many other important functions in the body. Vitamin D receptors gene and 25-OH vitamin D1α-hydroxylase gene receptors are expressed in monocytes and macrophages in presence of lipopolysaccharide or mycobacterium tuberculosis. This may explain the role of vitamin D in controlling infections. It has been shown that vitamin D level below 20 ng/ml impairs the activation of macrophage and monocyte generated innate immunity. 1–25-dihydroxy vitamin D3 leads to increased synthesis of cathelicidins, a peptide capable of destroying mycobacterium tuberculosis, and other infective agents. This may explain higher prevalence and a more aggressive course of tuberculosis in black population compared to white (Liu et al., 2006).

MULTIPLE SCLEROSIS AND INFLAMMATORY DISEASE

Multiple sclerosis, type I diabetes mellitus and inflammatory bowel diseases also have linked to vitamin D deficiency. These diseases are more prevalent in the population living in high altitude. If an individual resides 10 years of his early life below 35° latitude, the risk of multiple sclerosis is reduced by 50% (VanAmerongen et al., 2004). The risk of multiple sclerosis reduces by 42% in the women receiving 400 IU vitamin D daily (Munger et al., 2004). Risk of type I diabetes also decreases by increased intake of vitamin D by pregnant mothers as well as the child. In a study from Finland, 10,366 children were given 2000 IU vitamin D3 daily in the first year of life. At 31 years follow-up, the risk of type I diabetes was reduced by 80% (Hyppönen et al., 2001). In the children with vitamin D deficiency, the risk of diabetes increases by 200% (Chiu et al., 2004). Low level of vitamin D results in reduced insulin synthesis thereby increasing metabolic syndrome. The risk of type 2 diabetes mellitus also reduces by 33% by 1200 mg calcium and 800 IU vitamin D daily compared to those having less than 600 mg calcium and 400 IU vitamin D (Pittas et al., 2006).

Cancer: The incidence of prostate cancer, breast cancer and lymphoma is higher in the people living at high altitude compared to low (Holick, 2007). The role of vitamin D in reducing the incidence of cancer may be due to its effect on reducing angiogenesis (which reduces cell proliferation) and enhancing apoptosis. In population studies, it has been reported that if vitamin D is below 20 ng/ml, the risk of colon cancer, breast cancer and lymphoma increases by 30%–50% (Holick, 2007). In the Nurse's Health Study on 32,826 subjects, odds of colorectal cancer were inversely related to vitamin D level (Feskanich et al., 2004). Prospective studies have also revealed relative risk reduction from 1 to 0.53 when intake of vitamin D was increased from 6 to 94 IU daily to 233–652 IU daily (Gorham et al., 2005). In children, the risk of non-Hodgkin's lymphoma was reduced by 40% who were exposed to sunlight (Berwick et al., 2005). Similarly, men working outdoor develop cancer prostate 3–5 years later than those working indoor. Vitamin D deficiency has also been linked to hypertension, schizophrenia and respiratory dysfunction. The indications for vitamin D measurement are summarized in Table 7.5.

TREATMENT OF VITAMIN D DEFICIENCY

Rickets: To improve 1 ng/ml of serum vitamin D level, 100 IU of 25(OH)D2 or D3 are required. The requirement of vitamin D in infants and toddler with rickets is 2000 IU daily or 50,000 IU weekly for 6 weeks. Once serum vitamin D level reaches more than 30 ng/ml, the maintenance dose of vitamin D is 400–1000 IU daily (Holick et al., 2011). Rickets may also be treated by 600,000 IU intramuscularly orally or once a year (Gordon et al., 2008; Bischoff-Ferrari et al., 2009; Chibuzor et al., 2020). The yearly dosing may be appropriate for remote and resource poor setting with poor health infrastructure. In patients between 1 and 18 years of age with rickets, the recommended daily dose of vitamin D is 2000 IU daily or 50,000 IU weekly for 6 weeks. After this, the maintenance dose is 600–1000 IU daily if vitamin D level is more than 30 ng/ml. A combination of vitamin D and calcium is better than vitamin D alone in children of 6 months–14 years of age with nutritional rickets (Chibuzor et al., 2020).

Table 7.5 Indication for measuring vitamin D level

Suspected patients with
  Rickets
  Osteomalacia
  Osteoporosis
  Malabsorption syndrome: Inflammatory bowel disease, bariatric surgery, cystic fibrosis, radiation
    enteritis, Crohn's disease
Hepatic failure
Chronic renal failure
Hyperparathyroidism
Granulomatous disorder: Sarcoidosis, tuberculosis, histoplasmosis, coccidioidiomycosis, berylliosis,
  lymphoma
Pregnancy and lactation
Elderly with fall
Nontraumatic fracture
Body mass index >30 kg/m²
Drugs: First generation anticonvulsants, glucocorticoids, cholestyramine, antifungal (ketoconazole),
  antiretroviral drugs

Osteomalacia: The adults with osteomalacia are treated with 6000 IU daily or 50,000 IU weekly of vitamin D2 or D3 orally for 8 weeks. Once target vitamin D level is achieved (30 ng/ml), the maintenance dose of vitamin D is 1500–2000 IU daily (Holick et al., 2011) (Table 7.6). If serum vitamin D level is not improved, the underlying cause of malabsorption (coeliac disease, cystic fibrosis, etc.) should be investigated. Toxicity occurs if daily vitamin D dose exceeds 40,000 IU.

Granulomatous disease: In granulomatous diseases such as sarcoidosis, tuberculosis and lymphoma, the macrophages are activated and stimulate $1-25(OH)_2D3$. The active vitamin D increases the absorption of calcium from small intestine and mobilizes calcium from the skeletal system. This results in hypercalcemia and calciuria. These patients require maintenance of vitamin D deficiency. Over-dosing of vitamin D may result in hypercalcemia and hypercalciuria.

Hyperparathyroidism: The patients with primary hyperparathyroidism usually have high serum calcium and low vitamin D level. Their vitamin D level should be corrected with caution.

Obesity: The obese patient needs 2–3 times more vitamin D compared to nonobese vitamin D deficiency patients. The recommended dose of vitamin D is 6000–10,000 IU daily for 8 weeks followed by maintenance dose of 3000–6000 daily.

A systemic review on the role of vitamin D-raising intervention study in the functional outcome (pain, falls and quality of life) and cardiovascular risk (death and stroke) revealed definite benefit in falls but not in pain or quality of life. There was no consistent benefit in myocardial infarction, stroke, lipid levels, blood glucose level and blood pressure (Elamin et al., 2011).

GENETICALLY MEDIATED RICKETS OR OSTEOMALACIA

Rickets or osteomalacia may also occur in a number of hereditary disorders of vitamin D metabolism, vitamin D receptor mutations, renal tubular

Table 7.6 Recommended vitamin D for the treatment of rickets and osteomalacia

Rickets	Treatment	Maintenance
<1 year	• 2000 IU daily/50,000 weekly×6 weeks OR 600,000 IU yearly	• 400–1000 IU daily 600,000 IU yearly
1–18 years	• 2000 IU daily/50,000 weekly×6 weeks	• 600–1000 IU daily
Osteomalacia	• 6000 IU daily/50,000 IU weekly×8 weeks	• 1500–2000 IU daily

dysfunction (Fanconi syndrome) and phosphate absorption defect. Majority of these patients manifest during early life but may also manifest late depending on the severity of defect. Vitamin D dependent rickets (type 1) is due to impaired conversion of 25(OH)D3 to 1–25(OH)$_2$D3 in proximal renal tubules. Their serum 25(OH)D3 level is normal, but 1–25(OH)$_2$D3 level is low or undetectable. These patients respond to calcitriol. In vitamin D resistant rickets (type 2), serum 1–25(OH)$_2$D3 level is high and also have alopecia. These patients are resistant to calcitriol treatment and require daily infusion of calcium and phosphate. X-linked hypophosphatemia is due to defective phosphate reabsorption in the renal tubule. These patients have features of rickets or osteomalacia, but their serum vitamin D level is normal. Fanconi syndrome is an autosomal recessive disease with impaired absorption of amino acid, uric acid, phosphate, bicarbonate and glucose. Along with features of vitamin D deficiency, they have metabolic acidosis.

CONCLUSION

Vitamin D deficiency is a treatable and entirely preventable disease except hereditary causes of osteomalacia or rickets. Serum 25(OH)D2 or D3 level more than 20 ng/ml is considered sufficient. A level of <12 ng/ml is considered deficient and manifests with rickets in children and osteomalacia in adults. A serum level 12–20 ng/ml is considered insufficient and increases the risk of diabetes, hypertension, cancer and infection. Serum 1–25(OH)$_2$D3 should not be measured for diagnosis of vitamin D deficiency because it may be normal or elevated due to high parathormone hormone. Treatment of vitamin D deficiency requires high dose of 25(OH)D3 for 6–8 weeks followed by maintenance dose. Individuals with insufficient vitamin D should be supplemented. Community education regarding benefit of sun exposure and vitamin rich diet is useful.

REFERENCES

Abbas, M.A. 2017. Physiological functions of Vitamin D in adipose tissue. *The Journal of Steroid Biochemistry and Molecular Biology* 165(Pt B):369–381.

Askew, F. A., Bourdillon, R. B., Bruce, H. M., Jenkins, R. G. C., Webster, T. A. 1930. The distillation of vitamin D. *Proceedings of the Royal Society of London. Series B, Containing Papers of a Biological Character* 107(748):76–90.

Bauer, G. C. H., Carlsson, A., Lindquist, B. 1955. Evaluation of accretion, resorption and exchange reactions in the skeleton. *Kungl Fysiograf Sallskap I Lund Forh* 25:3–18.

Berridge, M.J. 2017. Vitamin D deficiency accelerates ageing and age-related diseases: A novel hypothesis. *The Journal of Physiology* 595(22):6825–6836.

Berwick, M., Armstrong, B. K., Ben-Porat, L., et al. 2005. Sun exposure and mortality from melanoma. *Journal of the National Cancer Institute* 97(3):195–199.

Bischoff-Ferrari, H. A., Dawson-Hughes, B., Staehelin, H. B., et al. 2009. Fall prevention with supplemental and active forms of vitamin D: A meta-analysis of randomised controlled trials. *BMJ (Clinical Research ed.)* 339:b3692.

Bischoff-Ferrari, H. A., Giovannucci, E., Willett, W. C., Dietrich, T., Dawson-Hughes, B. 2006. Estimation of optimal serum concentrations of 25-hydroxyvitamin D for multiple health outcomes. *The American Journal of Clinical Nutrition* 84(1):18–28.

Carlsson, A. R. V. I. D., Lindqvist, M., Magjrusson, T. 1952. Tracer experiments on the effect of vitamin D on the skeletal metabolism of calcium and phosphorus. *Acta Physiologica Scandinavica* 26:212–220.

Chibuzor, M. T., Graham-Kalio, D., Osaji, J. O., Meremikwu, M. M. 2020. Vitamin D, calcium or a combination of vitamin D and calcium for the treatment of nutritional rickets in children. *The Cochrane Database of Systematic Reviews* 4(4):CD012581.

Chick, H., Palzell, E.J., Hume, E.M. 1923. Studies of rickets in Vienna 1919–1922. Medical Research Council, Special Report No. 77.

Chiu, K. C., Chu, A., Go, V. L., Saad, M. F. 2004. Hypovitaminosis D is associated with insulin resistance and beta cell dysfunction. *The American Journal of Clinical Nutrition* 79(5): 820–825.

Cohen, M. C., Offiah, A., Sprigg, A., Al-Adnani, M. 2013. Vitamin D deficiency and sudden unexpected death in infancy and childhood: A cohort study. *Pediatric and Developmental Pathology: The Official Journal of the Society for Pediatric Pathology and the Paediatric Pathology Society* 16(4):292–300.

Dusso, A. S., Sato, T., Arcidiacono, M. V., et al., 2006. Pathogenic mechanisms for parathyroid hyperplasia. *Kidney International Supplement* 70(102):S8–S11.

EFSA NDA Panel (EFSA Panel on Dietetic Products, Nutrition and Allergies). 2016. Scientific opinion on dietary reference values for vitamin D. *EFSA Journal 14*(10):4547, 145 pp.

Elamin, M. B., Abu Elnour, N. O., Elamin, K. B., et al. 2011. Vitamin D and cardiovascular outcomes: A systematic review and meta-analysis. *The Journal of Clinical Endocrinology and Metabolism 96*(7):1931–1942.

Esvelt, R. P., Schnoes, H. K., DeLuca, H. F. 1978. Vitamin D3 from rat skins irradiated in vitro with ultraviolet light. *Archives of Biochemistry and Biophysics 188*(2):282–286.

Feskanich, D., Ma, J., Fuchs, C. S., Kirkner, G. J., Hankinson, S. E., Hollis, B. W., Giovannucci, E. L. 2004. Plasma vitamin D metabolites and risk of colorectal cancer in women. *Cancer Epidemiology, Biomarkers & Prevention: A Publication of the American Association for Cancer Research, Cosponsored by the American Society of Preventive Oncology 13*(9):1502–1508.

Gordon, C. M., Williams, A. L., Feldman, H. A., May, J., Sinclair, L., Vasquez, A., Cox, J. E. 2008. Treatment of hypovitaminosis D in infants and toddlers. *The Journal of Clinical Endocrinology and Metabolism 93*(7):2716–2721.

Gorham, E. D., Garland, C. F., Garland, F. C., et al. 2005. Vitamin D and prevention of colorectal cancer. *The Journal of Steroid Biochemistry and Molecular Biology 97*(1–2):179–194.

Holick, M.F. 2007. Vitamin D deficiency. *The New England Journal of Medicine 357*(3):266–281.

Holick, M. F. 2005. Vitamin D for health and in chronic kidney disease. *Seminars in Dialysis 18*(4):266–275.

Holick, M. F., Binkley, N. C., Bischoff-Ferrari, H. A., et al. 2011. Evaluation, treatment, and prevention of vitamin D deficiency: An Endocrine Society clinical practice guideline. *The Journal of Clinical Endocrinology and Metabolism 96*(7):1911–1930.

Hollis, B. W., Wagner, C. L. 2004. Vitamin D requirements during lactation: High-dose maternal supplementation as therapy to prevent hypovitaminosis D for both the mother and the nursing infant. *The American Journal of Clinical Nutrition 80*(6 Suppl):1752S–1758S.

Hulshinsky, K. 1919. Heilung von rachitis durch kunstlich hohen-sonne. *Deut. Med. Wochenscher* 45: 712–713; Z. Orthopad. Chir. 1920; 39:426 as described in Bills CE. In: Sebrell, Jr W.H., Harris, R.S. (Eds). *The vitamins. Vol. II.* New York: Academic Press, 1954, pp. 162.

Hyppönen, E., Läärä, E., Reunanen, A., Järvelin, M. R., Virtanen, S. M. 2001. Intake of vitamin D and risk of type 1 diabetes: A birth-cohort study. *Lancet (London, England) 358*(9292):1500–1503.

Irani, P. F. 1976. Electromyography in nutritional osteomalacic myopathy. *Journal of Neurology, Neurosurgery, and Psychiatry 39*(7):686–693.

Liu, P. T., Stenger, S., Li, H., et al. 2006. Toll-like receptor triggering of a vitamin D-mediated human antimicrobial response. *Science (New York, NY) 311*(5768):1770–1773.

Manna, P., Achari, A. E., Jain, S. K. 2017. Vitamin D supplementation inhibits oxidative stress and upregulate SIRT1/AMPK/GLUT4 cascade in high glucose-treated 3T3L1 adipocytes and in adipose tissue of high fat diet-fed diabetic mice. *Archives of Biochemistry and Biophysics 615*:22–34.

Marwaha, R. K., Tandon, N., Reddy, D. R., et al. 2005. Vitamin D and bone mineral density status of healthy schoolchildren in northern India. *The American Journal of Clinical Nutrition 82*(2):477–482.

Mellanby, E. 1919. An experimental investigation on rickets. *Lancet* 1:407–412.

Mellanby, E. 1976. Nutrition classics. The Lancet 1:407–12, 1919. An experimental investigation of rickets. Edward Mellanby. *Nutrition Reviews 34*(11):338–340.

Munger, K. L., Zhang, S. M., O'Reilly, E., et al. 2004. Vitamin D intake and incidence of multiple sclerosis. *Neurology 62*(1):60–65.

Nicolaysen, R., Eeg-Larsen, N., Malm, O. J. 1953. Physiology of calcium metabolism. *Physiological Reviews 33*(3):424–444.

Pearce, S. H., Cheetham, T. D. 2010. Diagnosis and management of vitamin D deficiency. *BMJ (Clinical Research ed.) 340*:b5664.

Pittas, A. G., Dawson-Hughes, B., Li, T., et al. 2006. Vitamin D and calcium intake in relation to type 2 diabetes in women. *Diabetes Care 29*(3):650–656.

Plotnikoff, G. A., Quigley, J. M. 2003. Prevalence of severe hypovitaminosis D in patients with persistent, nonspecific musculoskeletal pain. *Mayo Clinic Proceedings 78*(12):1463–1470.

Scheimberg, I., Perry, L. 2014. Does low vitamin D have a role in pediatric morbidity and mortality? An observational study of vitamin D in a cohort of 52 postmortem examinations. *Pediatric and Developmental Pathology: The Official Journal of the Society for Pediatric Pathology and the Paediatric Pathology Society 17*(6):455–464.

Steenbock, H., Hart, E. B. 1913. The influence of function on the lime requirements of animals. *Journal of Biological Chemistry 14*:59–73.

Thacher, T. D., Fischer, P. R., Strand, M. A., Pettifor, J. M. 2006. Nutritional rickets around the world: causes and future directions. *Annals of Tropical Paediatrics 26*(1):1–16.

VanAmerongen, B. M., Dijkstra, C. D., Lips, P., Polman, C. H. 2004. Multiple sclerosis and vitamin D: An update. *European Journal of Clinical Nutrition* 58(8):1095–1109.

Windaus, A., Lettre, H., Schenck, Fr. 1935. 7-Dehydrocholesterol. *Justus Liebigs Annalen der Chemie* 520:98–106.

Windaus, A., Bock, F. 1937. Über das provitamin aus dem Sterin der Schweineschwarte. *Zeitschrift für Physiologische Chemie* 245:168–170.

WHO. 2019. *Nutritional rickets: a review of disease burden, causes, diagnosis, prevention and treatment.* Geneva: World Health Organization.

Yuk, J. M., Shin, D. M., Lee, H. M., et al. 2009. Vitamin D3 induces autophagy in human monocytes/macrophages via cathelicidin. *Cell Host & Microbe* 6(3):231–243.

8

Vitamin E deficiency and its neurological effects

INTRODUCTION

Vitamin E consists of eight soluble compounds, four tocopherols (Tα, Tβ, TΥ and Tδ) and four tocotrienols (TEα, TEβ, TEΥ and TEδ). Tα is the most important form of vitamin E in the tissues. Vitamin E is considered as an antioxidant, and also it has anti-inflammatory and antidegeneration effects. In humans, vitamin E deficiency has been associated with ataxia, neuromuscular weakness and macular degeneration. Tα has also been used to prevent a number of degenerative and systemic disorders. Dietary vitamin E deficiency is rare and usually associated with fat malabsorption syndrome. Lately inherited genetic defects in vitamin E metabolism causing isolated vitamin E deficiency or in association with abetalipoproteinemia have been reported. In this chapter, pathophysiology, clinical manifestations and management aspects of vitamin E deficiency are presented.

HISTORICAL BACKGROUND

Herbert M. Evans and Katherine S. Bishop described a factor in the lipid extract of lettuce which was needed for reproduction of rats (Evans and Bishop, 1922). In 1924, this factor was named vitamin E (Barnett, 1924). The effect of vitamin E on neurological disorders was demonstrated in the offspring of vitamin E deficient rats. The affected pups had limb paralysis. This effect of vitamin E was attributed to its antioxidant action (Olcott and Mattill, 1931). In humans, the role of vitamin E deficiency in neurological disorders was reported in 1965 (Kayden et al., 1965). Though vitamin E was regarded as an antioxidant, alternative molecular mechanisms in cell signaling and inflammation have been reported in recent years (Mahoney and Azzi, 1988). Several genetic mutations have been reported which can result in vitamin E deficiency. Milestones in the discovery of vitamin E have been mentioned in Figure 8.1.

SOURCES OF VITAMIN E

Vitamin E is abundantly present in both vegetarian and nonvegetarian food. Fruits and vegetables have a lower amount of vitamin E compared to meat, nuts and cereals. Fruits mainly contain Tα. Among the nuts, Tα is found in peanuts, sunflower, and almonds, and TΥ is found in walnut, peanuts, pistachio and sesame seeds. Both Tα and TΥ are found in various oils derived from corn, soybean, peanuts and sunflower. Tδ is found in tomato seeds, rice germ and soybean oil. Tocotrienols are found in lower quantity in nuts but are mostly available in palm oil, barley, annatto and some cereals (Table 8.1). Since tocopherols are closely associated with oils, Tα found in plant oils is also rich in MUFA (monounsaturated fatty acid), and TΥ is found in nuts and nut oils and is rich in PUFA polyunsaturated fatty acid. Plasma level of TΥ suggests monounsaturated fat intake, and TΥ suggests polyunsaturated fatty acid intake.

STRUCTURE AND FUNCTIONS OF VITAMIN E

The natural form of vitamin E has eight types of lipophilic molecules (Tα, β, Υ, δ and TEα, β, Υ, δ). All these forms of tocopherols have a chromanol ring with 16 carbon phytyl-like side chains in which

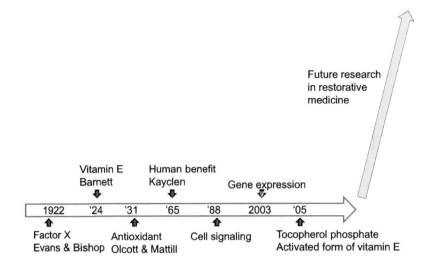

Figure 8.1 Milestones in the discovery of vitamin E and its biological functions.

Table 8.1 Dietary sources of vitamin E

Source	mg/100 mg food	Source	mg/100 g
Oils		**Fruits**	
Wheat germ oil	149	Olive	3.8
Hazelnut oil	47	Avocado	2.1
Sunflower oil	41	Cranberries	2.1
Almond oil	39	Kiwi	1.5
Nuts and seeds		Blackberries	1.2
Almond	26	Apricot	0.9
Hazelnut	15	Mango	0.9
Pine nut	9.3	Raspberries	0.9
Peanut	8.3	**Vegetables**	
Pistachio	2.9	Turnip green	2.9
Pumpkin seed	2.2	Mamey sapote	2.1
Cashew	0.9	Spinach	2.0
Nonvegetarian diet		Mustard green	1.8
Crayfish	15	Beet green	1.8
Octopus	12	Butternut squash	1.5
Fish roe	7.0	Broccoli	1.5
Snail	5.0	**Milk and milk product**	0.03–1.3
Abalone	4.0		
Rainbow trout	2.8		
Goose meat	1.7		
Atlantic salmon	1.1		
Lobster	1.0		
Meat & meat product	0.02–1.1		

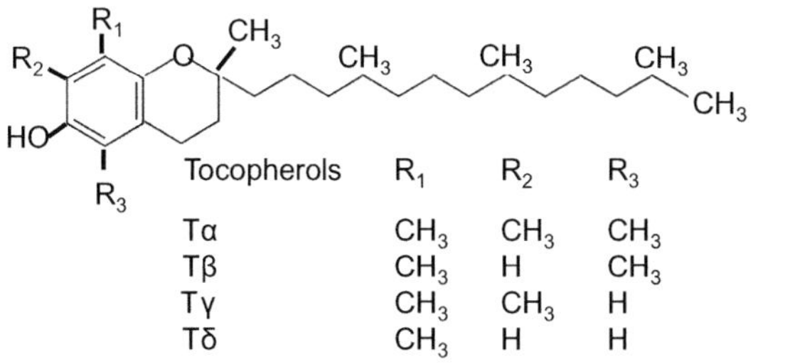

Figure 8.2 Schematic diagram showing the structure of tocopherol and its analogues.

Table 8.2 Daily requirement of vitamin E in different age groups

Age	mg/day
0–6 months	4
7–12 months	5
1–3 years	8
4–8 years	7
9–13 years	11
>13 years	15
Pregnancy	15
Lactation	19

tocopherols are saturated, and tocotrienols have 3 double bonds (Figure 8.2). Different isoforms of T and TE differ at five or seven position of chromanol ring with –H or –CH₃ group. Out of all these isoforms, Tα is the predominant form of vitamin E. Low intake of Tα may result in vitamin E deficiency. Animal and initial human data have revealed benefit of Tα in preventing atherosclerosis, inflammation and Alzheimer disease; however, subsequent human studies failed to support these findings, rather, there was an increased frequency of carcinoma prostate (Klein et al., 2011; Christen et al., 2015; Huttunen, 1995; Christen et al., 2010; Farina et al., 2017). Recent studies have therefore evaluated the effects of other isoforms of vitamin E.

Tocopherols are important substances and cannot be synthesized in humans; therefore, dietary intake is necessary. The recommended daily allowance for adults is 15 mg. There is no additional requirement in pregnancy; however, the recommended daily allowance in lactating mother is 19 mg. The recommended daily allowance for infants (0–6 months) is 4 mg, for 7–12 months of age 5 mg, for 1–3 years of age 6 mg, 4–8 years of age 7 mg and for 9–13 years of age 11 mg (Table 8.2; Traber and Manor, 2012).

ABSORPTION AND METABOLISM

About 20%–40% of dietary vitamin E is absorbed from the small intestine. Dietary vitamin E is hydrophobic; hence, it has to be stabilized by bile acid (micellar stabilization) so that it can flow through the aqueous environment of the intestine. Before absorption, it is hydrolyzed by the esterases secreted from the pancreas and intestinal mucosa. In the intestine, it is absorbed into the enterocyte through passive diffusion. Inside the enterocyte,

vitamin E is incorporated with dietary lipid and apolipoprotein into chylomicron and transported through mesenteric lymphatic to systemic circulation. Vitamin E is stored in liver as a rapid turnover depot and in the adipose tissue as slow turnover depot. About 8% of vitamin E is excreted in bile. Vitamin E circulates with HDL (high density lipoprotein) and LDL (low density lipoprotein). Vitamin E is hydrolyzed before entering the cell, and it enters the cell through LDL receptor. About 1% of vitamin E is excreted in urine (Figure 8.3).

In the liver, Tα binds to α-tocopherol transfer protein (αTTP). αTTP with ATP binding cassette transporter A1 (ABCA1) incorporates Tα with lipoprotein, which is released into circulation, and is available to the tissues (Traber, 2007; Manor and Morley, 2007). Tα has 100% affinity for αTTP but the other isoforms have lower affinity; Tβ 50%, TΥ 10%–30% and Tδ has 1% affinity for αTTP. The majority of unbound vitamin E is catabolized by cytochrome P450. There are other vitamin E binding proteins such as SEC14p and supernatant protein factor.

MECHANISM OF ACTION

Vitamin E has antioxidant and nonantioxidant mechanisms of actions. Antioxidant effects of vitamin E are mediated by peroxy radical scavenging and inhibition of lipid peroxidation. Vitamin C and glutathione maintain vitamin E in a reduced state (Figure 8.4; Traber and Manor 2012). The nonoxidant effects of vitamin E are being increasingly recognized, which include inhibition of protein kinase C, leading to decreased cell proliferation,

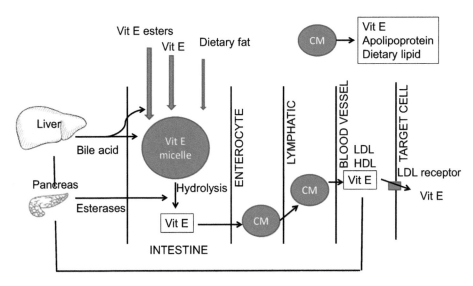

Figure 8.3 Schematic diagram showing absorption and distribution of vitamin E (Vit E). CM=chylomicron; HDL=high density lipoprotein; LDL=low density lipoprotein.

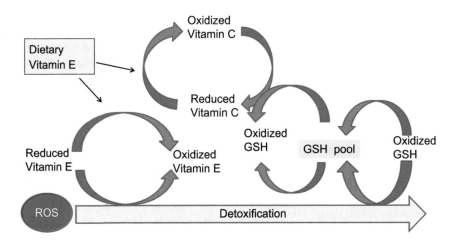

Figure 8.4 Antioxidative functions of vitamin E that help in scavenging ROS (reactive oxygen species). GSH=glutathione.

inflammation, atherosclerosis, diabetic vascular complication and platelet aggregation. It also affects prostaglandin synthesis and phospholipase A2. The transcription factors such as peroxisome proliferator-activated receptor ϒ, nuclear factor kB, nuclear factor erythroid-derived 2 – like 2, RAR-related orphan receptor α, hypoxia inducible factor 1α, pregnane X receptor and estrogen receptor β (Khadangi and Azzi, 2019). Vitamin E also regulates a number of genes such as xanthine oxidase, scavenger receptors SR-A, collagenase, CD36, tropomycin, αTTP and Cyp3a (Azzi et al., 2016).

VITAMIN E DEFICIENCY STATE

In humans, dietary vitamin E deficiency is extremely rare, and occurs in the following settings:

1. Along with fat malabsorption
2. Liver disease
3. Pancreatic disease
4. Intestinal resection
5. Genetic: abetalipoproteinemia and isolated α-tocopherol transporter (αTTP) deficiency.

Fat malabsorption occurs in cystic fibrosis, hepato-biliary disease and abetalipoproteinemia. Amongst the liver diseases, chronic cholestatic hepatobiliary disease is associated with vitamin E deficiency in 50%–70% of patients. The other liver diseases associated with vitamin E deficiency include biliary atresia, neonatal hepatitis, steatohepatic dysplasia and familial cholestatic syndrome. Resection of small intestine and bariatric surgery may also result in vitamin E deficiency after 10–20 years.

CLINICAL FEATURE OF VITAMIN E DEFICIENCY

Vitamin E deficiency may be due to fat malabsorption or isolated vitamin E deficiency. Fat malabsorption may be associated with deficiency of other fat-soluble vitamin (A, D and K). Both these groups of disorders have similar clinical manifestation. The clinical picture resembles spinocerebellar ataxia characterized by retinal degeneration, ptosis, ophthalmoplegia, ataxia, areflexia, proximal muscle weakness and loss of joint position and vibration. Touch and pinprick are minimally affected distally (Figure 8.5; Jung et al., 2019). Patients may have dysesthesia and distal sensory loss due to associated neuropathy (Sokol, 1988). Vitamin E deficiency neurological syndromes are well characterized in childhood cholestasis. These patients get five neurological signs at 2 years interval.

1. Hyporeflexia or areflexia
2. Truncal ataxia

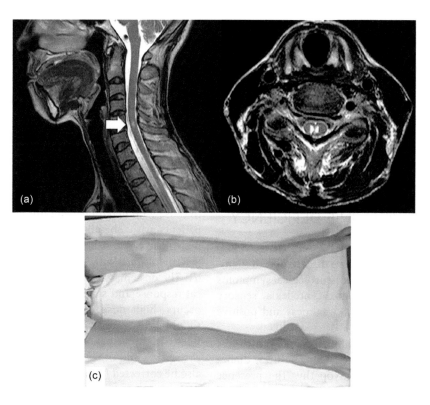

(a) (b) (c)

Figure 8.5 MRI and clinical photographs of a 50-year-old woman who presented with ataxia and myeloneuropathy following intestinal resection. (a) Spinal MRI shows T2 hyper intensity of cervical spinal cord. (b) Axial section shows T2 hyper intensity of posterior and lateral columns. (c) Generalized wasting. Her serum vitamin E level was low (3.71 mg/dl, normal 5–20 mg/dl), but serum vitamin B12, serum copper and ceruloplasmin levels were normal. (With permission from Jung, J. B., Kim, Y., Oh, K., et al. 2019. Subacute combined degeneration associated with vitamin E deficiency due to small bowel obstruction: A case report. *Medicine* 98(36):e17052.)

3. Limb ataxia
4. Ophthalmoplegia
5. Peripheral neuropathy.

Hyporeflexia is the earliest to appear by 2 years of age. Other symptoms appear by 2–4 years, and limb ataxia is the last to appear at 6 years (Sokol et al., 1985). Few patients may manifest in adulthood with psychomotor abnormality and chronic liver disease.

Vitamin E deficiency due to abetalipoproteinemia occurs due to defects in absorption of vitamin E in intestine and transportation in liver. Abetalipoproteinemia is a rare metabolic disorder occurring in less than 1 in 100,000 populations. It has multisystem manifestations characterized by fat malabsorption leading to diarrhea, acanthocytosis (Figure 8.4), retinitis pigmentosa leading to night blindness, spino-cerebellar ataxia, peripheral neuropathy and muscle weakness. Defective absorption of fat and fat-soluble vitamins results in failure to thrive. A majority of these patients manifest with neurological complaints by second decade, and if untreated succumb by third decade (Berriot-Varoquetux et al., 2000). Abetalipoproteinemia is attributed to mutations in microsomal triglyceride transfer protein (MTP) gene leading to defective absorption of vitamin E by intestinal mucosa and transport from liver to blood circulation due to low or absence of lipid molecule (Zamel et al., 2008).

ISOLATED VITAMIN E DEFICIENCY

Ataxia with isolated vitamin E deficiency (AVED) is a rare autosomal recessive disease, which manifests by second decade. The neurological symptoms include spinocerebellar ataxia, areflexia, sensory ataxia, dysarthria, muscle weakness and positive Babinski sign.

AVED resembles Friedreich ataxia but differs by the absence of skeletal abnormalities, diabetes mellitus and cardiomyopathy. The presence of titubation and dystonia are features of AVED which also help to distinguish from Friedreich ataxia. Since these patients do not have fat malabsorption, acanthocytosis is not present and helps in differentiation from abetalipoproteinemia. Several genetic mutations of αTTP gene have been reported (Di Donato et al., 2010). The phenotypic expression of different mutations is beyond the scope of this chapter.

INVESTIGATIONS

The diagnosis of vitamin E deficiency is based on clinical findings and low level of serum vitamin E (Tα) of 5 μg/ml or lower. The serum level of Tα should be interpreted in the light of clinical findings. Sometimes low serum levels do not have corresponding clinical signs. Plasma vitamin E is incorporated into the chylomicrons; therefore, its level depends on the level of plasma lipid; 0.8 mg Tα/g lipid or lower is considered abnormal (Russell, 2005). Stool fat is increased in fat malabsorption and serum lipid concentration, and other fat-soluble vitamins are also low suggesting a generalized state of malabsorption. Cerebrospinal fluid is normal. Nerve conduction study reveals distal sensory polyneuropathy, although motor conduction abnormality and features of demyelinating neuropathy has been reported (Puri et al., 2005). Somatosensory and visual evoked potentials are frequently abnormal. Magnetic resonance imaging reveals T2 hyper intensity in the spinal cord simulating subacute combined degeneration and copper deficiency.

TREATMENT

There is no consensus on the ideal dose of vitamin E (Tα), and a dose of 200 mg/day to 100 mg/kg/day has been tried. One mg Tα is equal to 10 IU of Tα. Following the treatment, improvement or stabilization of neurological status is possible even in those with hereditary vitamin E deficiency. The patients with abetalipoproteinemia may require high dose (5000–7000 mg/day). It has been suggested to start with 200–600 mg water miscible αT. The dose may be adjusted depending on clinical response and serum level. If no improvement occurs, high dose or parenteral administration should be tried (2 mg/kg/day intramuscularly). Bile salt supplementation in patients with malabsorption and other vitamin deficiencies should also be corrected (Russell, 2005).

VITAMIN E IN RESTORATIVE NEUROLOGY

Dietary vitamins and micronutrients are tried in the prevention and treatment of various age-related degenerative diseases either as a preventive or therapeutic measure. Vitamin E has also been used in these disorders in isolation or in combination.

Mortality benefit: Based on 78 randomized controlled trials including 296,707 participants aged 63 (18–103) years received antioxidants orally for 28 days to 12 years. The antioxidant group had morality benefit (11.7% vs 10.2%). However, the analysis of 56 trials with low risk of bias, the participants on antioxidants had increased mortality (12.8% vs 11.6%) especially with β carotene (13.8% vs 11.1%) and vitamin E (12% vs 10.3%) (Bjelakovic et al., 2012). These results have been questioned. Higher mortality in β carotene and vitamin E was due to inclusion of a Finish study, which had very high mortality because of a large proportion of smokers. Reanalysis of data in different subsets revealed that mortality was not significantly different in vitamin E group compared to placebo (Oliver and Myers, 2017).

Stroke: The association of stroke with vitamin E concentration in a meta-analysis on 3156 studies revealed that the increased dietary vitamin E intake was inversely related to stroke, and this benefit was present up to 10 years but not after 10 years. A nonlinear association between dietary vitamin E intake and stroke was also observed. A 17% reduction in stroke risk was present in those with high quantity of vitamin E intake (Cheng et al., 2018). The stroke prevention effect of vitamin E may be due to antioxidant property as it inhibits lipid peroxidation by scavenging reactive oxygen species, thereby protecting cell membrane. Atherosclerotic plaque stabilization, inhibition of platelet aggregation and prevention of thrombus formation has been reported by vitamin E. Four prospective trials, however, have not revealed a protective role of vitamin E in stoke of any type (Hirvonen et al., 2000; Keli et al., 1996; Marniemi et al., 2005; Ross et al., 1997). The role of dietary vitamin E in reducing stroke mortality in postmenopausal women and ischemic stroke in male smokers has also been reported (Vokó et al., 2003). High dietary vitamin E intake was associated with risk of intra-cerebral hemorrhage (Del Rio et al., 2011).

Dementia and cognitive impairment: Oxidative stress and excitotoxicity have been reported in the pathogenesis of Alzheimer disease (AD) and dementia; therefore, antioxidants and antiglutaminergic therapies have been tried in the treatment and prevention of dementia. In a meta-analysis, the role of vitamin E has been evaluated in 304 AD and 516 MCI (minimal cognitive impairment) patients from 4 randomized controlled trials. In AD, there was no benefit in cognitive measures over 6–8 months assessed by AD Assessment Scale – Cognitive Subscale but had less functional decline measured by AD Cooperative Study/Activity of Daily Living Inventory. There was no effect on neuro-psychiatric symptoms. Vitamin E did not have any effect in preventing cognitive decline in MCI patients (Farina et al., 2017).

Others: In muscular dystrophy, vitamin E and selenium have been tried. There was however no significant improvement in muscle power at 1 year (Gamstorp et al., 1986). In age-related macular degeneration, antioxidant (vitamin E, vitamin C and beta carotene) and zinc resulted reduction in progression of macular degeneration and to some extent improvement in visual acuity at 6.3 years follow up (AREDS, 2001).

Therefore, routine use of vitamin E is not recommended for prevention of neurological disease.

VITAMIN E TOXICITY

High dose vitamin E (>800 mg/day) reduces platelet aggregation and interferes with vitamin K metabolism and therefore should not be used with anticoagulants. A dose of 1 g/day or more may be associated with gastrointestinal disturbances.

CONCLUSION

Vitamin E is a fat-soluble vitamin comprising of four tocopherols and four tocotrienols. Vitamin E has antioxidative, antiinflammatory, antidegenerative and various nonoxidant activities for maintaining cell biology. Both vegetarian (fruits, vegetables, seeds and oils) and nonvegetarian foods contain vitamin E, but nonvegetarian food is a richer source. The causes of vitamin E deficiency are fat malabsorption, liver disease, pancreatic disease, intestinal resection and genetic disorders. Neurological presentation of vitamin E deficiency is rare and manifests with ataxia, peripheral neuropathy, neuromuscular weakness, ophthalmoplegia and macular degeneration. Vitamin E deficiency is diagnosed by the clinical presentation and low serum vitamin E level below 5 µg/ml. A wide range of dose has been tried ranging from 200 mg/day to 100 mg/kg/day. The role of vitamin E in preventing neurodegenerative and cardiovascular diseases is yet to establish.

REFERENCES

Age-Related Eye Disease Study Research Group. 2001. A randomized, placebo-controlled, clinical trial of high-dose supplementation with vitamins C and E, beta carotene, and zinc for age-related macular degeneration and vision loss: AREDS Report No. 8. *Archives of Ophthalmology (Chicago, IL: 1960)* 119(10):1417–1436. DOI: 10.1001/archopht.119.10.1417.

Azzi, A., Meydani, S. N., Meydani, M., Zingg, J. M. 2016. The rise, the fall and the renaissance of vitamin E. *Archives of Biochemistry and Biophysics* 595:100–108.

Barnett, S. 1924. Dietary requirements for reproduction: ii. The existence of a specific vitamin for reproduction. *Journal of Biological Chemistry* 58:693–710.

Berriot-Varoqueaux, N., Aggerbeck, L. P., Samson-Bouma, M., Wetterau, J. R. 2000. The role of the microsomal triglyceride transfer protein in abetalipoproteinemia. *Annual Review of Nutrition* 20:663–697.

Bjelakovic, G., Nikolova, D., Gluud, L. L., Simonetti, R. G., Gluud, C. (2012). Antioxidant supplements for prevention of mortality in healthy participants and patients with various diseases. *The Cochrane Database of Systematic Reviews* 3:CD007176. DOI: 10.1002/14651858.CD007176.pub2.

Cheng, P., Wang, L., Ning, S., et al. 2018. Vitamin E intake and risk of stroke: A meta-analysis. *The British Journal of Nutrition* 120(10):1181–1188.

Christen, W. G., Glynn, R. J., Chew, E. Y., Buring, J. E. 2010. Vitamin E and age-related macular degeneration in a randomized trial of women. *Ophthalmology* 117(6):1163–1168.

Christen, W. G., Glynn, R. J., Gaziano, J. M., et al. 2015. Age-related cataract in men in the selenium and vitamin e cancer prevention trial eye endpoints study: A randomized clinical trial. *JAMA Ophthalmology* 133(1):17–24. DOI: 10.1001/jamaophthalmol.2014.3478.

Del Rio, D., Agnoli, C., Pellegrini, N., et al. 2011. Total antioxidant capacity of the diet is associated with lower risk of ischemic stroke in a large Italian cohort. *The Journal of Nutrition* 141(1):118–123.

Di Donato, I., Bianchi, S., Federico, A. 2010. Ataxia with vitamin E deficiency: Update of molecular diagnosis. *Neurological Sciences: Official Journal of the Italian Neurological Society and of the Italian Society of Clinical Neurophysiology* 31(4):511–515.

Evans, H. M., Bishop, K. S. 1922. On The existence of a hitherto unrecognized dietary factor essential for reproduction. *Science (New York, NY)* 56(1458):650–651.

Farina, N., Llewellyn, D., Isaac, M., Tabet, N. 2017. Vitamin E for Alzheimer's dementia and mild cognitive impairment. *The Cochrane Database of Systematic Reviews* 4(4):CD002854.

Gamstorp, I., Gustavson, K. H., Hellström, O., Nordgren, B. 1986. A trial of selenium and vitamin E in boys with muscular dystrophy. *Journal of Child Neurology* 1(3):211–214.

Hirvonen, T., Virtamo, J., Korhonen, P., Albanes, D., Pietinen, P. 2000. Intake of flavonoids, carotenoids, vitamins C and E, and risk of stroke in male smokers. *Stroke* 31(10):2301–2306.

Huttunen, J. K. (Folkhaelsoinstitutet, Helsingfors (Finland)). 1995. Health effects of supplemental use of antioxidant vitamins. *Experiences from the Alpha-Tocopherol Beta-Carotene (ATBC) Cancer Prevention Study* 39(3):103–104.

Jung, J. B., Kim, Y., Oh, K., et al. 2019. Subacute combined degeneration associated with vitamin E deficiency due to small bowel obstruction: A case report. *Medicine* 98(36):e17052.

Kayden, H. J., Silber, R., Kossmann, C. E. 1965. The role of vitamin E deficiency in the abnormal autohemolysis of acanthocytosis. *Transactions of the Association of American Physicians* 78:334.

Keli, S. O., Hertog, M. G., Feskens, E. J., Kromhout, D. 1996. Dietary flavonoids, antioxidant vitamins, and incidence of stroke: The Zutphen study. *Archives of Internal Medicine* 156(6):637–642.

Khadangi, F., Azzi, A. 2019. Vitamin E – The next 100 years. *IUBMB Life* 71(4):411–415.

Klein, E. A., Thompson, I. M., Jr, Tangen, C. M., et al. 2011. Vitamin E and the risk of prostate cancer: The Selenium and Vitamin E Cancer Prevention Trial (SELECT). *JAMA* 306(14):1549–1556.

Mahoney, C. W., Azzi, A. 1988. Vitamin E inhibits protein kinase C activity. *Biochemical and Biophysical Research Communications* 154(2):694–697.

Manor, D., Morley, S. 2007. The alpha-tocopherol transfer protein. *Vitamins and Hormones* 76:45–65.

Marniemi, J., Alanen, E., Impivaara, O., et al. 2005. Dietary and serum vitamins and minerals as predictors of myocardial infarction and stroke in elderly subjects. *Nutrition, Metabolism, and Cardiovascular Diseases: NMCD* 15(3): 188–197.

Olcott, H. S., Mattill, H. A. 1931. The unsaponifiable lipids of lettuce. 3. Antioxidant. *Journal of Biological Chemistry* 93:65–70.

Oliver, C. J., Myers, S. P. 2017. Validity of a cochrane systematic review and meta-analysis for determining the safety of vitamin E. *BMC Complementary and Alternative Medicine* 17(1):408.

Puri, V., Chaudhry, N., Tatke, M., Prakash, V. 2005. Isolated vitamin E deficiency with demyelinating neuropathy. *Muscle & Nerve* 32(2):230–235.

Ross, R. K., Yuan, J. M., Henderson, B. E., Park, J., Gao, Y. T., Yu, M. C. 1997. Prospective evaluation of dietary and other predictors of fatal stroke in Shanghai, China. *Circulation* 96(1):50–55.

Russell, R. M. 2005. Chapter 61. Vitamin and trace mineral deficiency and excess. In: Braunwald, D., Fauci, A. S., Kasper, D. L., Hauser, S. L., Longo, D. L., Jameson, J. L., (Eds.) *Harrison's Principles of Internal Medicine*, 16th ed. New York: McGraw-Hill Inc., pp. 403–411.

Sokol R. J. 1988. Vitamin E deficiency and neurologic disease. *Annual Review of Nutrition* 8: 351–373.

Sokol, R. J., Guggenheim, M. A., Heubi, J. E., et al. 1985. Frequency and clinical progression of the vitamin E deficiency neurologic disorder in children with prolonged neonatal cholestasis. *American Journal of Diseases of Children* 139(12):1211–1215.

Traber M. G. 2007. Vitamin E regulatory mechanisms. *Annual Review of Nutrition* 27:347–362.

Traber, M. G., Manor, D. 2012. Vitamin E. *Advances in Nutrition (Bethesda, MD)* 3(3): 330–331. DOI: 10.3945/an.112.002139.

Vokó, Z., Hollander, M., Hofman, A., Koudstaal, P. J., Breteler, M. M. 2003. Dietary antioxidants and the risk of ischemic stroke: The Rotterdam Study. *Neurology* 61(9):1273–1275.

Zamel, R., Khan, R., Pollex, R. L., Hegele, R. A. 2008. Abetalipoproteinemia: Two case reports and literature review. *Orphanet Journal of Rare Diseases* 3:19.

9

Neurological manifestations of fluorosis

INTRODUCTION

Fluorosis occurs due to ingestion or inhalation of excessive fluoride and manifests with teeth, skeletal and ligament involvement. It is a crippling disease due to deposition of fluoride in hard and soft tissues of the body. Fluorosis is a public health problem because of high fluoride content in the soil and thereby in drinking water and vegetables. High water fluoride levels are found in the foot of high mountains and in the areas where sea has made geographical deposits. There are many fluorosis belts. The neurological manifestation in fluorosis is secondary to bone and ligament calcification leading to entrapment and compression.

HISTORY

The term fluorosis was first coined by Christiani and Gautier in 1925. Later Feil reported fluorosis as an occupational disease (Feil, 1930). Møller and Gudjonsson from Denmark described industrial fluorosis in cryolite miners (Møller and Gudjonsson, 1932). In India, endemic fluorosis was first reported by Shortt and colleagues in 1937 from Madras (Shortt et al., 1937; Reddy, 1979).

Earth crust contains about 85 million tons of fluoride, which is the 13th most common naturally occurring element. About 25 million tons of this element is in India. Fluorine is the most reactive halogen and the most electronegative; therefore, it is not found in a free state in the nature, but is bound as fluoride mineral complex. Fluorosis is endemic in India, China, Mexico and Argentina. A population of 66 million is at risk and six million mainly children are crippled by fluorosis.

EPIDEMIOLOGY

The main sources of fluoride are water, food and occupational exposure. The ground rich in phosphatic rocks is responsible for high fluoride content of ground water. The geographic fluoride belt extends from Turkey to China, and Japan through Iraq, Iran and Afghanistan (Figure 9.1; UNICEF, 1999). Contaminated groundwater though is the main source of fluorosis, contaminated cooking or drinking water, agricultural food products, industrial emissions and pollution as well as drugs and cosmetics may also contribute to fluorosis. The volcanic region has fluoride rocks. Water fluoride content of more than 1.5 ppm is considered toxic. Alkaline pH also increases fluoride absorption, whereas vitamin C, calcium and fresh fruits reduce fluoride absorption and its ill effects. Fluoride content of ground water varies in different geographical regions. The highest fluoride content of water is reported to be 95 mg/l in certain regions of South and North Africa. In India, the highest level of water fluoride has been reported from Haryana, up to 48.3 mg/l. Among the beverages, the high level of fluoride is reported in black tea (1 mg/cup), and excess drinking of tea can cause fluorosis (Whyte et al., 2008).

The environmental factors responsible for fluorosis are high ambient temperature, low rainfall and humidity, which may cause thirst leading to a large amount of water intake. Fluoride-rich subsoil rocks in the region, vegetable and fruits grown in fluoride-rich soil, fluoride-rich toothpaste, prolonged use of quinolones, voriconazole and indoor coal burning may also contribute to fluoride toxicity. About 40%–100% districts are affected in Rajasthan, Gujarat and Andhra Pradesh, about

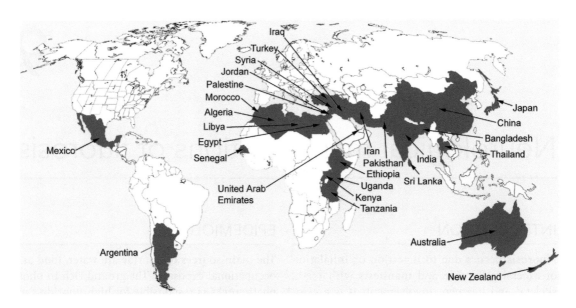

Figure 9.1 Global distribution of endemic fluorosis as per UNICEF in 1999.

40%–70% districts are affected in Haryana, Punjab, Madhya Pradesh and Maharashtra and less than 40% districts are affected in Tamil Nadu, West Bengal, Bihar and Uttar Pradesh (Figure 9.2; UNICEF, 1999; FRRDF, 1999).

The worldwide prevalence of fluorosis is 4.8%–47.5% (Datta and Datta, 2013), and it is a major health problem in 25 countries of Asia and Africa (Sellami et al., 2020). There are two major fluorosis belts: one that stretches from Kenya through Sudan, Algeria, Libya, Jordan and Syria and the other belt that stretches from China through Northern Thailand, India, Afghanistan, Iran, Iraq and Turkey. There are similar fluorosis belts in the Americas and Japan. Argentina and Mexico are also endemic for fluorosis. Fluorosis is uncommon in Europe and America. Children below 7 years manifest with dental fluorosis, and the adults with skeletal fluorosis. The development of skeletal fluorosis requires decades of fluoride exposure. The highest incidence of fluorosis is reported in the adults of 30–60 years of age. The males are more frequently affected than females. Malnutrition increases fluoride toxicity. Diet poor in calcium and vitamin C increases fluoride toxicity. In a study from China, fluorosis was less common in well-nourished individuals compared to poorly nourished (43.8% vs 69.2%). The deficient group consumed less than 400 mg of calcium and 20 g of protein daily (Liang and Cao, 1997). Magnesium reduces fluoride toxicity (Marier, 1969).

In the endemic areas, the main source of fluoride is water, but in China and India foods such as cereals and vegetables grown in fluoride rich fields are an important source of fluorosis. The laborers consuming 3000 calories diet have 54.66–75.76 mg of fluoride in their food which are above the recommended dose (Reddy, 1985).

ABSORPTION AND DISTRIBUTION

Fluoride is absorbed from gastrointestinal and respiratory tract. The absorption of fluoride depends on the solubility or whether it is in organic or inorganic form. Soluble form of fluoride is completely absorbed, whereas 60%–80% of less soluble inorganic or organic fluoride compounds are absorbed. Fluoride in water is absorbed by 90% and dietary fluoride by 30%–69%. The absorption of fluoride in gastrointestinal tract is influenced by dietary compositions. Presence of calcium, magnesium and aluminum in the diet reduces the solubility of fluoride, thereby reducing its absorption. Fluoride is absorbed by diffusion, circulates in the body and also enters the cells. It is excreted in stool, urine, sweat and breast milk. 10%–19% of fluid intake is excreted in the stool. Urinary excretion of fluoride depends on the pH and renal function. In chronic kidney disease, urinary excretion of fluoride is decreased, and these patients may develop fluorosis even at 1 mg/l of fluoride in drinking water.

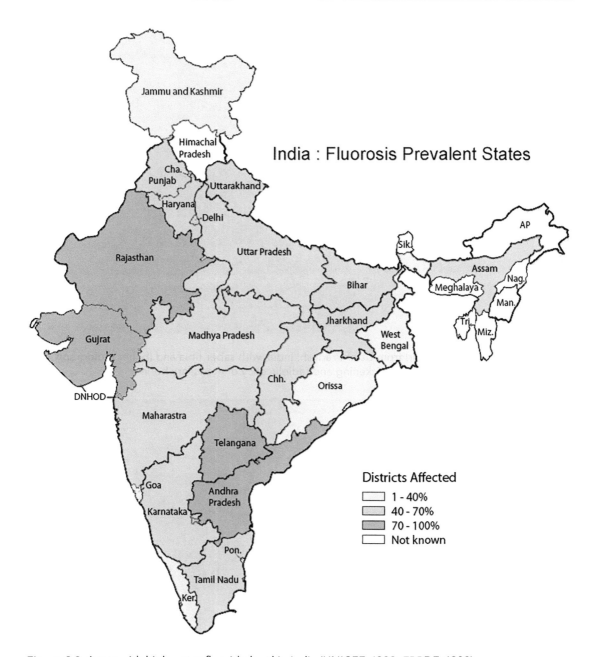

Figure 9.2 Areas with high water fluoride level in India (UNICEF, 1999; FRRDF, 1999).

PATHOPHYSIOLOGY

Fluoride is a bone-seeking element similar to calcium and magnesium. About 99% of fluoride is present in the bone. Uptake of fluoride is more in the actively growing end of the cancellous bone than compact mature bone. Fluoride is deposited in the bone as fluorapatite, and the bone becomes sclerosed (osteosclerosis). In children in South Africa, osteoporosis of the long bone has been reported especially in the lower limbs. The skeletal deformity simulates features of vitamin D deficiency such as bowed legs, genu valgum, saber tibia (Figures 9.3 and 9.4), widening of wrist and cubitus valgus (Jackson, 1962; Krishnamachari and Krishnaswamy, 1973). There is osteosclerosis of vertebra. The osteoporotic changes are more prominent in the areas with low dietary calcium, and it

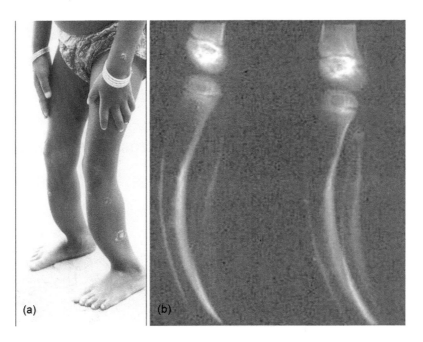

Figure 9.3 (a) A 6-year-old girl from Uttar Pradesh, India, with saber tibia and (b) her radiograph showing bowing of tibia, cortical thickening and radiolucency of medullary bone.

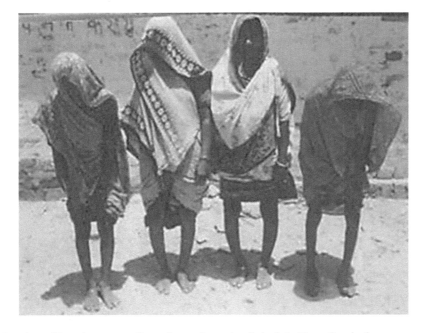

Figure 9.4 Bowing of legs in women from fluorosis endemic belt in Uttar Pradesh.

is postulated that secondary hyperparathyroidism due to hypocalcaemia might have mobilized bone calcium to the circulation because fluorapatite crystals are less soluble than hydroxyapatite. In India, the bony deformity of the lower limbs with osteoporosis is more prevalent in South India. In Punjab, these changes have not been reported although Haryana and Punjab have higher fluoride levels in drinking water. This may be due to higher calcium intake in their diet.

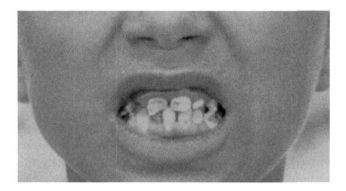

Figure 9.5 Dental fluorosis: pitting, brown pigmentation and hypoplastic teeth.

CLINICAL FEATURES

The clinical features of fluorosis may be described as dental, skeletal and miscellaneous. The neurological complications of fluorosis are rare and seen in advanced stage of skeletal fluorosis.

DENTAL FLUOROSIS

Exposure to high fluoride content before 7 years of age results in dental fluorosis. Dental fluorosis more commonly affects the permanent teeth, but in the endemic areas even the deciduous teeth may also be affected. Fluorosis mainly affects the enamel of the teeth. About 80% of the enamel is made of hydroxyapatite which is translucent. The fluoride replaces the hydroxyl part, and forms fluorapatite giving rise to chalk white color. Teeth lose their shining appearance and acquire chalky white patches mostly affecting the upper incisor teeth. These patches turn yellow to dark brown (Figure 9.5). Following loss of enamel, the teeth get corroded, and there is permanent loss of teeth. The severity of dental fluorosis is measured by Dean's index (Table 9.1). Community fluorosis index (CFI) measures both prevalence and severity of fluorosis (Table 9.2).

SKELETAL FLUOROSIS

Skeletal fluorosis occurs because of prolonged chronic ingestion of fluoride-rich water or diet above 1.5 mg/dl (Arlappa et al., 2013). The commonest age group for skeletal fluorosis is the third and fourth decade. In an endemic area, besides environmental factors, a number of genetic factors

Table 9.1 Dean's index for measurement of dental fluorosis

Subgroup	Manifestations
0	Normal enamel
0.5	Questionable fluorosis
	Slight alteration in translucency of enamel and occasional flake or spot
1	Very mild fluorosis
	White flake affects less than 25% of tooth area in 2 most affected teeth
2	More than 50% area in 2 most affected teeth
3	All enamel surface affected
	Discolored brown teeth
4	Severe hypo-plastic teeth with attrition and pitting, brown and black staining

Table 9.2 Community fluorosis index (FCI)

CFI: <0.4 is considered little or no public health problem
CFI: 0.4–0.5 Borderline fluorosis
CFI: >0.6 Excessive fluorosis

have been suggested for selective occurrence of fluorosis in some individuals. The possible candidate genes are matrix metallopeptidase 2, glutathione S-transferase pi-1, prolactin, vitamin D receptor and myeloperoxidase (Liu et al., 2016). Once fluoride enters the bone, it has a half-life of 7 years. Fluoride affects the bone strength in two ways: (a) 50% of fluoride forms fluorapatite hydroxide ion from hydroxyapatite crystal. (b) Fluoride increases bone turnover by regulating Runx-2 and RANKL (Pei et al., 2014). It affects expression of osteoprotegerin and osteocalcin leading to increased osteoblastic activity. Fluorapatite crystal is lager and has greater crystallinity; however, it has lesser solubility than hydroxyapatite crystal. This accounts for grater opacity of bone.

Most of the individuals with fluorosis are asymptomatic in the initial stage, but later may have vague pain, backache and pain in the hands, feet and joints due to stiffness. There is calcification of ligaments and tendinous attachment of muscles. There may be poker back deformity due to calcification of spinal ligaments. On examination, the spinal mobility is reduced. The patients are unable to extend the spine (Figure 9.6). They are unable to pick up any object from the floor (coin test) and unable to flex the neck to touch the chest by chin (chin test) and unable to extend the neck and shoulder (extension test) (Figure 9.6).

Radiological findings: The skeletal fluorosis can be diagnosed by the imaging findings and epidemiological data. Three stages of skeletal fluorosis have been described by Roholm in 1937.

1. Thick trabeculations and dense spans of axial bones resulting in a ground glass appearance of thoracolumbar vertebrae and iliac wings.
2. Loss of trabeculation and regular contours of the bone with ligament calcification such as paraspinous, sacrospinous and sacrotuberous ligaments along with tendinous insertion of muscles (Figure 9.7).
3. The bone becomes denser and opacified. There is periosteal thickening and cortex giving rise to marmoreal appearance of the skeleton. Radiograph of the bone reveals osteosclerosis, osteophytosis and ligamentous calcification of the pelvis and spine. The calcification of tendinous attachment to the bones looks like rose thorn. Calcification of interosseous membrane

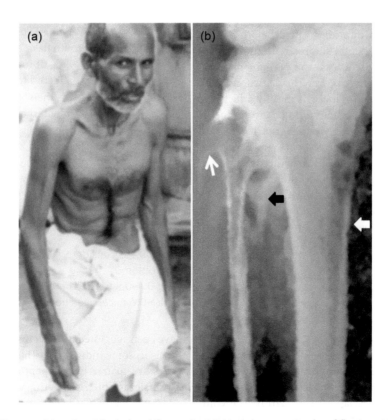

Figure 9.6 A 52-year-old male with skeletal fluorosis. (a) He is in an attitude of flexion. Unable to extend his back, touch chest by chin and extend his elbow. (b) Radiograph shows calcification of tendons at the origin of peroneal muscles (thin white arrow), interosseous membrane (thick black arrow) and periosteal thickening (thick white arrow).

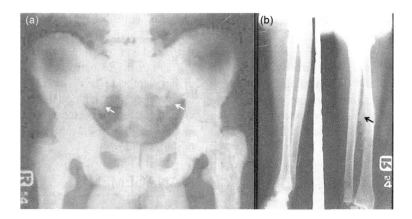

Figure 9.7 Radiograph of **(a)** pelvis showing calcification of ischio-tuberal ligament (white arrow). **(b)** Calcification of interosseous membrane of tibia and fibula (black arrow).

and posterior longitudinal ligament along with the opacification of axial bone is suggestive of skeletal fluorosis. The vertebrae have beak-like osteophyte and chalky white ground glass appearance more marked in the lumbar and cervical regions. Ossification and ligamentous calcification lead to spinal canal stenosis and foraminal narrowing resulting in spinal cord and root compression in the later stage. The other radiological features include coxa vara, genu valgum, genu varum, acetabular protrusion and reduction in vertebral height with corresponding increase in the width of the vertebra.

Computed tomography also reveals similar changes and is helpful in the evaluation of the patients with myelopathy, radiculopathy and rarely in vertebral artery occlusion. Spinal MRI also reveals the above mentioned changes but is specially indicated for soft tissue imaging and excluding other possibilities. In the later stage of skeletal fluorosis, there is restrictive lung disease because of stiff rib cage.

Bone mineral density is increased in fluorosis. 99mTc MDP scintigraphy reveals increased uptake of radiotracer in the axial bones and at the site of tendinous or ligamentous insertion

Histopathology of bone: Histology of compact bone reveals poorly formed Haversian system and disorganized lamellar system. Osteoid tissues extend to ligaments and muscle tendon.

Differential diagnosis: A number of conditions such as Paget's disease, ossification of posterior longitudinal ligament, diffuse idiopathic spinal hyperostosis (DISH), osteopetrosis, renal osteodystrophy and pseudohypoparathyroidism may also have osteosclerosis and ligamentous calcification which should be differentiated from fluorosis (Table 9.3).

Table 9.3 Differential diagnosis of skeletal fluorosis

Disease	Radiological findings		
	Bone density	Osteophytosis	Ligament calcification
Fluorosis	Diffuse ↑	+++	Diffuse
Paget's disease	Localized ↑	-	Diffuse
OPLL	-	=	PLL
DISH	-	+++	Diffuse
Osteopetrosis	Localized, multiple	-	-
Renal osteodystrophy	Diffuse ↑	-	-
Hypoparathyroidism	Localized ↑	-	-

OPLL, ossification of posterior longitudinal ligament; DISH, diffuse idiopathic skeletal hyperostosis; PLL, posterior longitudinal ligament.

NEUROLOGICAL COMPLICATIONS OF FLUOROSIS

The nervous system is not directly affected in endemic fluorosis, and the neurological complications are due to entrapment or compression of spinal cord, nerve root and/or peripheral nerve. The neurological complications are as follows:

1. Pain
2. Radiculopathy
3. Myelopathy
4. Entrapment neuropathy

Pain is the commonest complaint and is due to articular and ligament involvement. Rarely pain can be due to compression of nerve root or impairment in spinal mobility. Radiculopathy is associated with nerve root compression in upper limb with respective sensory motor deficit. Cervical myelopathy occurs due to cervical canal stenosis, and the patient presents with walking difficulty, weakness, sensory impairment, and bladder dysfunction occurs in the advanced stage of disease (Modi et al., 2019; Misra et al., 1988). There may be crippling deformity and flexor spasms. The peripheral nerves may be affected due to entrapment of peroneal, sciatic, ulnar or lateral cutaneous nerves. The nerve entrapment occurs due to calcification of ligament or tendon resulting in narrowing in of the tunnel through which the nerve passes. Rarely cranial nerve involvement occurs because of compression of 2nd and 8th cranial nerve. Vertebral artery compression in foramen transversarium may lead to vertebrobasilar ischemia or stroke. Vertebral arterial aneurysm has also been reported in fluorosis (Diao et al., 2018).

INVESTIGATIONS

The diagnosis of fluorosis is easy in the presence of dental or skeletal fluorosis in a fluorosis endemic area. Water fluoride level (>1.5 mg/l) provides additional help.

Urinary fluoride: Measurement of 24 h urinary fluoride is better than a spot value because of variability in the urinary excretion of fluoride. The reported range of 24 h fluoride in the patients with skeletal fluorosis is 0.5–13.0 mg/l (Reddy and Deme, 2016).

Serum fluoride has also wide variability. In normal individuals, it varies between 0.08 (0.03–0.13) mg/l, and in endemic fluorosis, it was 0.68 (0.04–0.20) mg/l. In 17 patients with skeletal fluorosis, urinary fluoride level was 3.28 (0.68–7.8) mg/l (Xiang et al., 2005). Blood fluoride in normal individuals has been reported to be less than 0.05 mg/l, and the level above 0.2 mg/l suggests a high chance of skeletal fluorosis.

MANAGEMENT

There is no specific treatment of fluorosis. Prevention or stopping the exposure is the most important management strategy. Skeletal fluorosis is treated by symptomatic treatment and nonsteroidal antiinflammatory drugs.

Dental fluorosis in children of 6–12 years of age is treated with a combination of calcium, vitamin D3 and vitamin C and has been reported to favor the regression of signs of skeletal fluorosis (Wang et al., 2007). For dental fluorosis, resin infiltration seems to be a promising treatment followed by bleaching and microabrasion (Nevárez-Rascón et al., 2020). Topical fluoride agents reduce dental caries in children compared to no fluoride supplementation (Zhang et al., 2020). Compressive myelopathy may be benefitted by decompressive surgery (Figure 9.8; Misra et al., 1988)

PREVENTION

Providing safe drinking water is the most important strategy to prevent fluorosis. Various materials such as activated alumina, serpentine, bone charcoal, alum and lime have been used for defluoridation of household water. Water supply source such as Nalgonda defluoridation project, India was undertaken to prevent fluorosis. The target of preventing dental fluorosis is that the water fluoride should be 0.2–0.4 mg/l. In the patients with kidney disease, the target should be lower. As per WHO, large-scale defluoridation plants have not been successful. It is recommended to harvest ground and surface water.

CONCLUSION

Fluorosis is a global health problem in Asia, Africa, Americas and Australia. Fluorosis is a crippling

(a) 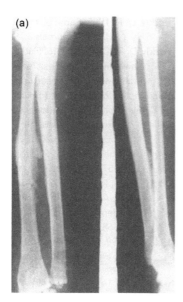 (b)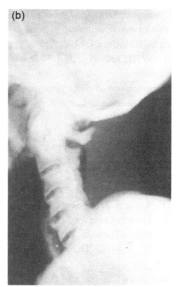

Figure 9.8 Radiograph of a patient with compressive cervical myelopathy due to skeletal fluorosis. **(a)** Forearm radiograph shows opacification of the interosseous membrane. **(b)** Cervical radiograph in lateral view after laminectomy reveals opacification of vertebra (osteosclerosis) and calcification of anterior and posterior longitudinal ligament. (With permission from Misra, U. K., Nag, D., Husain, M., Newton, G., Ray, P. K. 1988. Endemic fluorosis presenting as cervical cord compression. *Archives of Environmental & Occupational Health* 43(1):18–21. DOI: 10.1080/00039896.1988.9934368.)

disease resulting from deposition of fluoride in the bone and hard tissue of the body. Fluorosis is due to excessive intake of fluoride in drinking water, food or industrial pollution over a long period. Fluorosis mostly affects teeth, bone and ligaments. Dental fluorosis occurs in children and skeletal fluorosis in adults when water fluoride level is more than 1 mg/l especially in tropical countries. The patients manifest with stiffness and body ache. The neurological manifestations include myelopathy, radiculopathy, myeloradiculopathy and neuropathy because of compression of spinal cord, root or nerves. The neurological manifestations have been reported mainly from India. Fluorosis can be prevented by safe drinking water.

REFERENCES

Arlappa, N., Aatif, I. Q., Srinivas, R. 2013. Fluorosis in India: An overview. *Indian Journal of Public Health Research & Development* 1:97–102.

Christiani, H., Gautier, R. 1925. Emanations fluorees dex usines. Eude experimental de laction du fluor sur les vegetaux. *Annales d'Hygiene Publique (Paris)* 1:49–64.

Datta, P., Datta, P. P. 2013. Prevalence, etiology and clinical features of skeletal fluorosis: A critical review. *Innovare Journal of Medical Sciences* 1:5–6.

Diao, Y., Sun, Y., Wang, S., Zhang, F., Pan, S., Liu, Z. 2018. Delayed epidural pseudoaneurysm following cervical laminectomy and instrumentation in a patient with canal stenosis secondary to skeletal fluorosis: A case report. *Medicine (Baltimore)* 97(8):e9883. DOI: 10.1097/MD.0000000000009883.

Feil, A. 1930. Le fluorisme professionnel, intoxication professionnelle par l'acide fluorhydrique et les sels de fluor. *Paris Medecine* 2:242–248.

Fluorosis Research and Rural Development Foundation (FRRDF). 1999 *State of art report on the extent of fluoride in drinking water and the resulting endemicity in India*. New Delhi: Fluorosis Research and Rural Development Foundation.

Jackson, W. P. 1962. Further observations on the Kenhardt bone disease and its relation to flurosis. *South African Medical Journal* 36:932–936.

Krishnamachari, K. A., Krishnaswamy, K. 1973. Genu valgum and osteoporosis in an area of endemic fluorosis. *Lancet* 2(7834):877–879.

Liang, C.K., Cao, S.R. 1997. Epidemiological analysis of endemic fluorosis in China. *Environmental Carcinogenesis and Ecotoxicology Reviews* 15:123–138.

Liu, Q., Liu, H., Yu, X., Wang, Y., Yang, C., Xu, H. 2016. Analysis of the role of insulin signaling in bone turnover induced by fluoride. *Biological Trace Element Research* 171(2):380–390. DOI: 10.1007/s12011-015-0555-5.

Marier, J. R. 1969. The importance of dietary magnesium with particular reference to humans. *Fluoride* 2:185–187.

Misra, U. K., Nag, D., Husain, M., Newton, G., Ray, P. K. 1988. Endemic fluorosis presenting as cervical cord compression. *Archives of Environmental & Occupational Health* 43(1):18–21. DOI: 10.1080/00039896.1988.9934368.

Modi, J. V., Tankshali, K. V., Patel, Z. M., Shah, B. H., Gol, A. K. 2019. Management of acquired compressive myelopathy due to spinal fluorosis. *Indian Journal of Orthopaedics* 53(2):324–332. DOI: 10.4103/ortho.IJOrtho_570_17.

Møller, P. F., Gudjonsson, S. V. 1932. Massive fluorosis of bones and ligaments. *Acta Radiologica (Stockholm)* 1932(13):269–294.

Nevárez-Rascón, M., Molina-Frechero, N., Adame, E., et al. 2020. Effectiveness of a microabrasion technique using 16% HCL with manual application on fluorotic teeth: A series of studies. *World Journal of Clinical Cases* 8(4):743–756. DOI: 10.12998/wjcc.v8.i4.743.

Pei, J., Li, B., Gao, Y., et al. 2014. Fluoride decreased osteoclastic bone resorption through the inhibition of NFATc1 gene expression. *Environmental Toxicology* 29(5):588–595. DOI: 10.1002/tox.21784.

Reddy, D. R. 1979. Skeletal flourosis. In: Vinken, P. J., Bruyn, G. W. (Eds.) *Hand book of clinical neurology*. Amsterdam: North Holland Publishing Co., pp. 465–504.

Reddy, D. R. 1985. Some observations on fluoride toxicity. *NIMHANS Journals* 3:79–86.

Reddy, D. R., Dene, P. 2016. Fluorosis. In: Chopra, J. S., Sawhney, I. M. S. (Eds.) *Neurology in tropics*. 2nd ed. New Delhi: Elsevier, pp. 488–472.

Roholm, K. 1937. *Fluorine intoxication: A clinical hygienic study*. London: Lewis.

Sellami, M., Riahi, H., Maatallah, K., Ferjani, H., Bouaziz, M. C., Ladeb, M. F. 2020. Skeletal fluorosis: Don't miss the diagnosis! *Skeletal Radiology* 49(3): 345–357. DOI: 10.1007/s00256-019-03302-0.

Shortt, H. E., McRobert, G. R., Barnard, T. W., Mannadi Nayar, A.S. 1937. Endemic fluorosis in the Madras presidency. *Indian Journal of Medical Research* 25: 553–568.

UNICEF. 1999. Water front. A UNICEF publication on water, environment, sanitation and hygiene. Issue 12. FRR.

Wang, S. X., Wang, Z.H., Cheng, X. T., et al. 2007. Arsenic and fluoride exposure in drinking water: Children's IQ and growth in Shanyin county, Shanxi Province, China. *Environmental Health Perspectives* 115:643–647.

Whyte, M. P., Totty, W. G., Lim, V. T., Whitford, G. M. 2008. Skeletal fluorosis from instant tea. *Journal of Bone and Mineral Research: The Official Journal of the American Society for Bone and Mineral Research* 23(5): 759–769. DOI: 10.1359/jbmr.

Xiang, Q.Y., Chen, L.S., Chen, X.D., et al. 2005. Serum fluoride and skeletal fluorosis in two villages in Jiangsu Province, China. *Fluoride* 38(3): 178–184.

Zhang, J., Sardana, D., Li, K. Y., Leung, K., Lo, E. 2020. Topical fluoride to prevent root caries: Systematic review with network meta-analysis. *Journal of Dental Research* 99(5): 506–513. DOI: 10.1177/0022034520906384.

Iodine deficiency disorders and their neurological consequences

INTRODUCTION

Iodine has an atomic weight of 126.9 g per atom and is an essential element for thyroid hormone production by the thyroid gland. Most iodide is found in seawater and when oxidized, forms elemental iodine, a volatile substance which evaporates and returns back to soil by rain. Vegetables grown in soil contain iodine and maintain an iodine-food chain in iodine sufficient areas. Iodine deficiency belts are usually in inland, mountainous and flooding areas. Vegetables and plants grown in iodine deficient belt contain iodine 10 µg/kg, whereas in iodine sufficient areas, it is 1 mg/kg. Therefore, iodine supplementation or food from iodine sufficient belt should be made available. Iodine deficiency is the most important nutritional cause of impairment of brain development as well as the most important cause of preventable mental retardation. Children born in iodine deficiency belt are prone to suffer from mental retardation and other neurological disorders due to combined effect of maternal, fetal, neonatal and postnatal hypothyroxinemia.

HISTORY

Iodine is a Greek word, which means violet. During the period of Napoleon, Courtois observed violet vapors from seaweed ash, while preparing gunpowder. Gay Lussac named this element iodine. In 1895, iodine was demonstrated in thyroid by Baumann. In 1917, Marine and Kimball for the first time reported goiter in iodine deficiency state, following which iodine supplementation for goiter prevention was started in Switzerland and USA in the 1920s. In 1980, the World Health Organization (WHO) estimated 20%–60% people to have iodine deficiency state or goiter, which was more frequent in the developing countries. Since 1970–1990, most of the countries in the world practiced iodine supplementation for prevention of goiter. The discovery of neurological involvement in iodine deficiency is a by-product of iodine supplementation. Following iodine supplementation, not only goiter regressed but also the incidence of cretinism and mental retardation declined, and there was improvement in cognitive functions in the population. A number of conditions are included in iodine deficiency disorders (IDD).

EPIDEMIOLOGY

About 2 billion individuals in the world have insufficient iodine intake, and one-third of them are children (de Benoist et al., 2008; Zimmermann, 2009). As per WHO estimate in 2007, the worldwide prevalence of iodine deficiency is 30%, and the proportion of household iodized salt access is 70%. The prevalence of iodine deficiency is the highest in Europe 52% followed by eastern Mediterranean 47.2%, South-East Asia 30%, Western Pacific 21.2% and lowest in America 11% (WHO, 2007). Switzerland, Scandinavian countries, Canada, America and Australia have eliminated iodine deficiency by 1990. Iodine deficiency is still a public health problem in 47 countries. Household coverage of iodized salt in South-East Asia is 49%, and about 17 million babies are born annually in these areas are unprotected for iodine deficiency, and they constitute 40% of world's

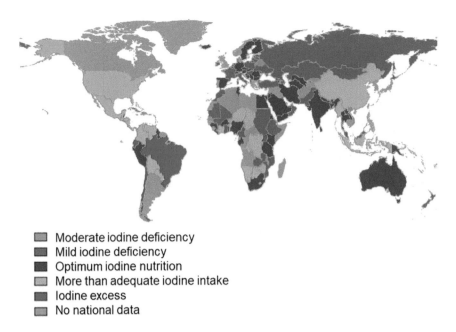

Moderate iodine deficiency
Mild iodine deficiency
Optimum iodine nutrition
More than adequate iodine intake
Iodine excess
No national data

Figure 10.1 Distribution of iodine status in different regions of the world based on urinary excretion. (With permission from Zimmermann, M. B., Jooste, P. L., Pandav, C. S. 2008. Iodine-deficiency disorders. *Lancet* (London, England) *372*(9645):1251–1262. DOI:10.1016/S0140-6736(08)61005-3.)

iodine unprotected children. Small-scale iodized salt production, lack of monitoring, lack of political commitment and low socioeconomic conditions are responsible for persistence of iodine deficiency in these countries. About 64% of households in sub-Saharan countries use iodized salt, but it is widely variable from country to country. In Sudan, Mauritania, Guinea Bissau and Gambia, only 10% households use iodized salt, whereas more than 90% households use iodized salt in Burundi, Kenya, Nigeria, Tunisia, Uganda and Zimbabwe. Nigeria has eliminated iodine deficiency. Iodine supplementation is politically appealing because of its direct intervention in humans as well as cognitive, social and economic advantages at a very low cost (Zimmermann et al., 2008). Worldwide distribution of iodine deficiency is shown in Figure 10.1.

SOURCES OF IODINE

The main source of iodine is sea food, seaweeds and fish, which contain large amounts of iodine. Meat is a poor source of iodine, and it depends on the feed provided. Other sources are dairy products, poultry, cereals and vegetables. Cooking, baking and food preservation by canning reduce the iodine content minimally (<10%). Erythrosine, a coloring agent of food, is a rich source of iodine. The iodine content of food is also affected by irrigation, fertilizer and livestock feed. Rock slat is a rich source of iodine. The important sources of iodine are presented in Table 10.1.

Table 10.1 Average iodine content in selected food items

Food item	Mean iodine level (µg/100g)
Bread	3
Cheese	
Whey	203
Cottage	27
Coffee	8
Egg	36
Fish	
Cod	180
Salmon wild	20
Salmon farm	3.8
Fruit and vegetable	0.7
Meat	4
Milk	16

ABSORPTION AND DISTRIBUTION

In healthy adults, iodine is rapidly and almost completely (>90%) absorbed in the stomach and duodenum. Before absorption, dietary iodine (iodate) is converted to iodine in the gut. Iodine is equally distributed in intracellular and extracellular compartments. It is cleared from circulation by thyroid and kidney. Little iodine is excreted in feces. In normal individuals, 10% of iodine is taken up by thyroid, but in chronic iodine deficient state, the uptake by thyroid may reach up to 80%. Iodine is secreted in breast milk. The half-life of circulating iodine is 10 h and is reduced in iodine deficiency state. Normal adults have 10–20 mg of iodine, 70%–80% of which is in thyroid gland (Chavasit et al., 2002). In chronic iodine deficiency, iodine concentration in thyroid may be below 20 µg (normal 60 µg). There is about 20–50 times concentration gradient of iodine between plasma and thyroid, which is maintained by sodium/iodine symporter (SIS) gene located on chromosome 19. Mutations of this gene may result in iodine transportation defect. In the thyrocyte, iodine is used for synthesis of thyroid hormone which is liberated into the circulation. The half-life of T4 is 5–8 days and that of T3 is 1–3 days. Subsequently, the hormone is degraded, and liberated iodine is taken up by the thyroid gland or excreted in the urine. Ultimately, 90% of ingested iodine is excreted in urine. Thyroid gland adapts for some time in a state of iodine deficiency by producing thyroid hormone. When iodine intake is less than 100 µg/ day, there is rise in TSH, which increases plasma inorganic iodine clearance by stimulating sodium/ iodine symporter. Thyroid stimulating hormone increases iodine uptake by thyrocyte, decreases renal excretion of iodine, increases synthesis and release of T3 by increasing the breakdown of thyroglobulin (TG). On Iodine intake up to 50 µg/ day, thyroid gland can maintain its iodine pool; however below this level, thyroid iodine is depleted leading to goiter (Delange, 2000).

Multi nodular goiter is a result of somatic mutation of monoclonal origin. In endemic iodine deficiency areas, children have high TSH, low T4, high or normal T3 level, and serum thyroglobulin is typically elevated. Cretinism and thyroid failure occurs in prolonged severe iodine deficiency state. Their circulating T3 and T4 levels are low, and TSH is very high. In endemic area, susceptibility for developing goiter may be due to both genetic and epigenetic factors.

Goitrogens: A number of dietary goitrogens may interfere with iodine uptake by thyroid gland. These include vegetables such as cabbage, cauliflower, kale, broccoli, turnip and rape seed. The other dietary goitrogens are lima beans, linseed, cassava, sorghum and sweet potato. Certain cyanogenic glucosides and thiocyanates of the cyanogenic glucosides compete with iodine uptake by the thyroid gland. Heavy smoking may also interfere with iodine uptake because of thiocyanates. Soy bread and infant formula without iodine fortification may produce hypothyroidism and goiter in infants. Deficiency of vitamin, iron and selenium may also aggravate iodine deficiency (Table 10.2).

DAILY RECOMMENDED DOSE OF IODINE

The World Health Organization recommends iodine intake 150 µg/day for men and women. The daily requirement is increased to 250 µg/day during pregnancy and lactation (WHO, 2001). The details of iodine requirement in different age groups as per WHO and US Institute of Medicine are presented in Table 10.3.

ROLE OF IODINE IN NEUROLOGICAL DEVELOPMENT

Iodine deficiency influences the growth and development and results in a wide variety of disorders which are included under the rubric of iodine deficiency disorders (IDD) (Table 10.4). In normal subjects, T4 is 50–100 µg and is more than T3. In iodine deficient state T4 is depleted, and T3 remains in the normal range for some time. In prolonged and severe iodine deficiency, T3 is also depleted. Therefore, T3 is a better index of severity of iodine deficiency, whereas maternal T4 is a better indicator of neurological development.

During pregnancy, iodine requirement increases by 50%. In an iodine deficient mother, since circulating T4 is low, she is unable to cope with the increased requirement which leads to further decrease in T4 level. This results in serious effects on neural development. Thyroid hormone

Table 10.2 Mechanism of iodine deficiency by different foods, nutrients and toxins

	Substance	Mechanism
A. Food		
Cassava, sweet potato, lima beans, sorghum, linseed	Cyanogenic glucosides	Compete with iodine uptake of thyroid
Millet, Soy	Flavonoids	Impair thyroid peroxidase activity.
Cruciferous vegetables (cabbage, kale, cauliflower, broccoli, turnip)	Glucosinolates	Compete with iodine uptake of thyroid
B. Nutrients		
Selenium deficiency	↑ Peroxides	Thyroid damage
	↓ Deiodinase	↓ Thyroid hormone synthesis
Iron deficiency	↓ Thyroperoxidase	Efficacy of iodine
Vitamin A deficiency	↑ TSH	Goiter
	↓ TSH β gene	
C. Toxins		
Perchlorate	Sodium/iodine symporter competitive inhibitor	↓ Iodine transport to thyroid ↓ Iodine uptake to thyroid
Disulphides	-	↓ Thyroidal iodine uptake
Smoking mother	Thiocyanate	↓ Iodine secretion in breast milk

Table 10.3 Recommendation of daily iodine intake

Age groups	World Health Organization (µg/day)	Age groups	US Institute of Medicine (µg/day)
0–5 years	91	0–12 months	110–130
6–12 years	120	1–8 years	90
>12 years	150	9–13 years	120
Pregnancy	250	>14 years	150
Lactation	250	Pregnancy	220
		Lactation	290

Table 10.4 Iodine deficiency disorders

Neurological:
   Neurological cretin (mental retardation, deaf mutism, strabismus, spastic diplegia, rigidity)
   Low intelligence and emotional quiescent
   Increased reaction time
Nonneurological:
   Myxedematous cretin
   Short stature/ growth retardation
   Endemic goiter
   Neonatal hypothyroidism
   Neonatal hyperthyrotropinemia
   Early and late pregnancy loss
   Increased perinatal and infant mortality

is important for cell migration, myelination and maturation of the nervous system (Stepien and Huttner, 2019).

In earlier studies, there was a controversy about trans-placental transfer of thyroid hormone to the fetus (Osorio and Myant, 1960; Fisher and Oddie, 1964). Subsequent studies, however, have revealed that the presence of T3 and T4 in the fetal tissues using radio-ligand studies (Obregón et al., 1984). T3 receptors in fetal brain have been demonstrated before fetus synthesizes thyroid hormone. Fetal thyroid gland starts producing T3 and T4 by 10–11 weeks of gestation, and TSH by 10 weeks (Norris, 1916; Shepard, 1967). Fetus depends on maternal thyroid hormone up to 10 weeks of gestation.

The degree of iodine deficiency affects maternal and fetal thyroid functions. There is no evidence of neurological involvement in mild iodine deficiency (50–99 μg/day). Aghini-Lombardi et al. reported delayed reaction time in 6–10 years of children whose daily iodine intake is 64 μg/day compared to those having 142 μg/day. The cognitive function however was normal (Aghini Lombardi et al., 1995). Children with moderate iodine deficiency (20–49 μg/day) with normal thyroid function manifest with low visuo-motor abilities, motor skill, perceptual and neuromotor abilities with low developmental and intellectual quotients (Delange, 2000). Severe iodine deficiency (<20 μg/day) manifests with more florid neurological and physical impairment.

Thyroid hormone deficiency in fetus results in irreversible brain damage (McCarrisson, 1908) and produces two polar forms of cretins:

A. Neurologic cretin
B. Myxedematous cretin.

Myxedematous cretin is more common in Africa and neurogenic cretin in other endemic areas.

(A) **Neurogenic cretin:** Neurologic cretin manifests with deafness, mutism, moderate to severe learning disability, spastic diplegia or quadriplegia and strabismus. The severity of these features is variable. The neurologic cretin simulates cerebral palsy. However, the spasticity in neurologic cretins is more proximal with hyperreflexia of biceps, knee and adductors, whereas ankle and wrist are relatively less affected. Neurogenic cretins are generally able to walk better than spastic cerebral palsy. About half the cretins have a complete sensory neural deafness (Figure 10.2). Memory

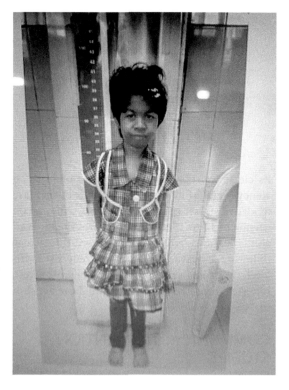

Figure 10.2 A 7-year-old girl having neurologic cretinism. She has mental retardation, deafness, speech abnormality and hyperreflexia. (Courtesy Prof D Sharma, Endocrinology Department, Guwahati Medical College.)

is relatively less affected and abstract thinking is more impaired. Bladder and bowel functions are spared. Thyroid function tests are normal.

(B) **Myxedematous cretin:** Myxedematous cretin manifests with florid features of hypothyroidism. Cognitive impairment is less severe. There is prominent growth retardation and impaired mentation. Myxedematous cretin has hypoplastic mandible, poor naso-orbital configuration, dry thick skin, dry hair, eyebrows and eye lashes and atrophic thyroid. Serum T3 and T4 levels are low, and TSH level is markedly elevated.

The prevalence of neurologic cretin in New Guinea, Thailand, China and Indonesia has been attributed to isolated iodine deficiency. Myxoedematous cretin in democratic Republic of Congo has been attributed to iodine deficiency in addition to selenium deficiency and high thiocyanate as a result of cassava-based diet. Iodine deficiency state results in over-stimulation of thyroid gland producing H_2O_2 and reactive oxygen species, which need an antioxidant (glutathione) for

Table 10.5 Neurological features of endemic cretin reported from China, Ecuador and Zaire

Clinical features	China (N = 247)	Ecuador (N = 67)	Zaire (N = 106)
Mental retardation	100%	87%	80%
Hearing impairment	87%	84% (deaf 48%)	38% (deaf 28%)
Speech abnormality	95%	95% (mute 73%)	48% (mute 28%)
Pyramidal/extrapyramidal	34% cerebral palsy	85% hyperreflexia	20% rigid
Inability to walk	20%	5%	4%

its clearance. Low selenium level results in deficiency of glutathione peroxidase there by increases oxidative stress. Low selenium also reduces conversion of T4 to T3 thereby increases the bioavailability of T4 to fetal brain. Increased thiocyanate following cassava consumption reduces iodine level. Neurological features of endemic cretin reported from China, Ecuador and Zaire are summarized in Table 10.5.

COMMUNITY INTERVENTION STUDIES

A number of iodine intervention studies have been conducted in severely and mildly affected areas in Africa, China, South America as well as other parts of the world. A double-blind placebo-controlled trial was conducted in Papua New Guinea in 1966. Iodized oil was injected intramuscularly to prevent cretinism and was compared with saline injection. Infants born between 1965 and 1972 were followed up for 10–15 years till 1982. In iodine-treated group at 4 years follow up, the risk reduction of cretinism was 0.27 and at 10 years 0.17. At 15 years follow up, the cumulative survival rate was better in iodine group. Motor and intellectual functions of the children born to the mother given iodine injection performed significantly better. This study highlights the importance of iodine in preventing cretinism as well as in improving cognitive and motor functions (Pharoah and Connolly, 1987). In a study from Zaire having a severe cretinism rate of 0.4%, 28 weeks pregnant women were allocated to iodized oil injection or placebo (vitamin). The offsprings were followed up at 72 months of age revealed much higher psychomotor developmental score compared to placebo (91 ± 13 vs 82 ± 14). (Zimmermann, 2009).

A study in severe iodine deficient region of China revaluated effect of iodine injection at different time points in pregnancy. The prevalence of moderate to severe neurological abnormalities in infants was 2% born out of mothers who received iodine in first and second trimester and 9% in third trimester; the latter was similar to those in no supplementation group. The mean development quotient was also improved in the treated group compared to children of untreated mother (90 ± 14 vs 75 ± 10). The newborn who received iodine for initial 3 years also had lower frequency of microcephaly compared untreated group (11% vs 27%) (Cao et al., 1994). A study in two villages of Ecuador with severe iodine deficiency was evaluated following iodine injection covering 90% of pregnant women, women in child-bearing age and children, and no intervention in the other village. Four yearly follow up was done for 20 years. No cretin was born in the treated village, and the children had 10 IQ points higher in the first and second grade school (Fierro-Benitez et al., 1988; Greene, 1994).

Intervention studies in mild to moderate iodine deficiency areas in Italy, Denmark and Belgium were conducted. Supplementation of iodized salt to the pregnant ladies in first, second and third trimester did not have any effect on maternal and childhood TSH, T3 and T4 levels (Berghout and Wiersinga, 1998; Zimmermann and Delange, 2004). The intervention studies revealed that iodine supplementation is beneficial in severe iodine deficiency areas, preconceptual supplementation is the best followed by first and second trimester supplementation. Supplementation in the third trimester is not beneficial. Iodine supplementation seems to have substantial effect in reducing the incidence of cretinism and microcephaly. The long-term effect on cognition and cognitive functions is not clear.

Infant mortality: Infant mortality is reduced by iodine supplementation in iodine deficient mothers. Maternal T4 level during pregnancy has an inverse relationship with death of offspring. In China, infant mortality and neonatal mortality rates were reduced following potassium iodide water irrigation for 2–4 weeks in three regions with severe iodine deficiency. The neonatal death reduced by 65% in the treated region (DeLong et al., 1997). In another study, iodized oil given to pregnant mothers at 28 weeks of gestation resulted in reduction of infant mortality rate (Thilly et al., 1994).

In Africa, the effect of iodized salt 1–3 months before conception was evaluated. There was reduced abortion, still births and prematurity in the treated group. The effect of iodine has also been evaluated in infants and school children. Infants were given 100 mg of iodized oil with oral polio vaccine at 6 months of age resulted in 72% reduction in death by 6 months of age (Chaouki and Benmiloud, 1994). In Indonesia, a cross-sectional study has shown the reduction in infant mortality rate and death by 5 years of age following iodized salt supplementation. Iodized salt supplementation in iodine deficient areas may reduce infant mortality rate by 50% (Cobra et al., 1997). Two meta-analysis have revealed the cognitive effects of iodine supplementation. In the group without iodine deficiency, the children had 13.5 IQ points higher than iodine deficient children (Bleichrodt and Born, 1994). In another meta-analysis including the Chinese studies revealed 12.5 IQ points improvement in children born after 3.5 years of iodine supplementation highlighting the importance of maternal iodine supplementation before conception (Qian et al., 2005).

Growth and development: Improvement in somatic growth has been reported in the children with normal iodine status as well as after iodine supplementation. The effect of iodine on somatic growth may be due to the effect of thyroid hormone on growth hormone secretion and modulation of growth hormone receptors. Insulin growth factor 1 (IGF 1) and insulin growth factor binding protein III are also dependent on thyroxin (Burstein et al., 1979; Näntö-Salonen et al., 1993). The role of growth hormone receptors is not well established (Zimmermann et al., 2007). Subclinical hypothyroidism due to iodine deficiency may be associated with thyroid atrophy, reduced scholastic performance, psychomotor retardation and poor learning.

MEASUREMENT OF IODINE STATUS

There are four methods to assess iodine status in the individual and in the community:

1. Urinary iodine
2. Goiter rate
3. Serum TSH
4. Serum thyroglobulin

These tests are complimentary. Urine iodine concentration is a sensitive indicator of iodine intake in recent few days, whereas thyroglobulin (TG) indicates iodine intake over weeks and months. Goiter is an indicator of chronic iodine deficiency status.

Measurement of thyroid size: Thyroid size measurement can be done by clinical examination (inspection or palpation) and thyroid ultrasonography (USG). Goiter survey is done in school-age children. If thyroid gland is more than the size of terminal phalanx of thumb, it is regarded as goiter. WHO classification of goiter is based on clinical examination is as follows (WHO, 2007):

0 = Not visible or palpable.
1 = Palpable but not visible in normal neck position.
2 = Thyroid gland is clearly visible in normal neck position.

Palpation of thyroid has poor sensitivity and specificity. Thyroid ultrasonography has been used for measurement of thyroid size in field survey. There are certain limitations of thyroid ultrasonography such as need of normative data, it is operator dependent and has high (4%–26%) inter-rater variability (Zimmermann et al., 2001, 2008). Thyroid size may not return to normal even after iodine supplementation. Goiter rate is an indicator of the severity of iodine deficiency in the community. In India, the prevalence of goiter in Maharashtra is 11.9%, West Bengal 9%, and Kerala, Tamil Nadu, Karnataka, Andhra Pradesh and Orissa is 4%. About 91% of households in India have access to iodized salt. The coverage of iodized salt is better in urban than rural areas (83.2% vs 66.1%) (UNICEF, 2009).

The WHO guidelines for measuring severity of iodine deficiency based on goiter rate are presented in the Table 10.6.

Table 10.6 Goiter rate and severity of iodine deficiency in the community (WHO, 2007)

Goiter rate (%)	Iodine deficiency
<5	Iodine sufficient
5–19.9	Mild iodine deficiency
20–29.9	Moderate iodine deficiency
>30	Severe iodine deficiency

Urinary iodine concentration: Urinary iodine concentration is a more reliable indicator of iodine intake because more than 90% of dietary iodine is excreted in urine. Urinary iodine can be measured by (a) a spot urine test, (b) ratio of urinary iodine to creatinine (µg of urinary iodine/g of creatinine) and (c) 24 h of urinary iodine excretion. Spot urine test is done in field surveys, but iodine excretion is variable in a day; therefore, a 24 h urinary excretion is a better indicator of iodine status. Ratio of iodine to creatinine may not be reliable as creatinine value may be low in malnourished, moreover iodine in spot urine is also variable at different time of the day. Low urinary iodine concentration suggests high probability of thyroid disorder. Urinary iodine level may be used for daily requirement of iodine intake (Table 10.7).

Table 10.7 Urinary iodine concentration and iodine status

Urinary iodine (µg/l)	Iodine status of subject
Children < 2 years	
< 100	Insufficient
> 100	Sufficient
School-aged children	
< 20	Severe iodine deficiency
20–49	Moderate deficiency
50–99	Mild deficiency
100–199	Sufficient
200–299	High (iodine-induced hyperthyroidism)
Pregnancy	
< 150	Insufficient
150–249	Adequate
250–499	More than adequate
> 500	Excessive
Lactation	
< 100	Insufficient
> 100	Adequate

Source: Modified from Zimmermann, M. B., Jooste, P. L., Pandav, C. S. 2008. Iodine-deficiency disorders. *Lancet* (London, England) 372(9645):1251–1262. DOI:10.1016/S0140-6736(08)61005-3; and World Health Organization. 2007. *Assessment of iodine deficiency disorders and monitoring their elimination: a guide for programme managers.* 3rd ed. Geneva: World Health Organization. https://apps.who.int/iris/handle/10665/43781.

$$BMI = Body\ weight\ in\ kg\ /height\ in\ meter^2$$

Thyroglobulin: Thyroglobulin is synthesized in the thyroid gland and is the most abundant intra thyroid protein. Iodine deficiency increases production of thyroglobulin due to high TSH and thyroid mass. Thyroglobulin correlates with iodine deficiency state. Normal thyroglobulin level is less than 10 µg/l (Institute of Medicine, Academy of Sciences, 2001). Following iodine supplementation thyroglobulin falls more rapidly than TSH. Spot test for thyroglobulin is available and may be used in community surveys.

Thyroid hormone and TSH: Thyroid hormones are a poor indicator of iodine status because T3 may remain unchanged or may be higher in iodine deficient population. T4 level however is low in iodine deficiency. TSH is a sensitive indicator of iodine deficiency in newborn, but in older children, it may remain in normal range even with iodine deficiency.

TREATMENT AND PREVENTION

Iodine deficiency can be treated by administering iodine either as drop, iodine solution or tablet.

The preventive strategies for iodine deficiency are:

1. Fortification of salt
2. Fortification of other food items e.g. bread, milk, water, etc.
3. Direct administration of iodine.

Iodized salt: Universal salt iodization has been widely practiced. Salt iodization is attractive because virtually everyone takes salt daily in fairly constant amount, salt iodization is simple, inexpensive and does not interfere with taste and flavor of food. The recommended dose is 20–40 mg iodine/kg salt (WHO/UNICEF/ICCIDD, 2007). For iodization, either potassium iodide (KI) or potassium iodate (KO$_3$) is used, but iodate is preferred because of greater stability (Diosady et al., 1997). If the iodized salt is stored in a humid environment or in porous bags, about 90% of iodine is lost in 1 year. Iodized salt was taken up in the 10th five-year plan in India with the goal of reducing the prevalence of IDD by less than 10%.

Iodization of drinking or irrigation water is expensive, and its monitoring is difficult. Some Western countries use iodophors in dairy industry especially in Switzerland and USA. In Finland, animal fodder is fortified with iodine to increase the iodine content of milk and meat. In inaccessible areas, iodized salt may not be available. In such situations, iodized oil orally or as intramuscular injection has been used in yearly dosing. Iodized oil is produced by esterification of unsaturated fatty acid in vegetable or seed oil. Infants below 6 months are recommended 100 mg/year and between 7–24 months 200 mg/year. School age children, pregnant or lactating mothers require 200–400 mg iodized oil yearly. Universal iodized salt supplementation has been achieved in Switzerland, Iran and China.

CONCLUSIONS

Iodine deficiency is prevalent in South East Asia and sub-Saharan Africa and results in a wide variety of disorders including mental retardation, deaf mutism, cognitive impairment, growth retardation, cretinism, goiter, hypothyroidism and increased fetal and infant mortality. Iodine deficiency can be prevented by supplementing iodine to mother before or during pregnancy, neonates and young children.

REFERENCES

Aghini Lombardi, F. A., Pinchera, A., et al. 1995. Mild iodine deficiency during fetal/neonatal life and neuropsychological impairment in Tuscany. *Journal of Endocrinological Investigation* 18(1):57–62. DOI: 10.1007/BF03349700.

Berghout, A., Wiersinga, W. 1998. Thyroid size and thyroid function during pregnancy: An analysis. *European Journal of Endocrinology* 138(5): 536–542. DOI: 10.1530/eje.0.1380536.

Bleichrodt, N., Born, M.P. 1994. A metaanalysis of research on iodine and its relationship to cognitive development. In: Stanbury, J.B. (Ed.) *The damaged brain of iodine deficiency*. New York: Cognizant Communication Corporation, pp. 195–200.

Burstein, P. J., Draznin, B., Johnson, C. J., Schalch, D. S. 1979. The effect of hypothyroidism on growth, serum growth hormone, the growth hormone-dependent somatomedin, insulin-like growth factor, and its carrier protein in rats. *Endocrinology* 104(4): 1107–1111. DOI: 10.1210/endo-104-4-1107.

Cao, X.Y., Jiang, X.M., Dou, Z.H., et al. 1994. Timing of vulnerability of the brain to iodine deficiency in endemic cretinism. *The New England Journal of Medicine* 331:1739–1744.

Chaouki, M.L., Benmiloud, M. 1994. Prevention of iodine deficiency disorders by oral administration of lipiodol during pregnancy. *European Journal of Endocrinology* 130:547–551.

Chavasit, V., Malaivongse, P., Judprasong, K. 2002. Study on stability of iodine in iodated salt by use of different cooking model conditions. *Journal of Food Composition and Analysis* 15(3):265–276.

Cobra, C., Muhilal, R.K., Rustama, D., et al. 1997. Infant survival is improved by oral iodine supplementation. *Journal of Nutrition* 127:574–578.

de Benoist, B., McLean, E., Andersson, M., Rogers, L. 2008. Iodine deficiency in 2007: global progress since 2003. *Food and Nutrition Bulletin* 29(3):195–202. DOI: 10.1177/156482650802900305.

Delange, F. 2000. Endemic cretinism. In: Braverman, L.E., Utiger, R.D. (Ed.) *The thyroid. A fundamental and clinical text*. Philadelphia, PA: Lippincott Publ, pp. 743–754.

DeLong, G. R., Leslie, P. W., Wang, S. H., et al. 1997. Effect on infant mortality of iodination of irrigation water in a severely iodine-deficient area of China. *Lancet* (London, England) 350(9080):771–773. DOI: 10.1016/s0140-6736(96)12365-5.

Diosady, L.L., Alberti, J.O., Venkatesh, M. MG, Stone, T.G. 1997. Stability of iodine in iodized salt used for correction of iodine-deficiency disorders. *Food and Nutrition Bulletin* 18:388–396.

Fierro-Benitez, R., Cazar, R., Stanbury, J. B., et al. 1988. Effects on school children of prophylaxis of mothers with iodized oil in an area of iodine deficiency. *Journal of Endocrinological Investigation* 11(5):327–335. DOI: 10.1007/BF03349050.

Fisher, D. A., Oddie, T. H. 1964. Comparison of thyroidal iodide accumulation and thyroxine secretion in euthyroid subjects. *The Journal of Clinical Endocrinology and Metabolism* 24:1143–1154. DOI: 10.1210/jcem-24-11-1143.

Greene, L.S. 1994. A retrospective view of iodine deficiency, brain development, and behavior from studies in Ecuador. In: Stanbury, J.B., (Ed.) *The damaged brain of iodine deficiency: cognitive, behavioral, neuromotor and educative aspects*. New York: Cognizant Communication Corporation, pp. 173–185.

Institute of Medicine (US) Panel on Micronutrients. 2001. *Dietary reference intakes for vitamin A, vitamin K, arsenic, boron, chromium, copper, iodine, iron, manganese, molybdenum, nickel, silicon, vanadium, and zinc*. Washington, DC: National Academies Press.

McCarrisson, R. 1908. Observations on endemic cretinism in the Chitral and Gilgit valleys. *Lancet ii*:1275–1280.

Näntö-Salonen, K., Muller, H. L., Hoffman, A. R., Vu, T. H., Rosenfeld, R. G. 1993. Mechanisms of thyroid hormone action on the insulin-like growth factor system: All thyroid hormone effects are not growth hormone mediated. *Endocrinology 132*(2): 781–788. DOI: 10.1210/endo.132.2.7678799.

Norris, E.H. 1916. The morphogenesis of the follicles in the human thyroid gland. *American Journal of Anatomy 20*: 411–448. DOI: 10.1002/aja.1000200306.

Obregón, M.J., Santisteban, P., Rodríguez-Peña, A., et al. 1984. Cerebral hypothyroidism in rats with adult-onset iodine deficiency. *Endocrinology 115*(2):614–624.

Osorio, C., Myant, N. B. 1960. The passage of thyroid hormone from mother to foetus and its relation to foetal development. *British Medical Bulletin 16*:159–164. DOI: 10.1093/oxfordjournals.bmb.a069817.

Pharoah, P.O.D., Connolly, K.J. 1987. A controlled trial of iodinated oil for the prevention of endemic cretinism: A long-term follow-up. *International Journal of Epidemiology 16*:68–73.

Qian, M., Wang, D., Watkins, W.E., et al. 2005. The effects of iodine on intelligence in children: A meta-analysis of studies conducted in China. *Asia Pacific Journal of Clinical Nutrition 2005*(14):32–42.

Shepard, T.H. 1967. Onset of function in the human fetal thyroid: Biochemical and radioautographic studies from organ culture. *The Journal of Clinical Endocrinology and Metabolism 27*(7):945–958. DOI: 10.1210/jcem-27-7-945.

Stepien, B. K., Huttner, W. B. 2019. Transport, metabolism, and function of thyroid hormones in the developing mammalian brain. *Frontiers in Endocrinology 10*:209. DOI: 10.3389/fendo.2019.00209.

Thilly, C., Swennen, B., Moreno-Reyes, R., et al. 1994. Maternal, fetal and juvenile hypothyroidism, birthweight and infant mortality in the etiopathogenesis of the IDD spectrum in Zaire and Malawi. In: Stanbury, J.B. *The damaged brain of iodine deficiency.* New York: Cognizant Communication Corporation, pp. 241–250.

UNICEF. Coverage Evaluation Survey. 2009. All India Report. Ministry of Health and Family Welfare, Government of India, New Delhi; 2010. Available from: http://www.unicef.org/india/health.html.

World Health Organization, United Nations Children's Fund, International Council for the Control of Iodine Deficiency Disorders. 2007. *Assessment of iodine deficiency disorders and monitoring their elimination.* 3rd ed. Geneva: WHO.

World Health Organization. 2001. *Assessment of iodine deficiency disorders and monitoring their elimination: a guide for programme managers.* 2nd ed. Geneva: World Health Organization. https://apps.who.int/iris/handle/10665/61278.

World Health Organization. 2007. *Assessment of iodine deficiency disorders and monitoring their elimination: a guide for programme managers.* 3rd ed. Geneva: World Health Organization. https://apps.who.int/iris/handle/10665/43781.

Zimmermann, M. B. 2009. Iodine deficiency. *Endocrine Reviews 30*(4): 376–408. DOI: 10.1210/er.2009-0011.

Zimmermann, M. B., Jooste, P. L., Pandav, C. S. 2008. Iodine-deficiency disorders. *Lancet (London, England) 372*(9645):1251–1262. DOI: 10.1016/S0140-6736(08)61005-3.

Zimmermann, M. B., Jooste, P. L., Mabapa, N. S., et al. 2007. Treatment of iodine deficiency in school-age children increases insulin-like growth factor (IGF)-I and IGF binding protein-3 concentrations and improves somatic growth. *The Journal of Clinical Endocrinology and Metabolism 92*(2):437–442. DOI: 10.1210/jc.2006-1901.

Zimmermann, M. B., Molinari, L., Spehl, M., et al. 2001. Toward a consensus on reference values for thyroid volume in iodine-replete schoolchildren: Results of a workshop on inter-observer and inter-equipment variation in sonographic measurement of thyroid volume. *European Journal of Endocrinology 144*(3):213–220. DOI: 10.1530/eje.0.1440213.

Zimmermann, M., Delange, F. 2004. Iodine supplementation of pregnant women in Europe: A review and recommendations. *European Journal of Clinical Nutrition 58*(7):979–984. DOI: 10.1038/sj.ejcn.1601933.

11

Neurological consequences of copper and zinc deficiency

INTRODUCTION

Copper and zinc are the two essential trace elements needed for a number of biological and enzymatic reactions. Copper store in an adult human is 100 mg and zinc store in a meager amount; hence, zinc has to be regularly consumed. Copper and zinc homeostasis is delicately maintained for a smooth body function. Copper deficiency and excess are usually uncommon because of a tight balance except in genetic copper transportation defects such as copper toxicity in Wilson disease due to ATP7B mutation and copper deficiency in Menkes disease due to ATP7A mutation. Dietary deficiency of zinc is common and manifests with skin, gonadal, gastrointestinal and neurological manifestation. A number of transporter defects can also result in zinc deficiency.

COPPER

History

Copper is one of the few metals available in nature, which can be directly used in a metallic form. Copper is in human use as far as 8000 BC. Copper was the first metal to be smelted from sulfide ores in 5000 BC. Copper was the first metal to be cast in mold in 4000 BC, and was the first metal to be used as alloy. Copper was mixed with tin to produce bronze in 3500 BC, which is even now used for carving sculptures. Copper was initially mined in Cyprus, a Mediterranean island, and was known as Cyprium (metal of Cyprus).

The Latin name *cuprum* became popular in old English and was called copper in 1530. Copper is used as bacteriostatic, fungicide, wood preservative and coloring agent.

Copper is an essential trace element for all living organisms and plants, and is utilized by aerobic organism for cellular respiration through mitochondrial respiratory chain cytochrome C oxidase. Copper is a redox metal and participates in various enzymatic reactions in cytosol as superoxide dismutase (SOD), in mitochondria as cytochrome C oxidase and in secretory compartment as tyrosinase and dopamine β-hydroxylase (Zucconi et al., 2007; Rinaldi, 2000; Kaler, 1998). Both low and high copper levels are hazardous for biological system; therefore, copper homeostasis is regulated at systemic, cellular and subcellular levels. Genetic dysregulation of copper metabolism results in Wilson disease, Menkes disease and aceruloplasminemia (ACP).

Absorption

Dietary copper is in cupric (Cu^{++}) form, which is converted to cuprous (Cu^{+}) form in the intestinal apical epithelium. The reduction of cupric form is mediated by ferroreductase, DCYTB and STEAP2 metalloreductase (El Meskini et al., 2003; Hardman et al., 2007). Copper is taken up by Ctr 1 in the intestinal apical membrane depending on the cellular copper concentration. Once the copper enters the intestinal cell, copper chaperon ATOX1, an antioxidant, transfers copper to copper transporter ATPase. ATP7A is located in trans-Golgi

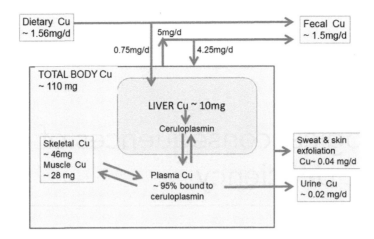

Figure 11.1 Schematic diagram showing maintenances of copper pool in the body.

network (TGN) and exports copper to the portal vein. ATP7A mutations result in Menkes disease. ATP7A also fuses with the basolateral membrane to export copper into the circulation. ATOX1 also transfers copper to ATP7B, which helps in binding copper to ceruloplasmin (CP) and transporting Cu to the systemic circulation. About 95% of serum copper binds to CP. The mutation of ATP7B gene results in Wilson disease. Excess copper in intestinal epithelial cells binds to metallothionein and glutathione to prevent copper-induced oxidative stress (Figure 11.1).

Dietary sources of copper

There was no reference value of dietary copper intake till UK reference values published in 1991. Subsequently, other countries also published their dietary reference values (Bost et al., 2016) (Table 11.1). Copper content in the diet is highly variable because it is determined by a number of local conditions such as soil concentration, manure, slurry, pesticide used on crops and emission from smelting and casting industry. Corrosion of plumbing pipes can also increase the copper level. The rich sources of copper are organ meat, nuts, cereals, fruits and vegetables. Milk and dairy products are not a rich source of copper. The copper intake in vegetarian diet is much higher than in the omnivorous diet. The bioavailability of vegetarian diet, however, is poor because of high phytate and fiber contents. The details of copper content in various dietary items are provided in Table 11.2.

Table 11.1 Recommended dietary copper value (mg/day) in different age groups

Age	Reference range of dietary copper intake
0–6 months	0.2–0.4
7–12 months	0.2–0.6
1–3 years	0.3–0.75
4–6 years	0.4–1.0
7–10 years	0.5–1.3
11–20 years	0.7–1.5
21–50 years	0.9–2.0
>50 years	0.9–1.7
Pregnancy	1.0–2.0
Lactation	1.3–2.0

The reference values are for USA, France, Australia, Nordic countries and UK (Boost et al., 2016).

Copper deficiency

Copper deficiency may be due to a number of genetic or acquired causes. The genetic causes are Menkes disease – which is due to ATP7A mutation – and ACP – due to the absence of CP synthesis. The acquired cause of copper deficiency may be due to nutritional deficiency and is seen in malnourished, low-body-weight newborns and infants. Copper deficiency is seen in gastrointestinal resection surgery, intractable diarrhea and prolonged enteral or parenteral nutrition without copper supplementation. Bariatric surgery is an important cause. Prolonged zinc therapy in Wilson disease may also result in copper deficiency. The causes of copper deficiency and excess are summarized in Table 11.3.

Table 11.2 Copper content in various food items

Vegetarian food	Copper (mg/kg)	Nonvegetarian	Copper (mg/kg)	Dairy product	Copper (mg/kg)
Cereals		Beef liver	157.0	Milk	0.1–0.88
Maize	0.6–16.6	Kidney	2.1–4.3	Fresh cheese	0.03
Wheat bread	2.9	Muscle	0.1–1.8	Processed cheese	0.025
Whole grain bread	3.4	Pork meat	0.1–9.1		
Vegetables		**Fish**			
Potato	0.48–16	Oyster	0.3–16		
Carrot	0.37–0.62	Tuna	0.1–1.2		
Broccoli	0.68–0.87	Salmon	0.5–0.8		
Peas	1.9–2.4	Shrimp	2–2.9		
Lettuce	0.1–2.9				
Tomato	0.1–3.4				
Cabbage	0.1–7.7				
Fruits					
Apple	0.1–2.3				
Banana	0.7–3.0				
Oranges	0.8–0.9				

Gastrointestinal secretion of copper plays an important role in the control of copper homeostasis with endogenous losses increasing from 0.45 to 2.46 µg/day when copper intake is increased from 0.7 to 6.6 µg/day.

Role of copper in cell injury

Copper is a redox metal and acts as a cofactor in many enzymatic actions that are essential for cell functioning (Table 11.4). Copper is carried by

Table 11.3 Causes of copper deficiency and excess

A. Causes of copper deficiency
  1. Genetic: Menkes disease, aceruloplasminemia
  2. Acquired:
     Malnutrition
     Malabsorption syndrome
     Inflammatory bowel disease: Cystic fibrosis, celiac disease, chronic diarrhea
     Gastrointestinal surgery: Gastrectomy, gastric bypass, small intestine resection, bariatric surgery
  3. Excessive use of copper-chelating agents
  4. Overuse of zinc, denture cream
  5. Total parenteral nutrition, jejunal feeding
  6. Diet low in copper

B. Causes of excess copper
  1. Genetic: Wilson disease
  2. Acquired:
     Indian childhood cirrhosis
     Non-Indian childhood cirrhosis
     Parenteral bolus administration of copper

Table 11.4 The action of main copper-requiring enzymes

Enzyme	Action
Ceruloplasmin	Oxidase activity, $Fe^{++} \rightarrow Fe^{+++}$
Superoxide dismutase	Superoxide radical metabolism $O_2^- + O_2^- + 2H^+ \rightarrow O_2 + H_2O_2$
Cytochrome c oxidase	Mitochondrial respiratory chain terminal enzyme complex of cytochrome a and a3
Lysyl oxidase	Elastin cross-linkage, collagen formation
Ascorbate oxidase	Oxidation of vitamin C
Tyrosinase	Melanin synthesis
Monoamine oxidase	Oxidative deamination
Dopamine β-hydroxylase	Epinephrine synthesis

a protein, CP, which oxidizes cuprous to cupric form and is subsequently bound to transferrin. Transferrin is another important element for copper–iron interaction in hephaestin, which is a copper-dependent ferroxidase and helps in iron absorption from the enterocyte. Absence or low level of copper therefore results in microcytic hypochromic anemia. Copper is also involved in cell division and protein synthesis. Copper also has an important role in the functioning of neurotransmitter pathways in central nervous system, e.g., melatonin, norepinephrine, dopamine, etc. For cellular respiration, copper helps in an electron transport through cytochrome 3 oxidase in the mitochondria. Copper is a cofactor in oxidative phosphorylation and SOD to prevent oxidative stress, cross-linking of collagen and elastin through lysyl oxidase. Low copper results in cerebral and peripheral demyelination simulating subacute combined degeneration. Excess of copper results in cirrhosis, cardiac dysfunction, pancreatic dysfunction, basal ganglia and brainstem degeneration.

Clinical effects of copper deficiency

Copper deficiency results in a variety of clinical manifestations, which include anemia, myelopathy, neuropathy, hair and cardiac involvement.

Hematological manifestations: The typical hematological effect of copper deficiency is anemia, which is usually microcytic hypochromic, but may as well be normocytic or macrocytic depending on the underlying cause of copper deficiency. Thrombocytopenia and neutropenia are unusual. Microcytic anemia is due to a decrease in

ferroxidase activity of CP and reduced iron oxidation. Anemia in copper deficiency may as well be due to an impaired iron transport. Haphaestin is a copper-containing ferroxidase enzyme and is present in the duodenal mucosa, which oxidizes iron and facilitates the iron transfer through the basolateral membrane into the circulation. Haphaestin also helps to transfer iron from the reticuloendothelial cells to plasma.

Microcytic anemia in malnourished infants, and those with chronic diarrhea and prolonged enteral or parenteral nutrition, may not only be due to iron deficiency but also be due to coexisting copper deficiency. Bone marrow may show the maturation abnormality of granulocyte and cytoplasmic vacuolation in RBC and WBC precursors. There may be features of myelodysplastic syndrome. Sideroblasts (rim granules around the nucleus of erythroblasts) are also present. Sideroblastic anemia may be due to abnormal cytochrome c oxidase, which fails to produce heme from ferric iron leading to the accumulation of iron.

Neurological manifestations: The neurological manifestations of copper deficiency involve spinal cord, peripheral nerve, dorsal root ganglia and optic nerve. The spinal cord involvement is similar to subacute combined degeneration in vitamin B12 deficiency. There is demyelination of posterior column and pyramidal tract. Peripheral nerve involvement manifests with distal symmetrical neuropathy. These patients manifest with ataxic paraparesis or quadriparesis with absent ankle reflex and prominent sensory ataxia. The spinal MRI reveals T2 hyperintensity of the posterior columns in cervical and dorsal regions (Figure 11.2). Involvement in copper deficiency has

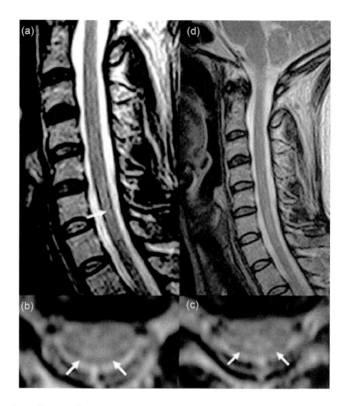

Figure 11.2 Cervicodorsal MRI of a patient with copper deficiency myelopathy. **(a)** Sagittal section on T2 sequence shows hyperintense signal changes in the cervical spinal cord. **(b) (c)** Axial section in the cervical spinal cord shows the involvement of dorsal cord (arrow). **(d)** The signal changes regressed after copper supplementation. (With permission from Zara G., Grassivaro F., Brocadello F., Manara R., Pesenti F. F. 2009. Case of sensory ataxic ganglionopathy-myelopathy in copper deficiency. *Journal of the Neurological Sciences*. 277(1–2):184–186. DOI:10.1016/j.jns.2008.10.017.)

two mechanisms: (a) impaired cytochrome c function leading to an impairment of electron transport resulting in spinal cord demyelination and (b) impairment in methylation cycle, i.e., methyl tetrahydrofolate transfers a methyl group to a wide range of macromolecule. This reaction occurs with the help of methionine synthase and copper, and produces myelin and purine, a component of DNA nucleotide bases. Impairment of this methylation process may result in myelin dysfunction. In seven patients with copper deficiency neurological syndrome, three were due to prolonged total parenteral nutrition, malabsorption syndrome, secondary to mastectomy, esophagectomy with jejunostomy, and bariatric surgery, and four were due to zinc-enriched dental cream. These patients presented with ascending paresthesia and gait ataxia was due to a posterior column impairment. They also had superficial hyoesthesia in feet, and all the patients had pyramidal signs. Nerve conduction was abnormal in four patients. Spinal MRI was abnormal in 4; T2 hyperintensity was present in the cervical region. Brain MRI revealed changes in three patients. Serum copper was low (1+1.2 μg/l) and urinary copper was normal in six patients. Serum and urinary zinc level was high in four patients. Six patients had normocytic normochromic anemia. The patients were treated with copper histidine 3.2+0.4 mg/day subcutaneously, and another received 6 mg monthly for 5 months. All the patients received oral supplementation. Six out of seven improved after 2 years. After 10 months, spinal MRI normalized though brain MRI was unchanged. Neurological improvement may occur in 2 months and MRI in 10 months (Poujois et al., 2018). In a Scottish study, 16 patients were detected in 5 years with copper deficiency, and 12 of whom had neurological manifestations. Sensory ataxia was the earliest symptom, and small-fiber neuropathy was common (Gabreyes et al., 2013).

Bone changes: The bone changes in copper deficiency are similar to rickets and scurvy, because of an impaired function of many copper-containing enzymes such as ascorbate oxidase and lysyl oxidase. There is an enlargement of epiphyseal bone with changes in the margins. Sometimes the bone may have osteoporotic changes.

Hair changes: The hair changes are rare in acquired copper deficiency, but in Menkes disease, the hairs are curled, rough and kinky (Figure 11.3). The concentration of copper is low in hair and nails.

Vascular complications: Blood vessel, especially in Menkes disease, may be tortuous with an enlarged lumen with increased capillary fragility.

Miscellaneous findings: There may be hypothermia, hypotonia, hepatosplenomegaly or achromatodermia. In Menkes disease, there may be convulsions and hypotonia along with cerebral and cerebellar degeneration (Figures 11.3 and 11.4). The CNS involvement in copper deficiency is attributed to an impaired functioning of dopamine β-hydroxylase and cytochrome c oxidase.

Diagnosis of copper deficiency state

Copper deficiency is rare, but in an appropriate clinical setting, it should be suspected. The diagnosis of copper deficiency is confirmed by serum copper and serum CP. Based on serum copper level, it is categorized as follows:

Mild deficiency: 60–80 μg/dl
Moderate deficiency: 40–59 μg/dl
Severe deficiency: <40 μg/dl

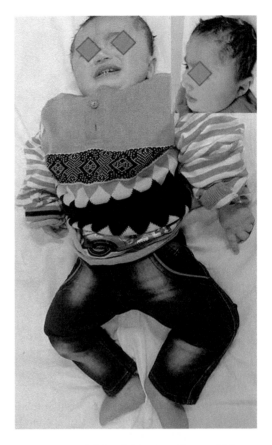

Figure 11.3 A child with Menkes disease. This 18-month very fair male baby was severely hypotonic (abducted hip) and had darks rough curly hair.

In copper deficiency, serum CP is low, and based on CP levels, the copper deficiency is categorized as follows:

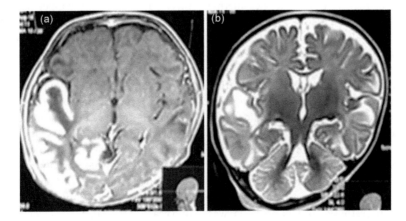

Figure 11.4 Cranial MRI of the same child with Menkes disease. (a) Axial section, T1 sequence shows hyperintense signal changes along the temporoparietal guri. (b) In T2 sequence, these lesions are isointense with hyperintensity just below the cortical mentle.

- Mild copper deficiency: serum CP level 10–20 mg/dl
- Moderate copper deficiency: serum CP levels 5–9 mg/dl
- Severe copper deficiency: serum CP levels <5 mg/dl
- Serum CP may be falsely low in the newborn and those with low birth weight.
- Copper level in hair and nails is also helpful in supporting the diagnosis.

Treatment

In acquired copper deficiency, oral copper is preferred in both low-birth-weight, newborn infants and children. If the child is not improving in 3 weeks, intravenous copper may be tried. The proposed doses of copper for the patients with copper deficiency are mentioned in Table 11.5.

Menkes disease: Menkes disease is an X-linked recessive disorder, and the defect lies on chromosome Xq13.7 with mutation of ATP7A gene. It is a rare disease affecting the boys, and its incidence is 1/100,000 to 1/200,000. Menkes disease manifests with neurological, collagen, hair and rarely hematological involvement. The newborns manifest with hypothermia, hypotonia and poor sucking. During infancy, the child may have seizures. Mild Menkes disease may manifest during 6–24 months with occipital horn syndrome and Ehler–Danlos syndrome IX. Extremely mild form of Menkes disease may manifest even during adolescence. The patients have extremely fair skin (achromodermia). and dark curly, rough and kinky hair (Figures 11.3 and 11.4). Microcytic hypochromic anemia is rare unlike acquired copper deficiency.

In Menkes disease, there may be diverticulae in urinary bladder. ATP7A gene is dominantly expressed in duodenum, upper part of small intestine and renal tubules. Copper deficiency in Menkes disease may be due to a reduced absorption from the intestine and kidney. Serum copper and CP levels are low. Cranial MRI may show cerebral and cerebellar atrophy, white matter T2 hyperintensity and tortuous intracerebral vessels on angiography. There may be subdural hygroma due to cerebral atrophy (Rangarh and Kohli, 2018). The diagnosis of Menkes disease is confirmed by ATP7A mutation study. There is no definite cure for Menkes disease. Intravenous or subcutaneous injection of copper is recommended but is not effective in advanced disease with neurological manifestations. Copper treatment is helpful in preventing infection and improving bone, skin and hair changes. Most children die by the age of 4 years.

Occipital horn syndrome: Occipital horn syndrome manifests with cutis laxa, hypermobile joints and bony prominence of occipital bone due to an impaired lysal activity leading to the disruption of collagen and elastin cross-linking. Due to the reduced dopamine β-hydroxylase activity, there is a reduced production of norepinephrine manifesting with post-ganglionic sympathetic dysfunction. Dysautonomia in occipital horn syndrome is characterized by bradycardia, postural hypotension and diarrhea. There is a reduced level of CSF catecholamine in both Menkes disease and occipital horn syndrome.

Aceruloplasminemia: ACP is an autosomal recessive disorder of iron metabolism due to a mutation in CP gene. ACP gene is located on chromosome 3q 24–25 spreading over 20 exons having 65 kb of DNA (Yoshida et al., 1995). CP can bind up to 6 atoms of copper, and it helps in the stability of copper in blood. There are two isoforms of CP: (a) soluble form is present in plasma and synthesized by hepatocyte, and (b) glycosyl phosphotidyl inositol-anchored membrane form is produced and expressed by various cells, including astrocytes, hepatocyte, pancreatic, retinal, epithelial cells and macrophages (Kono et al., 2010). CP is a ferroxidase and plays an important role in iron export from various cells mainly from astrocyte, neurons, hepatocyte, pancreatic and retinal cells. Because of an impaired iron transportation, erythropoiesis is also affected. These mechanisms result in iron deposition in the liver, pancreas and retina.

Clinical features: The clinical picture of ACP may be due to the iron deposition in the brain and

Table 11.5 Dose of copper in copper-deficient patients suggested by Akoi (2004)

Age groups	Oral dose	Parenteral (µg/kg/day)
Low-birth-weight neonate and infant	100–200 µg/kg/day	20–30
Infant and children	2.5–5.0 mg/day	20–35
Adolescent and adult	5–10 mg/day	15–20 (total 900–1500 µg/day)

other organs. ACP manifests during 40–60 years of age. About 65%–68% of patients with ACP manifest with neurological symptoms, including neuropsychiatric symptoms in 48%, cognitive impairment in 60%–80%, cerebellar signs in 62%–71% and extrapyramidal signs in 20%–64% of patients. Cerebellar signs include tremor, ataxia and dysarthria. Movement disorders include chorea, athetosis, dystonia, speech abnormality and walking difficulty. The movement disorders are due to the involvement of thalamus, basal ganglia and cerebellum. Cranial MRI reveals T2 hyperintensity of thalamus, basal ganglia, dentate nuclei of cerebellum and subcortical white matter. The clinical and radiological features of ACP resemble Wilson disease or neuronal brain iron accumulation (NBIA); however, the absence of Kayser–Fleischer ring and the presence of microcytic anemia help in differentiating ACP from Wilson disease. Iron deposition occurs in the liver but cirrhosis and liver failure are uncommon in ACP. Similarly, peripheral retinal degeneration occurs in 14%–76% but vision loss is uncommon (Figure 11.5) (He et al., 2007; Marchi et al., 2019).

The majority of patients with ACP are due to homozygous mutation but compound heterozygosity with milder symptoms has also been reported (Pelucchi et al., 2018; McNeill et al., 2008). The genotype and phenotype correlation has been reported. Some ACP phenotypes (Cys338Ser and IIe991Thr) are associated with the reduced ferroxidase activity with no or mild neurological impairment (Pelucchi et al., 2018). Homozygosity for Gly631Arg is associated with extra pyramidal features in Caucasians (Vroegindeweij et al., 2017).

Diagnosis: The diagnosis is suspected if there is a raised serum ferritin, microcytic anemia, reduced level of serum copper and absence of serum CP. The diagnosis is confirmed by genetic studies.

Treatment: Iron overload is treated by iron-chelating agents. Deferiprone crosses the blood–brain barrier and might be preferred in ACP. All iron-chelating drugs reduce serum ferritin and iron accumulation in the liver, but not in the brain. Clinical improvement, however, has been reported in some patients following chelating therapy but is not optimal (Dusek et al., 2016). Bloodletting for managing iron overload is not practiced because of associated anemia. Antioxidants such as vitamin E and zinc sulfate have been used for reducing iron-induced oxidative injury. Zinc sulfate resulted in the improvement of extrapyramidal features in anecdotal reports (Kuhn et al., 2007).

Copper toxicity

Acquired copper toxicity is rare because of a tight control of copper homeostasis. Up to 0.5 mg/kg/day of copper intake is considered safe. Copper in a

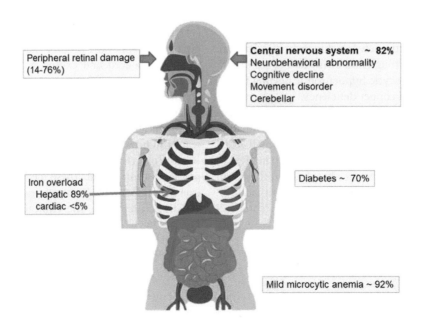

Figure 11.5 Schematic diagram shows clinical manifestations of aceruloplasminemia.

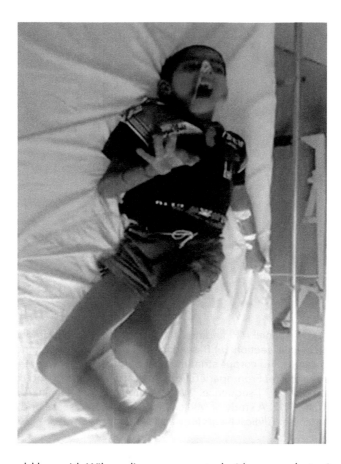

Figure 11.6 A 12-year-old boy with Wilson disease presented with severe dystonia.

dose of 10–15 mg/kg/day is associated with metallic taste, diarrhea and vomiting. Copper toxicity generally occurs in genetic disease like Wilson disease, an autosomal recessive disorder due to mutation of ATP7B in chromosome 13q 14.3 spanning over 21 exons. ATB7B is expressed in the liver, kidney, brain, heart, cornea etc. and is important for the incorporation of copper in CP. The patient with Wilson disease manifests with hepatic dysfunction in the first decade and neurological symptoms in the second decade. The neurological symptoms and signs include cognitive impairment, behavioral abnormality, movement disorders and spasticity (Figure 11.6). Cranial MRI reveals the involvement of corpus striatum, thalamus, and midbrain more frequently than the subcortical or cortical involvement (Figure 11.7; Ranjan et al., 2015). Seizure occurs in the late stage of the disease (Kalita et al., 2019). Wilson disease is treated with penicillamine, trientine, sodium thiomolybdate and zinc. Patients should also receive pyridoxine

and other symptomatic treatment for movement disorder and osteomalacia.

ZINC

Zinc is the 24th most abundant metal in the earth crust, and is abundantly found in Australia, Asia and USA. Zinc was used as an alloy with copper to make brass which was initially used in 3rd millennium BC. Pure metallic zinc was discovered by a German chemist Andreas Sigismund Marggraf in 1746. In 1800, Luigi Galvani and Volta described the electrical properties of zinc. Zinc is used as an alloy in brass, corrosive-resistant zinc plating for iron, battery, small nonstructural casting, dietary supplement, deodorant (ZnCl), anti-dandruff (zinc pyrethrins) and luminescent paint (zinc sulfide). The role of zinc in the growth of *Aspergillus niger* was reported by Raulin in 1869. Todd et al., (1934) demonstrated the role of zinc in the growth and development of rats. About 100 years later, Prasad

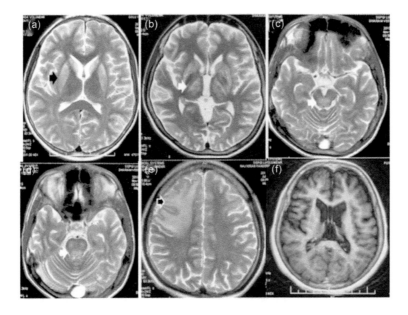

Figure 11.7 Representative cranial MRI findings in the patients with Wilson disease having neurological manifestation in axial section. (a) Basal ganglia T2 hyperintensity in putamen, caudate, globus pallidus. (b) Thalamus and corpus striatum T2 hyperintensity. (c) Midbrain T2 hyperintensity. (d) Pontine T2 hyperintensity. (e) Frontoparietal subcortical white matter and cortical T2 hyperintensity. (f) Cortical atrophy in T1 sequence. (With permission from Ranjan, A., Kalita, J., Kumar, S., Bhoi, S. K., Misra, U. K. 2015. A study of MRI changes in Wilson disease and its correlation with clinical features and outcome. *Clinical Neurology and Neurosurgery* 138, 31–36. DOI: 10.1016/j.clineuro.2015.07.013.)

and colleagues reported children with zinc deficiency from Persia who consumed clay (pica). The children manifested with anemia, hepatosplenomegaly, skin changes, physical and mental retardation. Later, zinc-specific malabsorption syndrome or autosomal recessive genetic disorder was reported by Neldner and Hambidge in 1975.

Zinc is needed for antenatal and postnatal development. About 2 billion people in the developing world are affected by zinc deficiency. About 1,40,000 patients are registered annually, 30% of whom are due to dietary Zn deficiency. Zinc is needed for about 1000 enzymatic reactions, and its deficiency results in growth retardation, diarrhea and susceptibility to infections.

Daily requirement and dietary sources of zinc

Human body contains about 2–4 g of zinc but plasma zinc concentration is only 12–16 μM, of which 60% is bound to albumin, 30% to α2 macroglobulin and 10% to transferrin (Rink and Gabriel, 2000). There is no storage of zinc in the body; therefore, daily intake of zinc is needed for maintaining a steady state. The requirement of zinc is age dependent: in an adult male 15 mg, females 12 mg and children 5–12 mg daily (Table 11.6).

The bioavailability of zinc is dependent on the composition of diet. The presence of phytate, phosphate and fibers reduces the bioavailability of

Table 11.6 Daily requirement of zinc in different age groups

Age groups	Zinc requirement (mg/day)
9–12 months	5
1–≤ 4 years	7
4–≤7 years	10
7–≤10 years	11
10–≤13 years	12
Adult and adolescent males	15
Adult and adolescent females	12
Pregnancy	15
Lactation	22

zinc. Other bivalent cations such as copper, iron, magnesium, cadmium and nickel also reduce the absorption of zinc. Iron supplementation during pregnancy may reduce zinc in both mother and fetus (Scholl et al., 1993). Zinc requirement increases during growth and pregnancy should be taken care of, because zinc has an important role in cell proliferation.

Dietary source of zinc

Zinc is widely available, and the rich sources are nonvegetarian food items such as meat, sea foods including oysters, shrimps, mussels and Alaskan crabs. Eggs have a moderate amount of zinc. A large egg contains 5% of daily requirement of zinc. Dairy products such as milk, curd and cheese also contain a moderate amount of zinc. The other sources of zinc are legume, chickpea, lentils and beans. Seeds of squash, pumpkins, sesame, nuts (pea nuts, cashew, almonds and pine) are medium sources of zinc. Poor sources of zinc are whole grain, wheat, rice, oats, quinoa and vegetables (potato, sweet potato, green pea and kale). The zinc content of different food items is mentioned in Table 11.7.

Absorption

About 16%–50% of dietary zinc is absorbed, and absorption depends on dietary composition and plasma zinc concentration. Zinc is mainly absorbed from the intestinal brush border in the duodenum and jejunum. Zinc absorption occurs by (a) a carrier-mediated mechanism and (b) saturable processes in a rate-limiting manner. If the luminal zinc is very high (200–1000 µM), zinc may be absorbed by a passive diffusion. Usually, zinc absorption depends on its dietary concentration. If there is low zinc concentration, the absorption is enhanced, and vice versa. Zinc absorption is better in aqueous solution compared to meals. Zinc is transported from the lumen to the enterocyte with the help of Zrt and Irt-like protein (ZIP). In the enterocyte, zinc remains in three forms: (a) bound to protein, (b) in the vesicle, or (c) in free form. Free zinc is available to tissues, for cell signaling and redistribution. In the cell, free zinc is maintained in a pico-molar concentration. Free zinc is regulated with the help of zinc-transporting protein.

Table 11.7 Zinc concentration in various dietary sources

Food items	Zinc (mg/100 g)
Nonvegetarian food	
Beef	2.5–6.0
Pork	1.3–3.8
Liver	4.0–6.0
Poultry (chicken, duck, turkey)	2.0–3.0
Egg	0.3–0.5
Fish	1.0–2.0
Oysters	20.0–150.0
Dairy products	
Milk	0.2–0.4
Cheese	1.0–5.0
Butter	0.1–0.15
Cereals	
Wheat flour	0.9
Whole meal flour	3.0
Beans and lentils	3.03–4.02
Rice	1.3
Sugar	0.1
Fruits	0.1–0.3
Seeds	2.48
Coconut	0.5
Vegetables	
Potato	0.2–0.3
Carrot	0.64
Radish	0.16
Cauliflower	0.23
Red cabbage	0.22
Sweet corn	0.12
Vegetable oil	0.12–0.2

Cellular biology of zinc

Zinc acts as a cofactor in more than 1000 enzymatic processes and more than 2000 transcription processes. Incorporation of zinc in the target cells is not well understood. Transferrin receptors for zinc influx have been reported. In the peripheral blood mononuclear cell, free zinc may reach up to 70% following the exogenous zinc administration. Zinc is important for the following reasons:

1. Structural integrity of cells,
2. Cell proliferation

3. Enzymatic activity,
4. Modulation of number of enzymes,
5. Immune modulation,
6. Growth and development.

Transcription and replication of fetal genes are regulated by zinc finger motif. Zinc deficiency therefore results in an impaired cell proliferation especially in the cells with high turnover rate such as reproductive cells and immune cells. Thymulin is secreted by thymocyte, which induces markers of differentiation in immature T cells. Zinc acts as a cofactor for thymulin. Thymulin helps in the release of cytokine from the peripheral blood mononuclear cells and increases the proliferation of CD8 cells with the help of IL2. Zinc is important for CNS functioning from intrauterine life. In the CNS, zinc regulates the expression of transcription factor, cell proliferation and myelination, and modulates synaptic activity and neuronal plasticity during the developing phase and adulthood. Zinc is also used by several key enzymes in neuronal metabolism and neurotransmitter formation (Table 11.8).

Clinical features of zinc deficiency

Zinc deficiency results in diverse clinical manifestations with large cell turnover rate. The clinical manifestations of acquired zinc deficiency are presented in Table 11.9.

The clinical features of zinc deficiency may be divided into mild, moderate and severe.

Mild zinc deficiency: It is due to dietary deficiency without premorbid conditions. The patient presents with hypogusia, weight loss, infertility or delayed gonadal maturation due to low testosterone levels.

Moderate zinc deficiency: It occurs with underlying malabsorption, liver or kidney disease or

Table 11.8 Enzymes in which zinc is a cofactor

Enzyme	Enzyme class
Alcohol dehydrogenase	Oxidoreductase
Aldolase II	Isomerase
Alkaline phosphatase	Hydrolase
Carbonic anhydrase	Lyase
RNA polymerase	Transferrase
tRNA synthetase	Ligase

Table 11.9 Clinical features of zinc deficiency

Gastrointestinal	Anorexia, diarrhea
Skin and hair	Bullous/ pustular dermatitis, erosive eczema, hyperkeratosis, skin atrophy, alopecia
Gonads	Delayed maturation, hypogonadism
Growth	Physical retardation
Immunity	Reduced immunity, susceptibility to infection
Neurological	Hypogusia, hyposmia, night blindness, pica, depression, emotional instability, ataxia, dementia
Others	Impaired glucose tolerance, coronary artery disease, cataract, cancer, abnormal pregnancy

severe malnutrition. These patients have additional features such as anorexia, growth retardation and impaired gonadal development or dysfunction, skin changes and night blindness.

Severe zinc deficiency: It usually occurs in patients on total parenteral nutrition, penicillamine therapy or genetic cause of zinc absorption defect (ZIP4 mutation). The patients manifest with severe pustular or bullous dermatitis starting from mucocutaneous junction (eye, anal, oral) to the periphery. The patient may also have diarrhea, alopecia, recurrent infections, and various neuropsychiatric and neurological manifestations.

Acrodermatitis enteropathica: Skin is the third most zinc-abundant tissue. Acrodermatitis enteropathica may be due to the zinc transporter defect or due to acquired zinc deficiency, including necrolytic migratory erythema, chronic diarrhea, pellagra, biotin deficiency, total perenteral nutrition or intestinal resection. Among the zinc transporter protein, ZIP4 (Zrt and Irt-like) mutation is responsible for acrodermatitis enteropathica. These transporter proteins are located in the intestinal epithelium and epidermal basal keratocyte. More than 30 mutations of ZIP4 have been reported in relation to inherited acrodermatitis enteropathica. The other clinical features of acrodermatitis enteropathica are similar to severe zinc deficiency.

The other diseases linked to zinc transporter defects are

1. Spondylo Cheiro dysplastic form of Ehler–Danlos syndrome in which ZIP 13 mutation has been demonstrated in the dermal fibroblast.
2. Transient neonatal zinc deficiency is due to ZnT2 mutation in the secretory vesicle of mammary gland.
3. Epidermodysplasia verruciferous is due to ZnT1 mutation in the epidermal keratinocyte. The skin manifestations depend on the type of dermal cell involvement.

Diagnosis of zinc deficiency

The diagnosis of zinc deficiency can be made by the following:

1. Low serum zinc level (normal serum zinc level is 84–159 µg/dl.)
2. Serum copper level (>120 µg/dl) is usually increased in zinc deficiency, and the copper/zinc ratio is 1.5 or more.
3. Improvement after zinc therapy.

Plasma or serum zinc may not reflect the intracellular zinc level, which is higher than plasma. If there is a clinical suspicion, and zinc level is normal, a therapeutic trial of zinc is justified. Serum zinc level has a diurnal variation, high in the morning and low in the evening. Serum zinc level is also affected by certain drugs: its level is decreased by glucocorticoiods, clofibrate and oral contraceptive pills, and it is increased by thiazide, loop diuretics and disulfiram. Neonate, infant and pregnant women have low zinc level, whereas seafood and stress are associated with high levels (Yanagisawa, 2004).

Treatment

The standard treatment of zinc deficiency is 2–3 mg/kg/day orally. It may be given in the form of zinc sulfate, zinc gluconate or zinc picolinate. The clinical features improve in 1–3 weeks. In acrodermatitis enteropathica due to ZIP4 mutation, lifelong treatment with zinc in a dose of 1–2 mg/kg/day is needed. In preterm infants with zinc deficiency, breastfeeding is sufficient and symptoms resolve in a week. If mother is deficient, she should be supplemented with zinc 1mg daily.

Zinc as a therapeutic option: Zinc has wide-ranging biological and immunological effects. Zinc is a standard treatment for acrodermatitis enteropathica, malabsorption syndrome, chronic diarrhea and bariatric surgery. In Wilson disease, zinc is used as a competitive inhibitor for copper absorption, and it increases metallothionein. Zinc has been recommended for neurological Wilson disease though it is not a primary disorder of zinc metabolism. Supplementation of zinc in pregnancy has reduced preterm birth but not fetal loss, congenital malformation, intrauterine growth retardation, low birth weight, prolong labor and pre- or post-term delivery (Chaffee and King, 2012). Zinc supplementation in children has shown a mild benefit in growth in malnourished children from underprivileged section, but there was no effect on the children with normal height and weight.

CONCLUSION

Copper and zinc are trace elements needed for cellular growth and development, and take part in several enzymatic reactions. Treatment of dietary zinc deficiency is rewarding, and dermatitis recovers within week. Copper deficiency takes a longer time to recover. Attention to clinical and biochemical changes may clinch the diagnosis.

REFERENCES

Bost, M., Houdart, S., Oberli, M., Kalonji, E., Huneau, J. F., Margaritis, I. 2016. Dietary copper and human health: Current evidence and unresolved issues. *Journal of Trace Elements in Medicine and Biology: Organ of the Society for Minerals and Trace Elements (GMS)* 35:107–115.

Chaffee, B.W., King, J.C. 2012. Effect of zinc supplementation on pregnancy and infant outcomes: A systematic review. *Paediatric and Perinatal Epidemiology* 26 (Suppl 1):118–137. DOI: 10.1111/j.1365–3016.2012.01289.x.

Dusek, P., Schneider, S. A., Aaseth, J. 2016. Iron chelation in the treatment of neurodegenerative diseases. *Journal of Trace Elements in Medicine and Biology: Organ of the Society for Minerals and Trace Elements (GMS)* 38: 81–92.

El Meskini, R., Culotta, V. C., Mains, R. E., Eipper, B. A. 2003. Supplying copper to the cuproenzyme peptidylglycine alpha-amidating monooxygenase. *The Journal of Biological Chemistry* 278(14):12278–12284.

Gabreyes, A. A., Abbasi, H. N., Forbes, K. P., McQuaker, G., Duncan, A., Morrison, I. 2013. Hypocupremia associated cytopenia and myelopathy: A national retrospective review. *European Journal of Haematology* 90(1):1–9.

Hardman, B., Michalczyk, A., Greenough, M., Camakaris, J., Mercer, J., Ackland, L. 2007. Distinct functional roles for the Menkes and Wilson copper translocating P-type ATPases in human placental cells. *Cellular Physiology and Biochemistry: International Journal of Experimental Cellular Physiology, Biochemistry, and Pharmacology* 20(6):1073–1084.

He, X., Hahn, P., Iacovelli, J., et al. 2007. Iron homeostasis and toxicity in retinal degeneration. *Progress in Retinal and Eye Research,* 26(6):649–673.

Kaler, S. G. 1998. Metabolic and molecular bases of Menkes disease and occipital horn syndrome. *Pediatric and Developmental Pathology: The Official Journal of the Society for Pediatric Pathology and the Paediatric Pathology Society* 1(1):85–98.

Kalita, J., Misra, U. K., Kumar, V., Parashar, V. 2019. Predictors of seizure in Wilson disease: A clinico-radiological and biomarkers study. *Neurotoxicology* 71:87–92.

Kono, S., Yoshida, K., Tomosugi, N., et al. 2010. Biological effects of mutant ceruloplasmin on hepcidin-mediated internalization of ferroportin. *Biochimica et Biophysica Acta* 1802(11):968–975.

Kuhn, J., Bewermeyer, H., Miyajima, H., Takahashi, Y., Kuhn, K. F., Hoogenraad, T. U. 2007. Treatment of symptomatic heterozygous aceruloplasminemia with oral zinc sulphate. *Brain & Development* 29(7):450–453.

Marchi, G., Busti, F., Lira Zidanes, A., Castagna, A., Girelli, D. 2019. Aceruloplasminemia: A severe neurodegenerative disorder deserving an early diagnosis. *Frontiers in Neuroscience* 13:325.

McNeill, A., Pandolfo, M., Kuhn, J., Shang, H., Miyajima, H. 2008. The neurological presentation of ceruloplasmin gene mutations. *European Neurology* 60(4):200–205.

Neldner, K. H., Hambidge, K. M. 1975. Zinc therapy of acrodermatitis enteropathica. *The New England Journal of Medicine,* 292(17):879–882. DOI: 10.1056/NEJM197504242921702

Pelucchi, S., Mariani, R., Ravasi, G., et al. 2018. Phenotypic heterogeneity in seven Italian cases of aceruloplasminemia. *Parkinsonism & Related Disorders* 51:36–42.

Poujois, A., Djebrani-Oussedik, N., Ory-Magne, F., Woimant, F. 2018. Neurological presentations revealing acquired copper deficiency: Diagnosis features, aetiologies and evolution in seven patients. *Internal Medicine Journal* 48(5):535–540.

Rangarh, P., Kohli, N. 2018. Neuroimaging findings in Menkes disease: A rare neurodegenerative disorder. *BMJ Case Reports 2018*: bcr2017223858.

Ranjan, A., Kalita, J., Kumar, S., Bhoi, S. K., Misra, U. K. 2015. A study of MRI changes in Wilson disease and its correlation with clinical features and outcome. *Clinical Neurology and Neurosurgery* 138:31–36.

Rinaldi, A.C. 2000. Meeting report: Copper research at the top. *Biometals* 13:9–13.

Rink, L., Gabriel, P. 2000. Zinc and the immune system. *Proceedings of the Nutrition Society* 59(4):541–552. DOI: 10.1017/s0029665100000781.

Scholl, T.O., Hediger, M.L., Schall, J.I., Fischer, R.L, Khoo, C.S. 1993. Low zinc intake during pregnancy: Its association with preterm and very preterm delivery. *American Journal of Epidemiology* 137:1115–1124.

Todd, N. R., Elvenhjcm. C. A., Hart, E. B. 1934. Zinc in the nutrition of the rat. *American Journal of Physiology* 107:146–156.

Vroegindeweij, L., Langendonk, J. G., Langeveld, M., et al. 2017. New insights in the neurological phenotype of aceruloplasminemia in Caucasian patients. *Parkinsonism & Related Disorders 36:* 33–40.

Yanagisawa, H. 2004. Zinc deficiency in clinical practice *JMAJ* 47(8): 359–364.

Yoshida, K., Furihata, K., Takeda, S., et al. 1995. A mutation in the ceruloplasmin gene is associated with systemic hemosiderosis in humans. *Nature Genetics* 9(3):267–272.

Zucconi, G. G., Cipriani, S., Scattoni, R., Balgkouranidou, I., Hawkins, D. P., Ragnarsdottir, K. V. 2007. Copper deficiency elicits glial and neuronal response typical of neurodegenerative disorders. *Neuropathology and Applied Neurobiology* 33(2):212–225.

12

Water as a nutrient in health and disease

INTRODUCTION

Water is an essential nutrient for all living beings. Without food, humans can survive for 4–6 weeks but without water not more than 2–4 days. Water constitutes 75% of body weight in infants, 60% in adults and 55% in the elderly. The water in human body is present in intracellular (55%–75%) and extracellular compartments (25%–45%; Figure 12.1). A 70-kg adult will have 42 l of total body water: 28 l in the intracellular and 14 l in the extracellular space (Wang et al., 1999). Of the extracellular fluid (ECF), 1 l will be in transcellular (cerebrospinal fluid, pleural, peritoneal, synovial and ocular) and 3 l in the blood as plasma, and 10 l as the interstitial fluid, including lymph. The fluid in the intracellular space should be constant for a proper cellular functioning. This constancy is due to homeostasis mechanism that regulates and monitors intracellular solutes, osmotic pressure, pH and temperature. Water homeostasis is maintained in a narrow range because of an intricate balance between neuroendocrine and renal system. Since there is a limited store of water in human body, it is excreted by kidney, skin, gastrointestinal tract and through respiration; therefore, water has to be taken daily. Water intake depends on ambient temperature, humidity as well as age and physical activity. Hypohydration and overhydration both can affect physical and mental functioning.

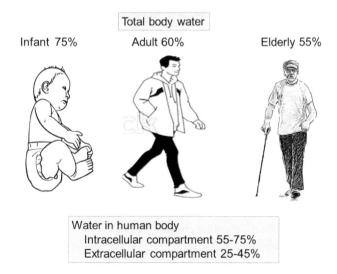

Total body water

Infant 75% Adult 60% Elderly 55%

Water in human body
Intracellular compartment 55-75%
Extracellular compartment 25-45%

Figure 12.1 Schematic diagram shows the total amount of water in human body, which reduces with increasing age.

HISTORY

Water is closely linked to life and human civilization. About 10,000 years ago when humans took to agrarian lifestyle, they settled along the river, spring, lake and sea. Jericho is the earliest urban civilization near a spring as early as 8000–7000 BC. In Egyptian civilization, about 3000 BC, there are evidences of wells, and in Mesopotamian civilization rain water stone channel (canals). In Mohenjo-Daro civilization, there are evidences of well, water pipes and toilets. The importance of safe drinking water was realized even in ancient period.

WATER HOMEOSTASIS

Water intake is partially controlled by the thirst. Hypohydration (output exceeding intake) results in the activation of hypothalamic osmoreceptors, thereby releasing antidiuretic hormone (ADH) from the posterior pituitary. Thirst is elicited by both ECF osmotic pressure and ADH release. The threshold for hypothalamic osmoreceptors for thirst is higher than for the osmoreceptors involved in ADH release; hence, ADH can act on the kidney to increase water reabsorption before the onset of thirst. This response is blunted in the elderly; therefore, they have a risk of dehydration in hot and humid environment (Phillips et al., 1984).

REGULATION OF FLUID INTAKE

All land animals drink water because of thirst, which prevents hypohydration. Humans are the only species to drink not only because of thirst but also for pleasure (Hedonic drinking). There are three sources of water: (a) beverages, (b) food and (c) metabolic. Drinking includes water and other drinks, which constitutes 85%–90% of water intake. However, food water constitutes 40%–80%, and this amount depends on the types of food. Fruits and vegetables have higher water content compared to cereals and pulses. The water content in different food items is presented in Table 12.1. The metabolic water (endogenous) refers to the water produced by the oxidation of macronutrients. In normal adults, 70%–80% of water is in the form of water and beverage, 20%–30% is from food and 10% from metabolic water. In the temperate region, a normal person drinks 1.5 l daily. Another 500–1000 ml is as a component of food and 200–300 ml as metabolic water, so the total fluid intake is 2–3 l. The amount of drinking water is influenced by climate (humidity and temperature) and physical activity.

OUTPUT

Water is mainly excreted by kidney, skin, respiratory and gastrointestinal tract. In a sedentary adult, daily urine output is 1–2 l. Sweating and

Table 12.1 Water content of different food items

Food item	Percentage of water
Water	100
Fat-free milk, watermelon, cantaloupe, strawberries, lettuce, cabbage, celery, spinach, pickles, squash (cooked)	90–99
Yogurt, fruit juice, apples, grapes, pears, pineapple, oranges, carrots, broccoli (cooked)	80–89
Avocados, bananas, cottage cheese, ricotta cheese, backed potato, cooked corn, cooked dal, shrimp	70–79
Cooked rice, legumes, pasta, ice cream, salmon, chicken breast	60–69
Cheese, cooked tenderloin steak, ground beef, hot dogs	50–59
Pizza	40–49
Bread, chapati, roti, paratha (wheat), cheddar cheese, bagels	30–39
Biscuits, cake, pepperoni sausage	20–29
Butter, margarine, raisins	10–19
Walnuts, roasted peanuts, chocolate, chip cookies, crackers, cereals, pretzels, taco shells, peanut butter	1–9
Sugar, oil	0

insensible loss is 450 ml, respiratory loss is 200–350 ml and fecal water loss is 100–200 ml, amounting to a total loss of 2–3 l, thereby balancing the intake. The water loss from the skin and respiratory tract depends on ambient temperature, humidity and physical activity. Sweating is an effective means of reducing body temperature in hot and humid climate. Sweat loss may be as high as 1–2 l/h, which may lead to hypohydration and hyperosmolality. Sweat is hypotonic (20–40 mmol/l) compared to the plasma and ECF (150 mmol/l). The intake and output of water in a healthy adult in temperate climate are presented in Table 12.2.

REGULATION OF WATER BALANCE

Coordination of sensitive detection of water volume and osmolality in the body is needed to maintain a constant water and mineral balance. The neural pathways act as integrative centers, specially hypothalamus and pituitary gland. These neural centers are sensitive to humoral factors such as ADH, atrial natriuretic peptide (ANP) and aldosterone leading to diuresis, natriuresis and blood pressure control. The signal from the integrative center comes to executive organs such as kidney, sweat gland and salivary gland. Homeostasis of water is maintained by a change in water volume within few 100 ml. Thirst manifests when plasma osmolality is increased to 288 mOsmol/Kg or ECF volume depletion is 1%–3% of body weight. In hypovolemic state, posterior pituitary releases ADH, which enhances the water absorption from renal tubules. Hyperosmolar state stimulates osmoreceptors of hypothalamus, which also induce thrust. Thrust is associated with firing of hypothalamic neurons. Restoration of water volume reduces the firing of hypothalamic neurons. Experimental study putting water on the tongue also has shown a reduction

in firing of hypothalamic neurons and thrust. This anticipatory reflex explains the relation of taste and hypothalamic thrust neurons. In hypovolemic state, kidney has to actively absorb water and produce concentrated urine to maintain euvolemia. There is increasing stress on kidney if intravascular volume is depleted and there is hyperosmolar state (Figure 12.2). It is therefore recommended to drink water before being thirsty.

The elderly are less thirsty on fluid depletion, and fluid intake may not increase even by highly palatable drinks. This is attributed to the impairment of osmo- and baroreceptors. Elderly individuals also have impaired renal fluid conservation mechanism and impaired response to hot and cold stress. During cold exposure, there is an impaired vasoconstriction, thereby resulting in the shift of fluid to the interstitial and intracellular space. This results in intravascular hypovolemia and hyperosmolar states. During hot weather, the sweating is also ineffective in the elderly.

HEALTH EFFECTS OF HYPOHYDRATION

Adequate hydration is important for proper body functioning in all age groups. There is, however, little objective evidence about daily water requirement in healthy individual. The effects of dehydration on different body systems are discussed in the following section.

Neurological effects

Hypohydration may result in headache, varying degree of cognitive impairment, delirium and coma.

Headache: It is a common belief that hypohydration is associated with headache, which may be associated with poor concentration and irritability.

Table 12.2 Intake and output of water in a healthy adult in temperate climate (modified from Jéquier and Constant, 2009)

	Input (ml/day)			Output (ml/day)	
	Average	Range		Average	Range
Beverages	1575	1400–1750	Urine	1600	1200–2000
Food	675	600–750	Skin	450	450–450
Metabolic water	300	250–350	Respiration	300	250–350
			Feces	200	100–300
Total	2550	2250–2850	Total	2550	2000–3100

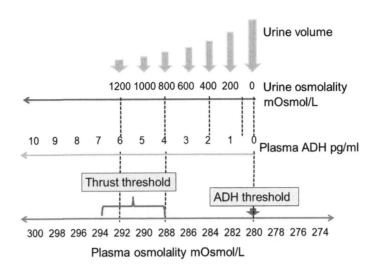

Figure 12.2 Schematic diagram shows the relationship of plasma osmolality with threshold for antidiuretic hormone (ADH) release and thrust, plasma ADH level, urinary osmolality and urine volume. (Adapted from Verbalis, J. G. 2003. Disorders of body water homeostasis. *Best Practice & Research. Clinical Endocrinology & Metabolism* 17: 471–503. DOI: 10.1016/S1521-690X(03)00049-6.)

Studies have revealed that hypohydration may trigger and perpetuate migraine, chronic daily headache or tension headache (Blau et al., 2004, Blau, 2005). If headache is the sole manifestation of hypohydration, it improves within 30 min to 3 h of fluid replacement. It is possible that the reduced plasma volume may induce intracranial dehydration or intracranial hypotension, which may account for headache. In a randomized controlled trial, the patients with migraine and tension headache were advised to take 1.5 l of additional water. In the treated group, there was a modest reduction in severity and duration of headache compared to the control group although the frequency of headache was not affected. This suggests that water has a limited role in migraine and tension headache prophylaxis (Spigt et al., 2005). Intravenous therapy is only indicated in migraine patients in emergency with features of dehydration. Headache with uncertain etiology should not be treated with intravenous fluid (IVF) (Naeem et al., 2018).

Delirium: In the elderly, hypohydration is an important risk factor for delirium. In a cross-sectional study, the predisposing factors for delirium in 155 patients with dementia were assessed. 109 (70.3%) of them had delirium, which was related to dehydration, pain, depression and preexisting behavioral disturbance, number of medications, fever and malnutrition (Voyer et al., 2008). This study suggests that modifiable risk factors such as dehydration, infection and electrolyte imbalance should be given due importance to prevent delirium in the elderly. In sick and elderly individuals, the thirst and kidney regulation mechanisms are impaired; therefore, these need special attention to prevent dehydration.

Cognition: Mild dehydration manifests with poor concentration, vigilance and impaired short-term memory (Bar-Or et al., 1980; Cian et al., 2001; Gopinathan et al., 1988; D'Anci et al., 2009; Suhr et al., 2004). Moderate dehydration is associated with impaired task performance, perceptual discrimination, arithmetic ability, visuomotor tracking and short-term memory (Cian et al., 2001; Gopinathan et al., 1988; D'Anci et al., 2009). Restoration of fluid in mild dehydration reverses the cognitive impairment (Meeusen and Decroix, 2018).

Muscle cramp: Muscle cramp is a transient severe painful involuntary contraction of skeletal muscle that can occur during or soon after exercise. The exact cause of cramp is uncertain, but has been attributed to disturbances of water and salt balance, sustained abnormal spinal reflex activity, result of fatigue of the affected muscles or underlying genetic channelopathies. In an earlier study, muscle cramp was evaluated in the workers in Hoover Dam and in steel mills of Youngstown, Ohio. The workers developing muscle cramps had higher frequency of dehydration, lower plasma sodium and chloride, little or no sodium or chloride in urine, elevated serum protein, increased red blood cell count and normal osmotic pressure (Dill et al., 1936). In an interventional study, dehydration has been attributed as a major cause of muscle cramp in athletes. Electrical stimulation or intense voluntary contractions of small muscles held in a shortened position have also been reported to produce cramp. This study suggests the role of dehydration in producing cramp (Maughan and Shirreffs, 2019).

Physical activity

The effect of dehydration on physical performance is evident from the athletes and military personal. As little as loss of 2% of body weight reduction due to dehydration is associated with reduced performance, reduction in endurance, increased fatigue, reduced motivation, increased perceived effort and impaired thermoregulation (Cheuvront et al., 2003, Paik et al., 2009). Rehydration can reverse these deficits and reduce oxidative stress. These effects are more apparent in sports like tennis and long-distance running compared to weight lifting and rowing (Vogelaere and Pereira, 2005; Kovacs, 2008; Cheuvront et al., 2007). Hypohydration may persist for a few hours if fluid intake after exercise is inadequate (Bar-Or et al., 1980). The risk of dehydration is more in un-acclimatized person, especially if there is a sudden change in weather or activity (Bergeron et al., 2005; Godek et al., 2005). Children may have greater risk of dehydration during exercise; hence, the coach should be educated about maintaining an adequate fluid intake. Children also take longer time than adults to acclimatize.

Skin

There is a pervasive myth in lay press that drinking 8–10 glasses of water daily results in glowing skin by removing toxins, but it is not supported by the evidence. Skin contains 30% water, which gives it elasticity, resilience and plumpiness. Stratum corneum and lipid layer of skin render it water proof. Loss of water from sweating occurs through both accrine and apocrine sweat glands rather than from the skin per se (Champion et al., 1992). Skin may be dry due to a prolonged hot water bath, scrubbing by soap, exposure to dry air, medications and diseases. Severe dehydration is associated with reduced turgor and tenting of skin. Adequate hydration may increase the skin thickness due to improved hydration. Wrinkling is a sign of aging and may also occur due to excessive sun exposure or genetic cause, and is not influenced by dehydration.

Cardiovascular effects

Loss of body water can result in a reduced blood volume. A slight change in intravascular volume leads to tachycardia, and a further reduction may result in postural hypotension and syncope. Rapid replenishment of water reduces heart rate and increases blood pressure due to its effect on baroreceptors. Following bloodletting, it is therefore important to replenish with water to prevent syncope (Lu et al., 2003). Rarely cold drinks may lead to bradycardia and syncope.

Renal functions

Kidney not only maintains water homeostasis but also excretes solutes to maintain serum osmolality. Kidney has an ability to dilute or concentrate urine from 40 to 1400 mOsmol/kg. The conservation of water by kidney is possible through ADH, renin–angiotensin–aldosterone and ANP. In the elderly, the ability to concentrate or dilute urine is reduced by 50% (80–700 mOsmol/kg). Kidney functions in severe dehydration are altered, resulting in acute renal failure.

Gastrointestinal functions

Water is mainly absorbed from the small intestine, and the rate of absorption depends on gastric emptying, and is faster if volume is large and of low osmolality. The capacity of small intestine to absorb water is 15 l and colon 5 l daily (Ritz et al., 2005). Constipation is often treated by increasing fluid intake; however, it is rarely effective in euhydrated individuals. A study in children with constipation did not show an improvement by increasing 50% water intake (Young et al., 1998). In the elderly, low water intake is an important cause of constipation (Robson et al., 2000).

Diarrhea and dysentery are important causes of dehydration and result in 1.5–2.5 million deaths in children annually. Oral rehydration is an important measure to prevent mortality due to diarrhea and dysentery.

RELATIONSHIP BETWEEN WATER CONSUMPTION AND ENERGY INTAKE

There are several studies about the role of beverages on health, but there is paucity of information on the role of water in reducing calorie intake and obesity. It is not known that consuming water is better than beverages. Beverages have calories, whereas water has none; therefore, drinking water with or before meal may help in the management of obesity. Consuming beverages before food did not reduce the calorie intake (Piernas et al., 2010a,b; Popkin et al., 2010). In the elderly, the mean energy intake is increased by 14.8% when premeal water was removed (Davy et al., 2008), but this effect was not present in nonobese young and middle-aged individuals (Daniels and Popkin, 2010). In a randomized controlled trial, school children supplemented by additional 1.1 glass of water reduced the risk of obesity by 31% (Muckelbauer et al., 2009).

WATER REQUIREMENT

The measurement of water intake in the community is a new concept, and such data are not available. Only a few countries regard water as a nutrient. Germany and USA have provided recommendations about water intake. It is not clear if water alone or in beverages (with sweet or with flavonoids) has the similar nutritional significance. Moreover, water is used in the preparation of food while cooking has also to be considered and may differ significantly in different cultures and regions. In USA, a normal adult consumes 2100 ml water daily, whereas in Europe, 500 ml only (Raman et al., 2004). The age-wise requirement of water is presented in Table 12.3. Water intake is related to calories. In the elderly, the calorie intake is less and water consumption is also low. Both body size and activity are considered for energy needs, and the same is true for water as well, ml/kg may be used for defining water requirement. Many beverages are sweet and may have calories, hence complicating the analysis. For 1000–1400 kcal, 1300 ml fluid intake is recommended amounting 1.23 ml water for 1 kcal. Relationship of water requirement and recommended energy requirement at different age groups and gender is presented in Table 12.4. A wide range of water intake is tolerated because of efficient water homeostasis. A number of variables such as temperature, humidity, physical activity, composition of food and associated medical condition influence the fluid intake. A physically active person in a hot and humid climate may require more water compared to a sedentary person in a temperate climate. Those consuming large amount of fruits and vegetables may require less water. On an average, a sedentary adult in normal condition would require 1.5 l water daily to maintain vital functions. Infants have a higher proportion of water in the body compared to the adults, but are vulnerable to dehydration because of the following reasons.

1. Higher surface area to body weight
2. Impaired thirst mechanism
3. Reduced ability to excrete dilute or concentrated urine.

Elderly are prone to hypohydration because of the reduction in ability to dilute or concentrate urine by kidney. Comorbidities in the elderly, including reduced mobility, visual

Table 12.3 Dietary intake of fluid in different ages (Institute of Medicine, 2004)

Age group	Male (l/day)			Female (l/day)		
	Total	Beverage	Food	Total	Beverage	Food
0–6 months	0,7	0.7	-	0.7	0.7	-
7–12 months	0.8	0.6	0.2	0.8	0.6	0.2
1–3 years	1.3	0.9	0.4	1.3	0.9	0.4
4–8 years	1.7	1.2	0.5	1.7	1.2	0.5
9–13 years	2.4	1.8	0.6	2.1	1.6	0.5
14–18 years	3.3	2.6	0.7	2.3	1.8	0.5
>19 years	3.7	3.0	0.7	2.7	2.2	0.5
Pregnancy				3.0	2.3	0.7
Lactation				3.8	3.1	0.7

Table 12.4 Relationship of water requirement and recommended energy requirement in different age groups and gender

Age (years)	Male			Female		
	EER (kcal/day)	AI fluid (ml/day)	AI/EER	EER (kcal/day)	AI fluid (ml/day)	AI/EER
2–3	1000–1400	1300	0.93	1000–1400	1300	0.93
4–8	1400–1600	1700	1.06	1400–1600	1700	1.06
9–13	1800–2000	2400	1.20	1600–2000	2100	1.05
14–18	2400–2800	3300	1.18	2000	2300	1.15
19–30	2600–2800	3700	1.32	2000–2200	2700	1.23
31–50	2400–2600	3700	1.42	2000	2700	1.35
>50	2200–2400	3700	1.54	1800	2700	1.50

Source: Adapted from Popkin, B. M., D'Anci, K. E., Rosenberg, I. H. 2010. Water, hydration, and health. *Nutrition Reviews* 68(8):439–458.
AI, adequate intake; EER, estimated energy requirements.

impairment, swallowing difficulty and intake of drugs such as diuretics and laxatives, render the elderly patients prone to dehydration. Dehydration in the elderly results in high frequency of falls, fractures, seizures and infection (Grandjean and Campbell, 2004).

Euhydration refers to a state in which water intake and output are balanced. Hypohydration refers to a state of negative water balance, and hyperhydration is a state of positive water balance. For the diagnosis of fluid status abnormalities subjective, noninvasive objective and laboratory tests are recommended.

TYPES OF DEHYDRATION

There are three types of dehydration

1. **Isotonic dehydration**: Isotonic dehydration occurs when salt loss and water loss are equal as occurs in severe diarrhea. In isotonic dehydration, extracellular volume (ECV) is reduced, and it is managed by normal saline.
2. **Hypertonic dehydration:** Hypertonic dehydration occurs when there is loss of water in excess of salt. This type of dehydration occurs when there is decreased thirst, impaired consciousness, and loss of excess water such as diabetes insipidus, osmotic diuresis, vomiting or excessive sweating in hot and humid climate.
3. **Hypotonic dehydration:** Hypotonic dehydration occurs in gastrointestinal loss in which the fluid replacement is done by water or fluid

containing low sodium or potassium. In such a situation, water shifts into the cells, thereby reducing ECF. The cells swell and isotonic dehydration ensues. It may require both hypertonic saline to restore sodium and normal saline to restore volume.

CLINICAL SIGNS OF DEHYDRATION

The clinical signs of dehydration have low sensitivity and specificity; however, dry mucus membrane of mouth, nose, and longitudinal furrows on the tongue have more than 80% sensitivity. Incoherent speech, limb weakness, dry axilla and sunken eyes have good specificity (Thomas et al., 2008). History of thirst, high colored urine, low urine output, negative fluid balance (difference in intake and output) and loss of weight may be early clinical indicators of hypohydration and help in early management. Body weight should be measured at the standard time, especially in the morning after passing stool and urine for reliable results. The signs of severe and moderate dehydration are presented in Table 12.5.

WORLD HEALTH ORGANIZATION (WHO) SCALE OF DEHYDRATION

Clinical dehydration scale: Clinical dehydration scale is recommended for children aged 1–36 months with gastroenteritis. Grading of dehydration is based on the score of appearance, eye sign, mentation and tear. A score of 0 is normal, 1–4 mild to moderate and 5–8 severe (Table 12.6).

Table 12.5 Clinical signs of dehydration

Severe	Moderate
Extreme thirst	Dry sticky mouth
Sleepiness, irritability, confusion	Lethargy, tiredness
Dry mouth, skin and mucus membrane, loss of skin turgor	Thirst
Little or no urine output, high colored urine	Reduced urine output
Sunken eyes	Reduced or no tears on crying
Hypotension, tachycardia	Weakness
Fever	Headache
Delirium, unconsciousness	Dizziness
	Light headedness

Subjective measures of dehydration: These parameters include thirst, skin turgor and dryness of mouth and eyes.

Noninvasive objective parameters: The noninvasive objective parameters of dehydration include body weight, pulse rate, systolic blood pressure and postural fall of blood pressure, intake output chart, constipation, temperature and respiratory rate.

Laboratory test: The laboratory tests of dehydration are hematocrit, hemoglobin, serum and urinary osmolality, serum creatinine and blood urea nitrogen.

Body mass: Acute change in body weight may reflect dehydration (1 ml water = 1 g); hence, a rapid change in body weight may be an indicator of water loss.

Blood indices: Hemoglobin and hematocrit are potential measures of change in hydration status provided the baseline values are known. Plasma serum sodium and osmolality will increase if there is water loss leading to dehydration. Osmolality and hematocrit may not change till there is a loss of 3%–5% of body mass.

Urine: Urine osmolality may increase in case of hypohydration. A body mass reduction of 1.9% after the fluid restriction may increase the urine osmolality to 900 mOsmol/kg (Shirreffs and Maughan, 1998).

Urine specific gravity may be used interchangeably with urine osmolality. Urine color is determined by the amount of urochrome; therefore, higher color of urine is consistent with hypohydration and increased specific gravity and osmolality. Urine color can be measured on an eight-colored scale (Armstrong et al., 2016). Urine markers may lag behind the serum markers.

Inferior vena cava (IVC) diameter: Ultrasonography-based IVC diameter below the diaphragm in supine position is used as a marker of volume status and volume responsiveness. Inferior vena cava diameter less than 10 mm suggests hypovolemia and more than 22 mm as hypervolemia. Diameter of IVC may be influenced by respiratory cycle and right heart function and volume status.

Central venous pressure (CVP): Central venous pressure is normally 8–12 cm of water, and if it is lower, it suggests hypovolemia. In ICU, CVP is often used to monitor fluid therapy. A meta-analysis evaluated the role of CVP in predicting volume response in 43 studies. The effect of 500 ml fluid challenge was evaluated on cardiac output and stroke volume. Overall 57.3%±1.3% had volume responsiveness; CVP in volume responders was 8.2±2.3 cm and in nonresponders 9.5±2.3 cm. Those who had low CVP responded to fluid challenge (Marik and Cavallazzi, 2013).

Table 12.6 Clinical dehydration scale in children (World Health Organization)

Parameter	0	1	2
Appearance	Normal	Lethargic, irritable	Drowsy, comatose
Eye	Normal	Sunken	Very sunken
Mentation	Normal	Sleepy	Comatose
Tear	Normal	Reduced	Absent

Score 0, no; 1–4, mild to moderate; 5–8, severe dehydration.

MANAGEMENT

The aim of treatment of hypovolemia is to restore euvolemia and prevent ongoing fluid losses.

Mild hypovolemia can be managed with normal diet and oral fluids. Moderate-to-severe hypovolemia needs IV fluids and management of underlying pathophysiology. Normal saline is the most appropriate fluid for the hyponatremic hypovolemia. Hypernatremic patients may require 5% dextrose or N/2 saline. The patients with acidosis and low HCO_3 may require sodium bicarbonate infusion in 5% dextrose. If the patient has anemia, RBC should be transfused.

FLUID MANAGEMENT IN RELATION TO EXERCISE

Exercise can result in a wide range of fluid loss because of sweating, which may range from 0.4 to 2 l/h. A soccer player may lose up to 8.8 l/day and a marathon runner up to 3.5 l/day. The rate of sweating in relation to running speed and duration is shown in Figure 12.3. The sweating is higher in tropics than in desert (Figure 12.4). It is important to exercise in a euhydrated state. The goal of hydration during exercise is not to lose more than 2% of body weight. Body weight measurement before and after the exercise may be an indicator of water loss, and should be assessed during the practice session. Pre-exercise hydration is ensured by taking 5–7

ml/kg beverages within 4 h of starting exercise. If the urine color is still high, the addition of 3–5 ml/kg fluid may be taken. During exercise, especially if exceeding 3 h, additional hydration by 0.4–0.8 l/h is needed. Post-exercise, one must drink beverages 1.5 l for each kg loss of body weight. It takes several hours for euhydration to be achieved after exercise; therefore, a repeat strenuous exercise should be avoided before 12 h. Too hot or too cold beverages may be avoided, and the recommended temperature is 15°C–21°C. Instead of plain water, the drink should contain NaCl (20–30 mEq/l), K (2–5 mEq/l) and carbohydrate (5%–10%) (Institute of Medicine, 1994). Salted snack or food with water may also suffice (American College of Sports Medicine et al., 2007).

FLUID THERAPY IN CRITICALLY ILL PATIENTS

Optimal IVF is not well defined, but a patient in shock is recommended to be given fluid challenge or a bolus of IVF. Fluid bolus refers to a therapeutic intervention in which 500 ml of fluid is administered in 15 min to correct hypotensive shock. Fluid challenge refers to a diagnostic infusion of 500–1000 ml crystalloid or 500 ml colloid in 30 min to evaluate the effect of fluid in optimizing tissue perfusion (Dellinger et al., 2013; Hoste et al., 2014). About 300 ml blood is stored in leg veins and passive leg raising introduces 300 ml without

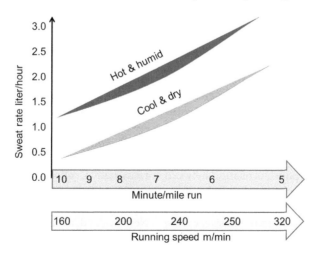

Figure 12.3 Schematic diagram shows the relation of sweat rate with running speed and distance in hot and humid as well as cool and dry region. (Adapted from Sawka, M. N. 1992. Physiological consequences of hydration: Exercise performance and thermoregulation. *Medicine & Science in Sports & Exercise* 24:657–670.)

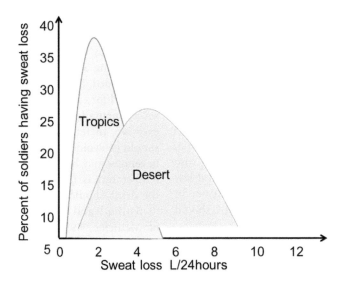

Figure 12.4 The sweat loss in tropical region and desert, which is more in tropics compared to desert. Percentage of soldiers showing the amount of sweat loss in tropics and desert. (Adapted from Molnar, G. W. 1947. Man in the tropics compared with man in the desert. In: Adolph, E. F., ed., *Physiology of man in the desert*. New York: Intersciences Publishers, pp. 315–325.)

increasing the blood volume and helps in assessing fluid responsiveness.

In a patient with septic shock, it is recommended to administer 30 ml/kg/h IVF to get a CVP of 8–12 cm of water, mean arterial blood pressure of more than 65 mmHg and urine output of more than 0.5 ml/kg/h.

In a study of fluid resuscitation in 406 episodes, in 334 patients, 52% were able to increase the cardiac output and stroke volume, whereas in 48% it did not provide benefit and added to volume overload (Michard and Teboul, 2002). The effect of fluid challenge can be monitored by static or dynamic measures. The static parameters of fluid responsiveness include CVP and pulmonary artery occlusion pressure (cardiac filling pressure). Central venous pressure measurement is not without limitations because the relation between CVP and volume is not linear but curvilinear. Rate of increase rather than absolute values of CVP may be more informative. A poor correlation between CVP and blood volume in hypovolemic shock has been reported (Shippy et al., 1984).

The dynamic markers of fluid responsiveness are available in the patients who are on artificial ventilation. During positive pressure, inspiration increases intrathoracic pressure, resulting in decreased preload and stroke volume. During expiration, the intrathoracic pressure decreases with increased venous return, preload and stroke volume. These dynamic changes in stroke volume in response to respiratory cycle may be used to assess fluid responsiveness. In patients who are fluid responsive, a variation in stroke volume during the respiratory cycle correlates with an alteration in pulse pressure. A significant variation in pulse pressure during respiration has been used for the prediction of fluid responsiveness (Michard et al., 1999, 2000). Doppler study of aortic blood flow measurement has been used as a surrogate marker of stroke volume. Inferior vena cava diameter and collapsibility have also been used as markers of fluid responsiveness (Feissel et al., 2004; Monnet et al., 2006).

TYPES OF FLUID

For IVF therapy, crystalloid and colloids are administered. In a study on 391 ICU patients requiring fluid resuscitation, colloids were given to 40%, crystalloids to 33% and blood products to 19%. Among the colloids, starch is mainly used in Canada, Europe and New Zealand, albumin in USA and gelatin in Hong Kong (Finfer et al., 2010).

Crystalloids: Salt-based fluid resuscitation has been practiced since early days. During cholera pandemic in 19th century, the first report of successful resuscitation of six cholera patients using sodium chloride and sodium bicarbonate solution was published. A number of electrolyte solutions are used such as Ringer lactate, plasmalyte and other fluids (Table 12.7). There are concerns about the other physiological ions in addition to sodium (such as potassium, calcium, magnesium, bicarbonate and phosphate) and effect on renal perfusion. A large amount of 0.9% saline may result in extracellular potassium shift leading to hyperkalemia (O'Malley et al., 2005). Chloride-rich solution can result in renal vasoconstriction and acute kidney injury, hyperchloremic metabolic acidosis and gastrointestinal dysfunction (Yunos et al., 2010; Chowdhury et al., 2012). Comparative usefulness of isotonic crystalloids for fluid resuscitation of critically ill ICU patients is based on a few observational studies and a single-center study. These studies demonstrated the association of balanced fluid like lactated Ringer's solution with reduced incidence of acute kidney injury and mortality and better outcome compared to normal saline (Shaw et al., 2012; Raghunathan et al., 2014; Yunos et al., 2012). In septic shock, balanced fluid improved the survival. A recent study compared normal saline with plasmalyte 148 in ICU fluid therapy (SPLIT) trial. This trial did not reveal any difference with respect to acute kidney injury, need for renal replacement therapy and mortality in the patients receiving normal saline or balanced salt solution. However, these patients were of mild severity – mostly surgical patients with few comorbidities, and the fluid received was only 2 l, which may be insufficient to demonstrate the effect of chloride-restrictive fluid

therapy on renal functions. Moreover, the incidence of acute kidney injury was less than 10% (Young et al., 2015).

Colloids: Colloids comprise a group of high-molecular-weight compounds suspended in a carrier vehicle. Colloids are retained in the intravascular compartment and provide oncotic pressure, thereby increasing plasma volume (Myburgh and Mythen, 2013). Albumin and starch compounds are commonly used colloids.

Albumin: Human albumin is a natural colloid; it is synthesized in the liver and accounts for 80% of intravascular osmotic pressure. Albumin is available as 4%–5% (iso-oncotic) and as 20%–25% (hyperoncotic) formulations, and is widely used as volume expander. In a meta-analysis, high mortality has been reported compared to those who did not receive albumin or crystalloid (Cochrane Injuries Group Albumin Reviewers, 1998). This study, however, was not supported by a subsequent meta-analysis (Wilkes and Navickis, 2001). Saline vs Albumin Evaluation (SAFE) study randomized 6997 patients to 4% albumin or 0.9% saline. There was no difference in 28-day mortality; however, 492 (7%) head injury patients had higher death in albumin arm compared to saline (OR 1.62, 95% CI 0.12–2.34; $P = 0.009$) and mortality was attributed to coagulopathy following albumin (Finfer et al., 2004). In ALBIOS trial in sepsis, 20% albumin did not result in a reduction of mortality, length of hospitalization and degree of organ dysfunction but there was no harm attributed to albumin (Caironi et al., 2014). Owing to high cost and lack of convincing reproducible benefit, Surviving

Table 12.7 Compositions of common intravenous fluids

Ingredient (mMol/l)	NaCl 0.9%	Ringer's lactate	Plasma-Lyte 148	Albumin 5%	Plasma
Sodium	154	131	140	130–160	140
Chloride	154	111	98	0	100
Potassium	0	5.4	5	≤2	5
Calcium	0	2	0	0	2.2
Magnesium	0	1	1.5	0	1
Bicarbonate	0	0	0	0	24
Acetate	0	0	27	0	0
Lactate	0	29	0	0	1
Gluconate	0	0	23	0	0
pH	5.4	6.5	5.5	7.4	7.4

Sepsis Campaign recommends albumin to those selected patients who have received substantial crystalloids (Dellinger et al., 2013).

Starch: Semisynthetic colloids prepared by hydroxylation of amylopectin from sorghum, corn or potatoes may be iso-oncotic (6%) or hyperoncotic (10%). First- and second-generation starch used high molecular weight, greater molecular substitution (0.5–0.7), which resulted in a prolonged intravascular volume expansion but was associated with toxic effects like coagulopathy, and deposition in skin, liver and kidney, leading to pruritus and organ dysfunction.

Hydroxyethyl starch (HES) is the third-generation starch that has low molecular weight (130 KD) and lower substitution, and is cheaper and easier to procure than albumin. Several trials have proven its safety and efficacy in reference to crystalloids. Crystalloid vs HES trial (CHEST) compared 6% HES with normal saline in 7000 critically ill patients requiring resuscitation. There was no difference in 90-day mortality. HES patients had double the adverse events compared to crystalloid arm, including skin rash, itching, requirement of renal replacement therapy (7% vs 5.6%, $P=0.004$) (Myburgh et al., 2012).

FLUID OVERLOAD

During IVF therapy, one should be cautious about volume overload as it has an important clinical and prognostic significance. Fluid overload is defined as 10% increase in body weight before starting IVF therapy. Fluid overload can also be suspected clinically by appearance of pitting edema, crepitation, pleural effusion or ascites or a positive fluid balance. Fluid overload is associated with high mortality across the studies. In a study on septic shock on vasopressors, the patients with positive fluid balance at 12 h and fourth day had higher mortality. The patients with CVP more than 12 cm water at 12 h after the fluid resuscitation had the highest mortality (Boyd et al., 2011). In a study on severe sepsis and septic shock, volume overload based on clinical criteria also revealed higher hospital mortality and need of paracentesis and diuretic therapy (Kelm et al., 2015). In a randomized controlled trial, 90-day mortality was also higher in the patients with volume overload before the renal replacement therapy (Vaara et al., 2012). In critically ill patients, it is important to follow the recommendations of Acute Dialysis Quality Initiative XII in which the fluid therapy has been divided into rescue, optimization, stabilization and de-escalation (Figure 12.5). During rescue stage, the focus is to use intravenous therapy to improve tissue perfusion; during optimization and stabilization phases, the emphasis is to maintain adequate perfusion avoiding volume over load. In the de-escalation phase, it is important to remove excess fluid used during resuscitation. A positive fluid balance more than 700 ml or less than 500 ml daily is associated with poor outcome. The position statements in different aspect of water intake, output, measures of volume status and resuscitation measure are presented in Table 12.8 (Sawka et al., 2015).

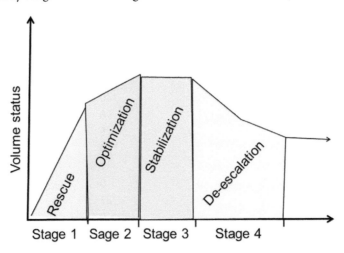

Figure 12.5 Schematic diagram shows the four stages of fluid replacement therapy as per the recommendation of Acute Dialysis Quality Initiative XII.

Table 12.8 Position statement on exercise and fluid replacement (American College of Sports Medicine)

Parameters	Level A evidence	Level B evidence
Fluid and electrolyte	1. Sustained exercise increases sweat rates, substantial water and electrolyte losses especially in warm-hot weather. 2. Water and electrolyte losses vary in individuals and in different activities. 3. Person dehydrates if sweat water and electrolyte losses are not replenished. 4. Men generally have higher sweating rates than women. 5. Older adults have decreased thirst sensitivity when dehydrated leading to lesser voluntarily effort to euhydration. 6. Older adults have slower renal responses to water leading to a greater risk of hyponatremia. 7. Meal consumption promotes euhydration. 8. Sweat electrolyte (sodium and potassium) losses need to replenish to reestablish euhydration.	1. Children have lower sweating rates than adults. 2. Caffeine intake does not markedly alter daily urine output or hydration status. 3. Alcohol intake can increase urine output and thereby delay full rehydration.
Hydration assessment	1. Change (loss) in body weight reflects sweat losses during exercise and can be used to calculate the amount of fluid replacement needs in specific exercise and environmental conditions.	1. Individuals can monitor their hydration status by employing simple urine and body weight measurements. 2. Individual with a first morning urine specific gravity $\leq$ 1.020 or urine osmolality $\leq$ 700 mOsmol/kg can be considered as euhydrated. 3. Several days of first morning body weight values can be used to establish baseline body weights that represent euhydration.

(Continued)

Table 12.8 (Continued) Position statement on exercise and fluid replacement (American College of Sports Medicine)

Parameters	Level A evidence	Level B evidence
Hydration effect	1. Dehydration increases physiologic strain and perceived effort to perform the same exercise task, and is more marked in warm-hot weather. 2. Dehydration (>2% loss in body weight) can degrade aerobic exercise performance, especially in warm-hot weather. 3. Dehydration is a risk factor for both heat exhaustion and exertional heat stroke. 4. Symptomatic exercise-associated hyponatremia can occur in endurance events. 5. Fluid consumption exceeding sweating leads to exercise-associated hyponatremia.	1. The degree of dehydration correlates with the physiologic strain and a decrease in aerobic exercise. 2. Dehydration (>2% loss of body weight) might degrade mental/cognitive performance. 3. Dehydration (3% loss of body weight) has a marginal influence on degrading aerobic exercise performance in cold environment. 4. Hyperhydration has equivocal benefits and several disadvantages. 5. Dehydration can increase the likelihood or severity of acute renal failure as a result of exertional rhabdomyolysis. 6. Large amount of sodium loss in sweat and small body weight (and total body water) can contribute to the exercise-associated hyponatremia.

Source: Adapted from Sawka, M. N., Burke, L. M., et al. 2007. American college of sports medicine position stand. Exercise and fluid replacement. Medicine & Science in Sports & Exercise 39(2):377–390. DOI:10.1249/mss.0b013e31802ca597.

A, recommendation based on consistent and good-quality experimental evidence (morbidity, mortality, exercise and cognitive performance, physiologic responses); B, recommendation based on inconsistent or limited quality experimental evidence.

WATER TOXICITY

Water toxicity is rare because of efficient water homeostasis. The clinical presentation of water toxicity is vague and includes nausea, vomiting, disorientation, confusion, altered mental status and coma. Excessive drinking of water may occur due to the following reasons: (a) drinking of a large quantity of water after a prolonged exercise without adding electrolyte, (b) excessive water drinking in competition or in prison torture, (c) psychogenic polydipsia and (d) water administration in the patients with high ADH levels.

Pathophysiology: Following excessive water drinking, the intravascular osmolality is decreased and water is shifted to the intracellular space, which has higher osmolality. This results in swelling of cells. In the central nervous system, swelling of neurons and glia leads to raised intracranial pressure, and symptoms such as headache, delirium, hallucination, delusion, lethargy, disorientation, drowsiness and if untreated seizures, coma and death (Cosgray et al., 1990).

Evaluation: History, intake output chart, increase in weight, serum sodium, serum and urinary osmolality and other measurements of volume status help in the diagnosis of water toxicity.

Treatment: The tenets of treatment of water toxicity are correction of hyponatremia and prevention of brain herniation. Aggressive correction of hyponatremia may result in osmotic demyelination and usually occur if sodium correction rate is more than 10–12 mEq/l in 24 h or 18 mEq/l in 48 h (Sterns, 1987). Sodium correction should be slower especially in chronic hyponatremia. The details of the treatment of hyponatremia are discussed in Chapter 13.

CONCLUSION

Water is an essential nutrient in health and disease. Human cannot survive without water for more than 4 days. The sources of water in human body are beverages, food and metabolic. Body water content is tightly regulated within a narrow range by the hypothalamus with the executor organs, including kidney, skin, respiratory tract and gastrointestinal tract. The thresholds for thirst and kidney regulation of water are blunted in elderly and young children; therefore, regular drinking should be practiced rather than when thirsty. The recommended water requirement is 1.23 ml for 1 kcal of energy intake. Dehydration amounting to more than 2% loss of body weight is associated with impaired neurocognitive functions and physical activity performance. Sweat rate is higher in hot and humid environment. Dehydration may be hypotonic, hypertonic or isotonic, and their management should be done accordingly. In critically ill patients, fluid management is life-saving.

REFERENCES

Adolph, E.F. (Ed.) 1947. *Physiology of man in the desert.* New York: Intersciences Publishers, pp. 315–325.

American College of Sports Medicine, Sawka, M. N., Burke, L. M., Eichner, E. R., Maughan, R. J., Montain, S. J., Stachenfeld, N. S. 2007. American College of Sports Medicine position stand. Exercise and fluid replacement. *Medicine and Science in Sports and Exercise* 39(2):377–390.

Armstrong, L. E., Johnson, E. C., McKenzie, A. L., Muñoz, C. X. 2016. An empirical method to determine inadequacy of dietary water. *Nutrition (Burbank, Los Angeles County, CA)* 32(1), 79–82.

Bar-Or, O., Dotan, R., Inbar, O., Rotshtein, A., Zonder, H. 1980. Voluntary hypohydration in 10- to 12-year-old boys. *Journal of Applied Physiology: Respiratory, Environmental and Exercise Physiology* 48(1):104–108.

Bergeron, M. F., McKeag, D. B., Casa, D. J., et al. 2005. Youth football: Heat stress and injury risk. *Medicine and Science in Sports and Exercise* 37(8):1421–1430.

Blau, J. N., Kell, C. A., Sperling, J. M. 2004. Water-deprivation headache: A new headache with two variants. *Headache* 44(1):79–83.

Blau J. N. 2005. Water deprivation: A new migraine precipitant. *Headache* 45(6):757–759.

Boyd, J. H., Forbes, J., Nakada, T. A., Walley, K. R., Russell, J. A. 2011. Fluid resuscitation in septic shock: A positive fluid balance and elevated central venous pressure are associated with increased mortality. *Critical Care Medicine* 39(2):259–265.

Caironi, P., Tognoni, G., Masson, S., et al. 2014. Albumin replacement in patients with severe sepsis or septic shock. *The New England Journal of Medicine* 370(15):1412–1421.

Champion, R.H., Burton, J. L., Ebling, F. J. G. (Eds.), 1992. *Textbook of dermatology (Rook).* Oxford: Blackwell.

Cheuvront, S. N., Carter, R., 3rd, Sawka, M. N. 2003. Fluid balance and endurance exercise performance. *Current Sports Medicine Reports* 2(4):202–208.

Cheuvront, S. N., Montain, S. J., Sawka, M. N. 2007. Fluid replacement and performance during the marathon. *Sports Medicine (Auckland, NZ)* *37*(4–5):353–357.

Chowdhury, A. H., Cox, E. F., Francis, S. T., Lobo, D. N. 2012. A randomized, controlled, double-blind crossover study on the effects of 2-L infusions of 0.9% saline and plasma-lyte® 148 on renal blood flow velocity and renal cortical tissue perfusion in healthy volunteers. *Annals of Surgery* *256*(1):18–24.

Cian, C., Barraud, P. A., Melin, B., Raphel, C. 2001. Effects of fluid ingestion on cognitive function after heat stress or exercise-induced dehydration. *International Journal of Psychophysiology: Official Journal of the International Organization of Psychophysiology* *42*(3):243–251.

Cochrane Injuries Group Albumin Reviewers, 1998. Human albumin administration in critically ill patients: Systematic review of randomised controlled trials. *BMJ (Clinical Research Ed.)* *317*(7153):235–240.

Cosgray, R. E., Hanna, V., Davidhizar, R. E., Smith, J. 1990. The water-intoxicated patient. *Archives of Psychiatric Nursing* *4*(5):308–312.

D'anci, K. E., Vibhakar, A., Kanter, J. H., Mahoney, C. R., Taylor, H. A. 2009. Voluntary dehydration and cognitive performance in trained college athletes. *Perceptual and Motor Skills* *109*(1):251–269.

Daniels, M. C., Popkin, B. M. 2010. Impact of water intake on energy intake and weight status: A systematic review. *Nutrition Reviews* *68*(9):505–521.

Davy, B. M., Dennis, E. A., Dengo, A. L., Wilson, K. L., Davy, K. P. 2008. Water consumption reduces energy intake at a breakfast meal in obese older adults. *Journal of the American Dietetic Association* *108*(7):1236–1239.

Dellinger, R. P., Levy, M. M., Rhodes, A., et al. 2013. Surviving sepsis campaign: International guidelines for management of severe sepsis and septic shock: 2012. *Critical Care Medicine* *41*(2):580–637.

Dill, D. B., Bock, A. V., Edwards, H. T., Kennedy, P. H. 1936. Industrial fatigue. *Journal of Industrial Hygiene and Toxicology* *18*:417–431.

Dellinger, R. P., Levy, M. M., Rhodes, A., et al. 2013. Surviving Sepsis Campaign Guidelines Committee including the Pediatric Subgroup (2013). Surviving sepsis campaign: International guidelines for management of severe sepsis and septic shock: 2012. *Critical Care Medicine,* *41*(2):580–637. DOI: 10.1097/CCM.0b013e31827e83af.

Feissel, M., Michard, F., Faller, J. P., Teboul, J. L. 2004. The respiratory variation in inferior vena cava diameter as a guide to fluid therapy. *Intensive Care Medicine* *30*(9):1834–1837.

Finfer, S., Bellomo, R., Boyce, N., French, J., Myburgh, J., Norton, R., SAFE Study Investigators, 2004. A comparison of albumin and saline for fluid resuscitation in the intensive care unit. *The New England Journal of Medicine* *350*(22):2247–2256.

Finfer, S., Liu, B., Taylor, C., et al. 2010. Resuscitation fluid use in critically ill adults: An international cross-sectional study in 391 intensive care units. *Critical Care (London, England)* *14*(5):R185.

Godek, S. F., Godek, J. J., Bartolozzi, A. R. 2005. Hydration status in college football players during consecutive days of twice-a-day preseason practices. *The American Journal of Sports Medicine* *33*(6):843–851.

Gopinathan, P. M., Pichan, G., Sharma, V. M. 1988. Role of dehydration in heat stress-induced variations in mental performance. *Archives of Environmental Health* *43*(1):15–17.

Grandjean, A. C., Campbell, S. M. 2004. *Hydration: Fluids for life. A monograph by the North American Branch of the International Life Science Institute.* Washington, DC: ILSI North America.

Hoste, E. A., Maitland, K., Brudney, C. S., et al. 2014. Four phases of intravenous fluid therapy: A conceptual model. *British Journal of Anaesthesia* *113*(5):740–747.

Institute of Medicine (US) Committee on Military Nutrition Research, Marriott, B. M. (Eds.). 1994. *Fluid replacement and heat stress.* Washington, DC: National Academies Press (US).

Institute of Medicine. 2004. Dietary reference intakes for water, potassium, sodium, chloride, and sulfate. Washington, DC: Institute of Medicine.

Jéquier, E., Constant, F. 2010. Water as an essential nutrient: the physiological basis of hydration. *European Journal of Clinical Nutrition* *64*, 115–123. DOI: 10.1038/ejcn.2009.11

Kelm, D. J., Perrin, J. T., Cartin-Ceba, R., Gajic, O., Schenck, L., Kennedy, C. C. 2015. Fluid overload in patients with severe sepsis and septic shock treated with early goal-directed therapy is associated with increased acute need for fluid-related medical interventions and hospital death. *Shock (Augusta, GA)* *43*(1):68–73.

Kovacs M. S. 2008. A review of fluid and hydration in competitive tennis. *International Journal of Sports Physiology and Performance* *3*(4):413–423.

Lu, C. C., Diedrich, A., Tung, C. S., et al., 2003. Water ingestion as prophylaxis against syncope. *Circulation* *108*(21):2660–2665.

Marik, P. E., Cavallazzi, R. 2013. Does the central venous pressure predict fluid responsiveness? An updated meta-analysis and a plea for some common sense. *Critical Care Medicine* *41*(7):1774–1781.

Maughan, R. J., Shirreffs, S. M. 2019. Muscle cramping during exercise: Causes, solutions, and questions remaining. *Sports Medicine (Auckland, NZ)* 49(Suppl 2):115–124.

Meeusen, R., Decroix, L. 2018. Nutritional supplements and the brain. *International Journal of Sport Nutrition and Exercise Metabolism* 28(2): 200–211.

Michard, F., Teboul, J. L. 2002. Predicting fluid responsiveness in ICU patients: A critical analysis of the evidence. *Chest* 121(6): 2000–2008.

Michard, F., Boussat, S., Chemla, D., et al. 2000. Relation between respiratory changes in arterial pulse pressure and fluid responsiveness in septic patients with acute circulatory failure. *American Journal of Respiratory and Critical Care Medicine* 162(1):134–138.

Michard, F., Chemla, D., Richard, C., et al. 1999. Clinical use of respiratory changes in arterial pulse pressure to monitor the hemodynamic effects of PEEP. *American Journal of Respiratory and Critical Care Medicine* 159(3):935–939.

Molnar, G. W. 1947. Man in the tropics compared with man in the desert. In: Adolph, E. F., ed., *Physiology of man in the desert.* New York: Intersciences Publishers, pp. 315–325.

Monnet, X., Rienzo, M., Osman, D., et al. 2006. Passive leg raising predicts fluid responsiveness in the critically ill. *Critical Care Medicine* 34(5):1402–1407.

Muckelbauer, R., Libuda, L., Clausen, K., Toschke, A. M., Reinehr, T., Kersting, M. 2009. Promotion and provision of drinking water in schools for overweight prevention: Randomized, controlled cluster trial. *Pediatrics* 123(4):e661–e667.

Myburgh, J. A., Mythen, M. G. 2013. Resuscitation fluids. *The New England Journal of Medicine* 369(13):1243–1251.

Myburgh, J. A., Finfer, S., Bellomo, R., et al. 2012. Hydroxyethyl starch or saline for fluid resuscitation in intensive care. *The New England Journal of Medicine* 367(20):1901–1911.

Naeem, F., Schramm, C., Friedman, B. W. 2018. Emergent management of primary headache: A review of current literature. *Current Opinion in Neurology* 31(3):286–290.

O'Malley, C. M., Frumento, R. J., Hardy, M. A., et al. 2005. A randomized, double-blind comparison of lactated Ringer's solution and 0.9% NaCl during renal transplantation. *Anesthesia and Analgesia* 100(5):1518–1524.

Paik, I. Y., Jeong, M. H., Jin, H. E., et al., 2009. Fluid replacement following dehydration reduces oxidative stress during recovery. *Biochemical and Biophysical Research Communications* 383(1): 103–107.

Phillips, P. A., Rolls, B. J., Ledingham, J. G., et al. 1984. Reduced thirst after water deprivation in healthy elderly men. *The New England Journal of Medicine* 311(12):753–759.

Piernas, C., Popkin, B. M. 2010a. Snacking increased among U.S. adults between 1977 and 2006. *The Journal of Nutrition* 140(2):325–332.

Piernas, C., Popkin, B. M. 2010b. Trends in snacking among U.S. children. *Health Affairs (Project Hope)* 29(3):398–404.

Popkin, B. M., D'Anci, K. E., Rosenberg, I. H. 2010. Water, hydration, and health. *Nutrition Reviews* 68(8):439–458.

Raghunathan, K., Shaw, A., Nathanson, B., et al. 2014. Association between the choice of IV crystalloid and in-hospital mortality among critically ill adults with sepsis. *Critical Care Medicine* 42(7):1585–1591.

Raman, A., Schoeller, D. A., Subar, A. F., et al. 2004. Water turnover in 458 American adults 40–79 yr of age. *American Journal of Physiology. Renal Physiology* 286(2):F394–F401.

Ritz, P., Berrut, G. 2005. The importance of good hydration for day-to-day health. *Nutrition Reviews* 63(6 Pt 2):S6–S13.

Robson, K. M., Kiely, D. K., Lembo, T. 2000. Development of constipation in nursing home residents. *Diseases of the Colon and Rectum* 43(7):940–943.

Shaw, A. D., Bagshaw, S. M., Goldstein, S. L., et al. 2012. Major complications, mortality, and resource utilization after open abdominal surgery: 0.9% saline compared to Plasma-Lyte. *Annals of Surgery* 255(5):821–829.

Shirreffs, S. M., Maughan, R. J. 1998. Urine osmolality and conductivity as indices of hydration status in athletes in the heat. *Medicine and Science in Sports and Exercise* 30(11):1598–1602.

Shippy, C. R., Appel, P. L., Shoemaker, W. C. 1984. Reliability of clinical monitoring to assess blood volume in critically ill patients. *Critical Care Medicine* 12(2):107–112.

Spigt, M. G., Kuijper, E. C., Schayck, C. P., et al., 2005. Increasing the daily water intake for the prophylactic treatment of headache: A pilot trial. *European Journal of Neurology* 12(9):715–718.

Sawka, M. N. 1992. Physiological consequences of hydration: Exercise performance and thermoregulation. *Medicine & Science in Sports & Exercise* 24:657–670.

Sawka, M. N., Burke, L. M., et al. 2007. American college of sports medicine position stand. Exercise and fluid replacement. *Medicine & Science in Sports & Exercise* 39(2):377–390.

Sawka, M. N., Cheuvront, S. N., Kenefick, R. W. 2015. Hypohydration and human performance: impact of environment and physiological mechanisms. *Sports Medicine (Auckland, N.Z.)*, 45 (Suppl 1):S51–S60. DOI: 10.1007/s40279-015-0395-7.

Sterns, R. H. 1987. Severe symptomatic hyponatremia: treatment and outcome. A study of 64 cases. *Annals of Internal Medicine* 107(5):656–664.

Suhr, J. A., Hall, J., Patterson, S. M., Niinistö, R. T. 2004. The relation of hydration status to cognitive performance in healthy older adults. *International Journal of Psychophysiology: Official Journal of the International Organization of Psychophysiology* 53(2):121–125.

Thomas, D.R., Cote, T.R., Lawhorne, L., et al. 2008. Understanding clinical dehydration and its treatment. *Journal of the American Medical Directors Association* 9(5):292–301.

Vaara, S. T., Korhonen, A. M., Kaukonen, K. M., et al. 2012. Fluid overload is associated with an increased risk for 90-day mortality in critically ill patients with renal replacement therapy: Data from the prospective FINNAKI study. *Critical Care (London, England)* 16(5):R197.

Verbalis, J. G. 2003. Disorders of body water homeostasis. *Best Practice & Research. Clinical Endocrinology & Metabolism* 17: 471–503. DOI: 10. 1016/S1521-690X(03)00049-6.

Vogelaere, P., Pereira, C. 2005. Thermoregulation and aging. *Revista portuguesa de cardiologia: orgao oficial da Sociedade Portuguesa de Cardiologia = Portuguese Journal of Cardiology: An Official Journal of the Portuguese Society of Cardiology* 24(5):747–761.

Voyer, P., Cole, M. G., McCusker, J., St-Jacques, S., Laplante, J. 2008. Accuracy of nurse documentation of delirium symptoms in medical charts. *International Journal of Nursing Practice* 14(2):165–177.

Wang, Z., Deurenberg, P., Wang, W., Pietrobelli, A., Baumgartner, R. N., Heymsfield, S. B. 1999. Hydration of fat-free body mass: Review and critique of a classic body-composition constant. *The American Journal of Clinical Nutrition* 69(5):833–841.

Wilkes, M. M., Navickis, R. J. 2001. Patient survival after human albumin administration. A meta-analysis of randomized, controlled trials. *Annals of Internal Medicine* 135(3):149–164.

Young, P., Bailey, M., Beasley, R., et al. 2015. Effect of a buffered crystalloid solution vs saline on acute kidney injury among patients in the intensive care unit: The SPLIT randomized clinical trial. *JAMA* 314(16):1701–1710.

Young, R. J., Beerman, L. E., Vanderhoof, J. A. 1998. Increasing oral fluids in chronic constipation in children. *Gastroenterology Nursing: The Official Journal of the Society of Gastroenterology Nurses and Associates* 21(4):156–161.

Yunos, N. M., Bellomo, R., Hegarty, C., Story, D., Ho, L., Bailey, M. 2012. Association between a chloride-liberal vs chloride-restrictive intravenous fluid administration strategy and kidney injury in critically ill adults. *JAMA* 308(15):1566–1572.

Yunos, N. M., Bellomo, R., Story, D., Kellum, J. 2010. Bench-to-bedside review: Chloride in critical illness. *Critical Care (London, England)* 14(4):226.

13

Electrolytes in health and disease

INTRODUCTION

Electrolyte is a substance that produces electrical conductivity when dissolved in water. In the dissolved state, the electrolytes are dispersed as anions and cations. The cations are attracted to the electrodes which have abundant electrons, whereas anions are attracted to the electrodes having deficiency of electrons. The movement of anions and cations is in opposite directions, which determines the amount of current. The important electrolytes are salts, acids, bases and some gases like hydrochloric acid. The electrolyte can also be formed by the dissolution of DNA, polypeptides and polystyrene sulfonates. All the electrolytes have a capacity to conduct electricity. Sodium, potassium, calcium, magnesium, bicarbonate and phosphate are important electrolytes in humans, animals and plants. Electrolytes are essential for body functioning, maintaining intracellular neutrality, generation and conduction of action potentials in nerves and muscles. Abnormalities in sodium, magnesium, calcium and bases may result in central nervous system (CNS) abnormalities in the form of altered sensorium and seizures, whereas abnormalities in potassium and calcium may result in neuromuscular weakness. All the electrolytes are closely linked to cellular excitability; therefore, these may be associated with cardiac and gastrointestinal abnormalities. Both increase and decrease in electrolytes beyond the physiological limits may pose health hazards. Homeostasis of electrolytes is efficiently maintained by the kidney and neuroendocrine system. In this chapter, the common electrolyte abnormalities and their clinical management are presented

HISTORY

The word "electrolyte" is derived from the Greek word (*Electro*=related to electricity, *Lytos*=ability to unite or loosen). Svante Arrhenius in 1884 demonstrated dissociation of solid crystalline salt into pairs of charged particles when dissolved. He was awarded Nobel Prize in Chemistry in 1903. Many years earlier, Michel Faraday named ions and postulated that ions are produced by electrolysis. The term sodium is derived from the Latin word *Natriun*. Sodium is the sixth most abundant element in earth crust and was first isolated by Sir Humphry Davy in 1807. Humphry Davy also discovered potassium in the same year when he passed current through wet potash. Potash is known for centuries, and is the only element present the nature in ionic form. The symbol of potassium "K" is derived from Latin word *Kalium*. Sodium chloride is the commonest form of chlorine used as early as 6000 BC as rock salt. Chlorine gas was recognized in 1613 by a Flemish chemist Jan Baptist van Helmont and was studied in detail by a Swedish chemist Carl Wilhelm Scheele in 1774. In 1810, Sir Humphry Davy discovered chloride as an element. Calcium was named after the Latin word *Calx* (lime) which was also isolated by Davy in 1808. Calcium compounds were known from ancient times, but their chemistry was unknown. Calcium is the fifth most abundant element in the human body. Magnesium originates from the Greek word *Magnetes*, which refers to the location of a tribe. In 1618, a farmer at Epson in England noticed that cows refused to drink water from a well because of bitter taste. However, this water was able to heal scratches and rashes. This became famous as Epson salt and eventually was recognized as magnesium sulfate. Magnesium was also discovered by Sir Humphry Davy in 1808 in England. It is the ninth most abundant element in the universe and 11th most abundant in the human body and participates in more than 300 enzymatic reactions.

Hennig Brand was a German merchant, pharmacist and chemist in Hamburg who had an elusive goal to create a philosopher's tomb. For this purpose, he heated a mixture of sand, charcoal and tar-like substance produced by boiling 1200 gallons of urine. This mixture was heated at the highest possible temperature in a furnace. A white vapor was formed after several hours which condensed to a thick and glittering drop. Brand named it phosphorous (*Latin = emitting light*).

SODIUM

The human body needs a small amount of sodium to generate nerve impulses and contracting and relaxing muscles, and to maintain the proper balance of water, minerals and tonicity. It is estimated that humans need only 500 mg of sodium daily for these vital functions. The 2015–2020 Dietary Guidelines for Americans recommend daily consumption of less than 2.3 g as a healthy eating pattern, but an average intake of an American is more than 3.4 g daily. World Health Organization recommends a maximum of 5 g/day (WHO, 2012), and the salt intake in India is much higher than the recommended dose, about 11 g/day. High salt intake is associated with hypertension and increases the risk of cerebrovascular and cardiovascular complications. The salt content in various food items is summarized in Tables 13.1 and 13.2.

Serum sodium and osmolality: Solute and particle concentrations refer to osmolality expressed as mOsmol/kg or mMol/l. Water is easily diffusible across the membrane and allows maintaining equilibrium between intracellular and extracellular fluid osmolality. The solutes in the extracellular and intracellular space however differs, and the gradient is maintained by ion channel transporters and ATP-dependent membrane pump. Sodium and its accompanying anions (Cl, HCO_3) are the major components of extracellular fluid (ECF), whereas potassium and organic phosphate esters (ATP, phospholipid, creatine phosphate) are the components of intracellular fluid (ICF). The tonicity of ICF and ECF is determined by the concentration of solutes, which are restricted in the respective compartment. Urea is an ineffective osmol as it does not lead to water shift across the membrane.

Sodium homeostasis: Water intake, vasopressin and absorption of water and solute by kidney

Table 13.1 Sodium content in various food items

Food	Sodium content mg/10 g
Table salt, baking powder, baking soda	3800
Bouillon cubes, powdered broths, soups, gravies	2000
Soy sauce	700
Snacks (cheese puffs, popcorn), Bacon	150
Sauces and spreads	120
Cheese, hard	80
Processed vegetables	60
Butter/margarine	50
Cheese(soft), processed fish	40
Cereals and its products (breakfast cereals, bread, biscuits, cakes, pastries)	25
Fish (raw or frozen)	10
Eggs	8
Milk and cream	5
Vegetables (fresh or frozen)	1
Fruits (fresh or frozen)	0.5

100 mg = 4.35 mmol

Table 13.2 Salt content in various raw and process foods

Vegetarian food	Sodium (mg/100 g)	Nonvegetarian	Sodium (mg/100 g)
Bran		**Beef**	
Bran, wheat	28	Topside, roast, lean and fat	48
Bran flakes	1,000	Corned beef, canned	950
Cheese		**Crab**	
Hard cheese, average	620	Boiled	370
Processed	1,320	Canned	550
Chickpeas		**Cod**	
Dried, boiled in unsalted water	5	Cod, in butter, fried in blended oil	100
Canned, re-heated, drained	220		
		Fish fingers, fried in blended oil	350
New potatoes		**Salmon**	
Raw, boiled in unsalted water	9	Raw, steamed	110
Canned, re-heated, drained	250	Canned	570
		Smoked	1,880
Peanuts		**Tuna**	
Plain	2	Raw	47
Dry roasted	790	Canned in oil, drained	290
Roasted and salted	400	Canned in brine, drained	320
Peas			
Raw, boiled in unsalted water	Trace		
Canned, re-heated, drained	250		
Potato chips			
Homemade, fried in blended oil	12		
French fries, oven chips, frozen, baked	53		
Sweet corn			
On-the-cob, whole, boiled in unsalted water	1		
Kernels, canned, re-heated, drained	270		

maintain body fluid osmolality in a narrow range of 280–295 mOsm/kg. Vasopressin is released from magnocellular neurons of hypothalamus and their axons project to posterior pituitary which release arginine vasopressin (AVP) in the circulation. The magnocellular neurons have osmoreceptors which determine the synthesis of AVP. These osmoreceptor neurons are very sensitive to osmotic changes. A rise of osmolality from 280 to 285 mOsm/kg results in release of AVP, and thirst is generated between 288 and 294 mOsm/kg. Volume status is an important determinant of AVP release. Hypovolemia triggers AVP release, and hypervolemia inhibits. Certain nonosmolar stimuli such as nausea, intra-cerebral angiotensin II, serotonin and several drugs may also trigger AVP release.

Sodium is filtered by glomeruli, which is sequentially reabsorbed by the renal tubules with the help of the renin–angiotensin–aldosterone system under the influence of sympathetic activity. Sodium absorption is associated with absorption of chloride which may exchange with bicarbonate. In 24 h, glomeruli filter about 180 l of fluid and 25,200 mM of sodium in a person having serum sodium of 140 mEq/l. This amounts to 1.5 kg salt which is 10 times the salt present in extracellular space. About 99.6% of this glomerular filtrate is reabsorbed, 75% in the proximal convoluted tubule and the remaining in the loop of Henle and distal collecting tubules. Hyponatremia is a disorder of water balance in which there is relative excess of body water compared to sodium and potassium.

DEFINITION AND CAUSES OF HYPONATREMIA

Normal serum sodium ranges between 135 and 145 mEq/l. Hyponatremia is defined when serum sodium is less than 135 mEq/l. Hyponatremia is the commonest electrolyte abnormality. A systematic analysis evaluating the pooled estimated means of hyponatremia over four decades revealed the prevalence of mild hyponatremia in hospitalized geriatric population in 22.2%, in nongeriatric patients in 6% and in critical care setting in 17.2%. The prevalence of severe hyponatremia (< 125 mEq/l) is 4.5% in geriatric, 0.8% in nongeriatric and 10.3% in ICU populations (Mannesse et al., 2013). In ambulatory population, hyponatremia has been reported in 4%–7%, which increases in the individuals residing in nursing homes. Hyponatremia, even mild, is associated with high mortality; therefore, it is important to diagnose and treat (Mistry et al., 2016; Braun et al., 2015).

ETIOLOGY

Hyponatremia is not a disease but a syndrome of low serum sodium associated with a variety of underlying causes such as cardiac failure, renal failure, cirrhosis, diarrhea, vomiting, endocrinal and iatrogenic etiologies (Table 13.3).

The elderly patients are more prone to develop hyponatremia due to associated comorbidities, multiple medications, and age-related impairment of thirst, renal and neurological functions. Acute central nervous system (CNS) diseases such as stroke, meningitis, encephalitis and subarachnoid hemorrhage and neurosurgical procedures are important causes of hyponatremia. In hospitalized neurological patients, the frequency of hyponatremia is about 43% in stroke, 36% in subarachnoid hemorrhage, 22.7% in viral encephalitis, 44.3% in tuberculous meningitis, 32% in pyogenic meningitis and 19% in aseptic meningitis (Chen et al., 2019;

Mapa et al., 2016; Misra et al., 2016; Misra et al., 2019; Karandanis and Shulman, 1976; Czupryna et al., 2014; Kalita et al., 2017).

PATHOPHYSIOLOGY

The osmolality is primarily dependent on serum sodium and its associated anions. It is important to understand the concept of total osmolality and effective osmolality. Total osmolality refers to the concentration of all the solutes in a given weight of water mOsm/kg regardless of solutes' capability to cross the biological membrane. Effective osmolality or tonicity refers to the number of osmoles that contribute to water movement across intracellular and extracellular compartment. Osmotic pressure gradient is dependent on effective solute. Generally, hyponatremia is associated with hypotonicity of intravascular space leading to cellular edema and if severe with clinical manifestations. Rarely isotonic hyponatremia may occur due to serum glucose or mannitol. Hyponatremia leads to hypotonicity of ICF resulting in shift of water from plasma to intracellular space, leading to swelling of neurons, glia and other cells. Brain is covered by a rigid skull; therefore, any increase in volume results in raised intracranial pressure and brain herniation much before other organ dysfunctions manifest. In chronic hyponatremia, brain adapts by extruding potassium and organic solutes to extracellular space, thereby reducing osmotic gradient.

Osmoregulation and release of vasopressin: Plasma osmolality is maintained by a coordinated function of hypothalamus, pituitary and kidney. Antidiuretic hormone (ADH) is released from the posterior pituitary due to stimulation of osmoreceptor of the hypothalamus in response to high plasma osmolality, which increases water reabsorption from renal tubule, thereby reducing serum osmolality. The reverse occurs when plasma osmolality is low. Osmoreceptors are present in the anterior hypothalamus. Decrease in stretch of neurons

Table 13.3 Causes of hyponatremia

Systemic diseases: heart failure, renal failure, cirrhosis of liver
Endocrinal: Addison disease, hypothyroidism, hypopituitarism, hypoaldosteronism, syndrome of inappropriate secretion of antidiuretic hormone (SIADH)
Gastrointestinal: diarrhea, vomiting
Excessive water drinking
Latrogenic: diuretics, nonsteroid anti-inflammatory drugs, antidepressants, amphetamine

increases their firing rate leading to release of AVP from the posterior pituitary gland and generation of thirst. The threshold for AVP release is lower than that of thirst. Change in serum osmolality regulates the release of vasopressin. The central osmoreceptors [transient receptor potential vanil-lodi 1 (TRPV1)] and peripheral osmoreceptors (TRPV4) give information about serum osmolality. TRPV1 is expressed in the vasopressin producing magnocellular cells and circumventricular organ in response to osmolality. TRPV4 is present in dorsal root ganglia innervating the blood vessels and is able to sense hyperosmolar shift in blood (Lechner et al., 2011; Liedtke et al., 2000).

CLINICAL FEATURES

The symptoms of hyponatremia depend on the rapidity of onset and severity of hyponatremia. Acute hyponatremia refers to development of hyponatremia within 48h and chronic if it evolves after 48h. Rapidly developing hyponatremia has more severe clinical manifestations because brain has little time to adapt to hypotonic environment. On the other hand, chronic hyponatremia has milder symptoms even with relatively lower serum sodium level because of adaptation. The adaptation is due to endogenous intracellular production of osmotically active solutes, e.g., potassium and organic solutes. Based on the serum sodium level, the severity of hyponatremia can be categorized into (Spasovski et al., 2014):

Mild: 130–134 mM/l
Moderate: 129–120 mM/l
Severe: < 120 mM/l

The symptoms of hyponatremia are nonspecific and can range from mild confusion to deep coma. A majority of patients with mild hyponatremia remain asymptomatic but may have subtle findings. The patient with hyponatremia may present with polydipsia, muscle cramps, confusion, headache, obtundation, altered sensorium, coma, seizure and status epilepticus. Chronic hyponatremia may result in gait abnormality, osteoporosis and fracture. The clinical features of hyponatremia are presented in Table 13.4.

CLASSIFICATION OF HYPONATREMIA

Hyponatremia may be classified based on volume status into hypovolemic, euvolemic and hypervolemic, the causes of which are summarized in Table 13.5. It is however difficult to assess the volume status using clinical and laboratory markers. The sensitivity of clinical signs and symptoms for diagnosis of hyponatremia is low.

Hypovolemic hyponatremia: Hypovolemic hyponatremia occurs in cerebral salt wasting (CSW), diuretic use, diarrhea, vomiting, Addison disease, pituitary failure, hypothalamic failure, osmotic diuresis, nephropathies, burn and in bowel obstructions. These patients usually manifest with hypovolemic state such as tachycardia, vomiting, diarrhea and elevated blood urea nitrogen to creatinine ratio. Urinary sodium usually is below 20 mEq/l, unless there is renal cause of sodium loss. In the patients receiving diuretics, urinary urea may be a better indicator as these patients may have diuretic induced natriuresis. Fractional excretion of urea less than 35% is more sensitive and specific for the diagnosis of pre-renal azotemia (Carvounis et al., 2002). The treatment of hypovolemic hyponatremia is volume replacement using normal saline or oral salt supplementation. The underlying cause should be treated. Intake output monitoring is important for volume correction.

Table 13.4 Clinical features of hyponatremia

Mild	Moderate	Severe
Asymptomatic	Nausea	Vomiting
Nonspecific	Headache	Cardiorespiratory distress
	Confusion	Confusion
		Somnolence
		Obtundation
		Seizure
		Coma

Table 13.5 Causes of euvolemic, hypovolemic and hypervolemic hyponatremia

Euvolemic	Hypovolemic	Hypervolemic

Endocrinal
  Hypothyroidism
  Adrenal insufficiency
	Diabetes, corticosteroid
	  withdrawal
		Heart failure

Hypertonic fluid administration	Sweating, burn	Chronic renal failure

Syndrome of inappropriate
  secretion of antidiuretic
  hormone
	Ketonuria	Cirrhosis of liver

	Iatrogenic (hypotonic fluid)	Iatrogenic (hypertonic solution)

	Cerebral salt wasting	Syndrome of inappropriate
		  secretion of antidiuretic
		  hormone

Euvolemic hyponatremia: Euvolemic hyponatremia occurs in SIADH, hypothyroidism, glucocorticoid deficiency and amphetamine ecstasy. Diagnosis is based on clinical examination, low serum uric acid, normal BUN to creatinine ratio and spot urine sodium >20mEq/l. One must enquire the history of diuretic use and low salt diet which may facetiously elevate or reduce urinary sodium concentration. Treatment is fluid restriction by 500 ml less than the urinary output in the previous 24h. Patients should be allowed to take salt and protein. The patients with a urinary osmolality of more than 500 mOsm/kg, 24h urine volume less than 1.5 l, slow correction rate of serum sodium (<20 mEq/l) in 48h and serum sodium concentration lower than sum of urinary sodium and potassium concentration are unlikely to respond adequately (Verbalis et al., 2013). In difficult situations, volume expansion by 500 ml normal saline infusion may help in diagnosing SIADH, in which serum sodium will be decreased from baseline.

Hypervolemic hyponatremia: Hypervolemic hyponatremia occurs in cirrhosis of liver, heart failure, nephrotic syndrome and acute or chronic renal failure. Clinically, the patient has hypervolemic state, e.g., engorged neck veins, edema, central venous pressure more than 6cm of water, inferior vena cava diameter >21 mm and urinary sodium less than 20 mEq/l. If hypervolemic state is due to heart failure, fluid restriction to 1 l/day and diuretics are useful. The management of primary state depends on the underlying cause.

There are two important causes of hyponatremia in neurology practice: SIADH and CSW.

SIADH is attributed to inappropriate secretion of antidiuretic hormone (ADH) resulting in low serum osmolality and increase in water absorption. This leads to expansion of extracellular volume and delutional hyponatremia despite normal renal sodium handling. SIADH is a volume expanded state, but most patients do not show clinical evidence of hypervolemia because only one-third of total retained water is in extracellular space. Release of ADH in SIADH is attributed to a large number of conditions: CNS (meningitis, encephalitis, stroke, subarachnoid hemorrhage and trans-spheroidal surgery), pulmonary diseases (pneumonia, lung cancer), malignant conditions, surgery and drugs (carbamazepine, oxcarbazepine, SSRI and cyclophosphamide).

Cerebral salt wasting refers to a primary natriuresis leading to hyponatremia and volume depletion without a known stimulus for natriuresis. Cerebral salt wasting is attributed to a number of natriuretic factors such as ANP (atrial natriuretic factor), BNP (brain derived natriuretic factor from ventricle), and C type natriuretic factor following a dysregulated sympathetic response. The level of ANP and BNP does not help in differentiation of CSW and SIADH because of the compensatory mechanism. In SIADH, hyponatremia is aggravated by 100 ml normal saline infusion, whereas it leads to improvement of serum sodium in CSW. Frusemide 20 mg IV may improve serum sodium in SIADH but not in CSW. The safety and reliability of these tests however have not been validated (Casulari et al., 2004). SIADH and CSW may have overlapping clinical and laboratory features such as hyponatremia, low serum osmolality, high urinary sodium and osmolality. The most reliable differentiating feature is evidence of low extra cellular volume in CSW and is normal or increased in SIADH.

Some authors therefore do not differentiate between CSW and SIADH, and have suggested a term "hyponatremia natriuretic syndrome" (Narotam et al., 1994) or "cerebral salt wanting syndrome" (Sterns and Silver, 2008). We however feel comfortable in differentiating CSW and SIADH using the following simple bedside criteria.

Diagnosis of cerebral salt wasting: Cerebral salt wasting syndrome should be considered in the presence of the following features:

Essential: (all required)

1. Polyuria (24 h urine output > 3 l for at least 2 consecutive days).
2. Hyponatremia: serum sodium < 135 mEq/l on two occasions 24 h apart.
3. Exclusion of secondary causes of hyponatremia such as endocrine abnormalities, renal, cardiac or hepatic failure, or diuretics.

Supportive criteria: At least three out of five of the following:

1. Clinical evidence of hypovolemia such as hypotension, dry mucous membrane, tachycardia or postural hypotension.
2. Persistent negative fluid balance as revealed by intake output chart and/or weight loss.
3. Laboratory evidence of dehydration such as elevated hematocrit, hemoglobin, serum albumin or blood urea nitrogen.
4. Central venous pressure (CVP) < 6 cm of water.
5. Urinary sodium > 40 mEq/l or urine osmolality > 300 mOsm/l in two consecutive occasions (Misra et al., 2018).

MANAGEMENT OF HYPONATREMIA

Urgent treatment of hyponatremia is lifesaving, although a proper assessment of the patient may not be possible because of shock, sedation, primary CNS disease or mechanical ventilation in the ICU. The treatment depends on the severity of hyponatremia. Mild chronic hyponatremia may be treated with additional 5–12 g salt/day. Severe acute symptomatic hyponatremia should be urgently treated as it may result in brain edema, brain herniation and respiratory arrest. Caution should be taken not to overcorrect serum sodium. Treatment is initiated with 3% saline at a rate of 0.5–2 ml/kg/h till symptoms resolve.

The rate of sodium correction should not exceed by 10 mEq/l in first 24 h, and 8 mEq/l in the next 24 h. An increase in serum sodium of 4–6 mEq/l is sufficient to reduce symptoms of acute hyponatremia (Braun et al., 2015; Sterns et al., 2009). As per European Guideline, 150 ml of 3% saline is administered in 20 min and serum sodium is checked every 20 min; 3% saline should be repeated till symptoms improve and target rise of serum sodium of 5 mEq/l is achieved (Spasovski et al., 2014). Rapid correction of serum sodium can result in osmotic demyelination. Over correction is typically caused by rapid diuresis secondary to reduction of ADH. Frequent monitoring of serum sodium may prevent over correction. In a study of 25 patients with severe hyponatremia below 120 mEq/l revealed that administration of weight adjusted 3% saline and 1–2 mg of desmopressin 6–8 hourly resulted in serum sodium correction of 3–7 mEq/l/h without overcorrection (Sood et al., 2013). In another study, 3% saline bolus in 10 min improved serum sodium at a rate of 1.5–2 mEq/l/h without overcorrection (Sood et al., 2013; Verbalis et al., 2013). In the resource poor setting where the facilities for frequent serum sodium measurement are not possible, 100–150 ml of 3% saline may be administered in 1–2 h, and if there is symptomatic improvement further correction is possible by IV normal saline and oral salt 5–12 g orally or through Ryles tube and serum sodium may be checked as frequently as possible. In cerebral salt wasting in tuberculous meningitis and subarachnoid hemorrhage, additional use of fludrocortisone or hydrocortisone may normalize serum sodium and volume status early (Misra et al., 2018; Mistry et al., 2016).

Vaptans (conivaptan, lixivaptan, satavaptan and tolvaptan) are vasopressin receptor antagonists (VRAs) and are tried in the treatment of hypervolemic or euvolemic form of hyponatremia. A review of 20 trials including 2900 patients comparing VRA vs placebo in mild to moderate hyponatremia did not reduce death. A subgroup analysis, however, revealed insignificant increased risk of death in the patients with hypervolemia (Rezen-Zvi et al., 2010). Updated analysis of trials after that by Rezen-Zvi revealed that VRA increased serum sodium at 3–7 days (MD 4.3, 95% CI 3.51–4.95 mM/l) and at 7 months (MD 3.49, 95% CI 3.59–5.02); there was no difference in adverse events, but the risk of rapid increase in serum sodium was 60% higher in VRA group compared to placebo (RR 1.61, 85% CI 1.11–2.33) which was consistent in various VRAs. Subsequently, there were reports of osmotic demyelination leading to neurological sequelae in patients receiving tolvaptan (Di Benedetto and See, 2013) leading to drug safety communication by FDA (Torres et al., 2012). Moreover, there are concerns about high alanine aminotransferase (4.4% vs 1%) (U.S. Food and Drug Administration, 2013).

HYPERNATREMIA

Hypernatremia is defined as serum sodium more than 145 mM/l and is associated with high mortality in hospitalized patients (Leung et al., 2013; Gankam-Kengne et al., 2013). Hypernatremia can occur due to excessive water loss or poor water intake and rarely following high intake of sodium. The patients with poor thirst and those with low water intake as in impaired consciousness, mechanical intubation and old age are prone to hypernatremia.

Pathophysiology: Hypernatremia invariably increases plasma osmolality thereby resulting in cellular dehydration due to shift of water from intracellular space to extracellular space. On the first day of hypernatremia, brain volume is restored due to shift of water from CSF to the cell. There may be increase in interstitial fluid. In chronic hypernatremia, the cellular tonicity is maintained initially by shift of sodium and potassium and replacing these intracellular solutes by organic solutes (idiogenic osmoles). The animal and cell culture studies have revealed that organic solutes found in the brain cells are similar to the other cells for regulation of volume. These solutes are myoinositol, taurine, glyceryl phosphoryl choline and betaine. The organic solutes are taken up with the help of sodium-dependent co-transporter. In the brain, organic solute is mostly composed of myoinositol and amino acids (glutamine and glutamate). Myoinositol is taken up by sodium-myoinositol-cotransporter of the cell membrane.

Causes of hypernatremia: Hypernatremia occurs following excessive loss of water (pure water or hypotonic water) or gain of sodium due to sodium overloading or iatrogenic causes. The common causes of hypernatremia are presented in Table 13.6. The rise of sodium normally is proportional to the rise of osmolality resulting in increased thirst. In a situation, when the thirst is reduced such as in elderly, children intubation and mechanical ventilation or patients with altered sensorium may develop hypernatremia.

Symptoms of hypernatremia: The symptoms of hypernatremia can differ in infants and adults. Infants with hypernatremia may have tachycardia, restlessness, muscle weakness, shrill cry, insomnia, lethargy and coma. Seizures are less common in hypernatremia and occur following rapid rehydration. In adults, the symptoms of hypernatremia

Table 13.6 Causes of hypernatremia in reference to plasma volume

Hypovolemic	Euvolemic	Hypervolemic
Skin: burn, sweating	Poor water intake	Cushing syndrome
GI tract: diarrhea, vomiting, fistula	Extra renal loss: tachypnea, mechanical ventilation sweating with fever	Hyperaldosteronism
Renal: diuretic, mannitol, glucose, urea, intrinsic renal disease	Resetting of osmostat: essential hypernatremia	Hemodialysis
Post obstruction	Drugs: amphotericin B, phenytoin, lithium	Iatrogenic: salt tablet, saline infusion, IV bicarbonate infusion, enteral feeding
Head injury	Renal loss: nephrogenic diabetes insipidus, central diabetes insipidus	
	Sickle cell disease	
	Pituitary tumor	

are milder and include lethargy, weakness, restlessness, nausea and vomiting. Severe symptoms in hypernatremia occur if there is rapid rise of serum sodium level more than 160 mEq/l. Hypernatremia may result in brain shrinkage leading to vascular rupture; thereby intra-cerebral or subarachnoid hemorrhage. The clinical features of hypernatremia are summarized in Table 13.7.

Diagnosis: History and physical examination often give a clue to the underlying cause of hypernatremia. The diagnosis of hypernatremia is done by serum sodium above 145 mEq/l. The causes of hypernatremia are different based on the serum osmolality (Table 13.6).

Treatment: Treatment of the underlying cause is most important, and correcting the water deficit is the first step in the management of hypernatremia. If possible oral or enteral water should be used to correct the water deficit. Rapid correction of serum sodium can result in brain edema; therefore, lower than the calculated deficit of water should be used. In the patients with rapid development of hypernatremia, serum sodium can be corrected with 5% dextrose without increasing the risk of cerebral edema. Sodium correction at a rate of 1 mEq/l/h is considered safe (Pfennig et al., 2012; Reynolds et al., 2006). In the patients with chronic hypernatremia, the rate of correction of serum sodium should be 0.5 mEq/l/h with no more than 8–10 mEq/l/24 h (Reynolds et al., 2006; Adrogue and Madias, 2000; Vaishya et al., 2012). The target serum sodium should be 145 mEq/l. In case of central diabetes insipidus, desmopressin nasal spray or oral tablet may be used with close monitoring for water intoxication. In nephrogenic diabetes insipidus, offending drugs may be withdrawn, and in selected cases, thiazide dietetics or nonsteroidal anti-inflammatory drugs may be tried. The following formula is used for calculation of water deficit:

Water deficit = Current body water x weight x (serum Na/140–1)

It is practical to use 10% less than the value of body water at that particular age. In a 60 kg man with serum sodium of 160 mEq/l and current body water at 60 years is considered 45% (considering 10% less), the body water deficit is calculated as follows

Water deficit = 0.45 × 60 × (160/140–1) = 3.78 l

While supplementing fluid, one should add insensible, urinary and fecal loss. In a patient with hypernatremia, isotonic saline is not preferred as it does not significantly lower serum sodium. Moreover in patient with ongoing hypotonic fluid loss, normal saline may aggravate hypernatremia. It is therefore better to use 5% dextrose intravenously, and if patient can drink, free water can be given orally or through nasogastric tube. Caution should be exercised not to over correct water to prevent water intoxication. As in hyponatremia, serum sodium should be frequently monitored to avoid over and rapid correction.

Prognosis: Hypernatremia is associated with high mortality (10%–70%). In children, acute hypernatremia may have mortality up to 70%, and two-third of the survivors have neurological sequelae. In adults, hypernatremia above 160 mEq/l is associated with 75% mortality. Chronic hypernatremia however has a mortality of 10% (Adrogue and Madias, 2000).

POTASSIUM

Introduction

Potassium is an important intracellular cation, and all the cells maintain intracellular potassium gradient through the help of $Na^+-K^+-ATPase$ pump by which sodium is extruded and potassium enters into the cell. The potential difference between intracellular and extracellular compartment is necessary for generation of action potential and cellular function. About 2% of potassium is in extracellular fluid giving a concentration of 3.5–5 mEq/l. Potassium helps in cell division and growth by catalyzing many enzymatic reactions. Intracellular potassium also regulates acid–base balance by exchanging hydrogen ion and regulating rate of renal ammonia production. High

Table 13.7 Signs and symptoms of hypernatremia

Neurological: intense thirst, irritability, focal neurological deficit, altered sensorium, coma, seizure (rare), spasticity, rigidity
Systemic: fever, nausea, vomiting, tachypnea, signs of volume depletion (sunken eye, loss of skin turgor, tenting of skin)

extracellular potassium reduces membrane potential whereas hyperkalemia results in hyperpolarization of membrane (Kardalas et al., 2018). Imbalance of potassium can result in disruption of cardiac rhythm, muscle weakness and sudden cardiac death.

POTASSIUM HOMEOSTASIS

Daily potassium intake is about 100 mEq (1800 mg); of which 90% is excreted in the urine and, 10% in the feces; thus potassium level is intricately balanced (Figure 13.1). The common food items rich in potassium are mentioned in Table 13.8. Potassium content in muscle, bone, liver, RBC and extracellular fluid affect the internal potassium balance. Kidney plays an important role in maintaining total body potassium balance. Renal potassium excretion is a slow process requiring several hours; therefore, the initial buffering of extracellular potassium occurs by shifting of potassium in or out of muscles. The shift of potassium across the muscle membrane depends on intracellular potassium, insulin and catecholamine level. Increase in extracellular potassium concentration stimulates aldosterone secretion via angiotensin II, which increases urinary excretion of potassium. Two important determinants of potassium excretion are mineralocorticoid activity and distal delivery of water and sodium. Aldosterone is the main mineralocorticoid hormone and is responsible for renal sodium absorption and, renal potassium excretion

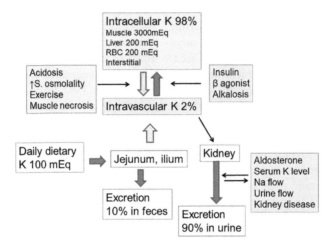

Figure 13.1 Schematic diagram showing potassium (K) homeostasis.

Table 13.8 Foods rich in potassium

Food	mg of K/100 g of food
Nuts	600
Beans and peas	1300
Salmon	628
Large white beans	561
Avocados	485
Green vegetables	550
Potatoes	535
Acorn squash	437
Milk	150
Button mushroom	356
Banana, papaya, dates	300
Tomatoes, pumpkin, cucumber	300

in the distal convoluted tubule and collecting duct. Aldosterone also shifts potassium from extracellular to intracellular space by stimulating Na^+-K^+-ATPase pump in the basolateral membrane. Aldosterone also increases renal sodium absorption thereby restoring extracellular fluid (ECF) volume. In hyperkalemic state, aldosterone release is modulated by direct effect on the cell zona glomerulosa. In hypovolemia, aldosterone results in absorption of sodium without potassium excretion whereas in hyperkalemic state, there is increased excretion of potassium without increased sodium excretion, which is known as *aldosterone paradox* (Wang and Giebisch, 2009).

Potassium is filtered by glomeruli, and all the filtered potassium is absorbed in proximal renal tubule and loop of Henle by a passive process of sodium and water reabsorption. In distal renal tubule and collecting duct, potassium is absorbed through potassium channel. H^+-K^+-ATPase system helps in hydrogen ion secretion and potassium absorption. Hyperkalemia therefore is common in renal failure especially if glomerular filtration rate is less than 20 ml/min.

HYPOKALEMIA

Potassium disorders are common. Hypokalemia is defined as serum potassium below 3.5 mEq/l, and occurs in up to 21% in hospitalized patients and 2%–3% in outpatient population (Paice et al., 1986; Lippi et al., 2010; Liamis et al., 2013). Hyperkalemia is defined as serum potassium more than 5 mEq/l in adults, more than 5.5 mEq/l in children and more than 6 mEq/l in neonates. Hyperkalemia occurs in 6% of hospitalized and 1% of outpatient population (Paice et al., 1986; Liamis et al., 2013).

Causes of hypokalemia: Hypokalemia occurs due to excessive loss or intracellular shift of potassium. Excessive loss of potassium either through kidney or GI tract is the commonest cause. Inadequate intake is a rare cause of hypokalemia. Diuretics are the commonest cause of hypokalemia mainly following thiazide, chlorthalidone or loop diuretics. About 80% individual on diuretic therapy develop hypokalemia which is dose dependent and generally mild (3–3.5 mEq/l) unless associated with other causes. Various endocrinal, renal and GI causes may result in hypokalemia (Table 13.9).

Clinical features: The clinical features of hypokalemia depend on the severity and rapidity of hypokalemia. Patients are usually symptomatic if serum potassium is less than 3 mEq/l. The cardiac patients on digitalis therapy may be symptomatic at higher serum potassium level. Patients may develop metabolic acidosis, tubulo-intestinal disease and renal cyst formation. The neurological manifestations include muscle cramps, muscle paralysis and sometime there may be rhabdomyolysis in severe metabolic acidosis. Gastrointestinal

Table 13.9 Causes of hypokalemia

Increased potassium loss	Trans-cellular shift of potassium	Inadequate intake
Gastrointestinal: chronic vomiting, diarrhea, bentonite (clay) ingestion, villious adenoma of colon	Drugs: insulin, beta agonist, decongestant, xanthine, amphotericin B, verapamil, chloroquine, barium, cesium	Anorexia, diarrhea, starvation
Drugs: diuretic, laxative, corticosteroid	Alkalosis, refeeding syndrome, diabetes insipidus, head injury, myocardial infarction, sympathetic stimulation, thyrotoxicosis, hypothermia	Pseudohypokalemia: Delayed estimation, Leukocytosis>75,000/mm^3
Renal: osmotic diuretic, renal tubular acidosis, aldosteronism, Bartter syndrome, Gitelman syndrome, Liddle syndrome, Fanconi syndrome, hypomagnesemia, dialysis, plasmapheresis	Familial hypokalemic periodic paralysis	

Table 13.10 Clinical features of hypokalemia

1. Mild hypokalemia:
   Asymptomatic or mild symptoms in elderly or cardiac patients
2. Moderate to severe hypokalemia:
   Neurological: Cramp, paralysis, rhabdomyolysis
   Cardiovascular: ECG changes (U waves, T wave flattening, ST-segment changes),
     cardiac arrhythmias, heart failure, sudden death
   Gastrointestinal: Constipation, paralytic ileus
   Renal: Metabolic acidosis, tubular interstitial nephritis, nephrogenic diabetes insipidus
   Respiratory: Respiratory paralysis due to muscle weakness or metabolic acidosis

symptoms include constipation, and paralytic ileus in severe cases. Patients may have ECG changes initially (U wave, flat T wave, ST segment changes) followed by cardiac arrhythmia and sudden death in severe hypokalemia (Table 13.10).

Laboratory investigation

The aim of investigation is to find out severity of hypokalemia and underlying cause because treatment aims not only at restoration of serum potassium level but also associated acid–base, magnesium and other biochemical abnormalities. The basic investigations include serum chemistry (serum potassium, sodium, magnesium, calcium, and creatinine, blood urea nitrogen, glucose, and thyroid stimulating hormone), urine potassium and chloride, arterial or venous blood gas analysis and ECG. The other specific tests should be guided by clinical history, family history and evidence of hypertension.

Urinary potassium 15 mEq/l/day or spot urine potassium/creatinine ratio more than 1.5 mEq/mmol suggest renal loss of potassium. In the next step, arterial or venous blood gas analysis, serum chloride, magnesium and bicarbonate give indication of underlying etiology as follows (Kardalas et al., 2018; Viera and Wouk 2018):

1. Asymptomatic/mildly symptomatic hypokalemia and low urinary potassium excretion with metabolic acidosis suggest lower GI loss (villious adenoma of colon or laxative use).
2. Low urine potassium excretion with metabolic acidosis occurs in bulimic patients.
3. High urine potassium excretion with acidosis suggests diabetic ketoacidosis or renal tubular acidosis (type I or II).

4. High urinary potassium excretion, metabolic alkalosis and normal blood pressure suggest diuretic use, vomiting, Bartter syndrome and Gitelman syndrome. Normal urine chloride suggests Bartter syndrome and Gitelman syndrome.
5. Hypertensive patient developing spontaneous hypokalemia or on diuretic, plasma aldosterone to renin activity should be measured.

Abdominal CT or PET may help to detect hormone secreting tumor. If no hyperplasia or adrenal tumor is detected, various genetic tests are indicated (Figure 13.2).

Treatment of Hypokalemia

The aim of treatment is to (a) replenish potassium, (b) remove offending drugs to reduce potassium loss and (c) treatment of non-iatrogenic causes of potassium loss.

The offending drugs such as diuretic, laxative, β-agonist, sympathetic stimulant and control of blood sugar are important. If diuretic is needed, potassium sparing diuretic may be used. For mild to moderate hypokalemia, oral route is preferred, and intravenous potassium chloride is indicated only in severe hypokalemia or with ECG changes. The patients on digitalis, myocardial infarction or heart failure, need higher serum potassium level and attention should be paid for early and rapid correction in them. For every 0.3 mEq/l lower level of serum potassium is equivalent to 100 mEq reduction in total body potassium. If expected serum potassium level is 3.8 mEq/l and the patient is having 2.6 mEq/l, the total body deficit of potassium will be 400 mEq. This amount should be added to the ongoing loss. In nonurgent situation, hypokalemia

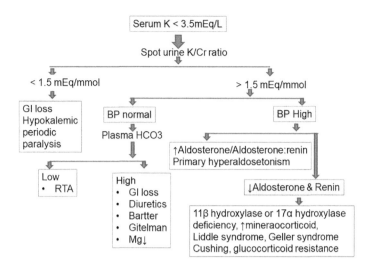

Figure 13.2 Schematic diagram showing methods of evaluation of a patient with hypokalemia. BP, blood pressure; GI, gastrointestinal; RTA, renal tubular acidosis.

is treated with potassium chloride 40–100 mmol/day in 3–4 divided dose with plenty of water (100–250 ml). In severe hypokalemia, 20–40 mmol potassium chloride should be mixed with normal saline and rate of correction should not exceed more than 20 mmol/h. Intravenous correction of potassium needs ECG monitoring, and frequent serum potassium measurement to avoid overcorrection. There is a possibility of rebound hyperkalemia, therefore, IV correction should be stopped once patient's ECG changes and muscle weakness improve, and if indicated oral supplementation may be continued. Refractory hypokalemia may be due to hypomagnesemia, which should be corrected. The rate of correction in children may be 0.5–1 mmol/l/kg in 1 h (~40 mmol). The treatment of hypokalemia is summarized in Table 13.11.

HYPERKALEMIA

Hyperkalemia is potentially a life-threatening condition and requires urgent management as it can cause muscle paralysis and cardiac arrhythmia. Hyperkalemia refers to serum potassium more than 5 mEq/l in adults, 5.5 mEq/l in children and more than 6 mEq/l in neonates. Hyperkalemia occurs in 10% of hospitalized and 1% of outdoor patients (Shemer et al., 1983; Paice et al., 1983). Hyperkalemia is attributed to increased intake, impaired excretion or transcellular shift. In practice, there are often multiple causes of hyperkalemia such as renal impairment, offending drugs and hyperglycemia which may be present in the same patient. Since healthy individuals can maintain normal serum potassium by increasing urinary

Table 13.11 Treatment of hypokalemia

Severity of hypokalemia	Clinical	Treatment
Mild (3–3.4 mEq/l)	Asymptomatic	Remove offending drugs Oral potassium 70 mmol/day
Moderate (2.5–2.9 mEq/l)	Asymptomatic or mild symptoms	Oral potassium 100 mmol/day
Severe (<2.5 mEq/l)	Symptomatic: monitor cardiac and respiratory	IV KCl 10–20 mmol/h Check serum Mg–if low, 8 mmol $MgSO_4$ in 10 ml normal saline infusion over 20 min

IV correction in mild to moderate hypokalemia is only indicated if oral potassium could not be tolerated.

Table 13.12 Causes of hyperkalemia

A. Renal:

1. Renal tubular secretory defect: Renal tubular acidosis type I, sickle cell disease, systemic lupus erythematous, renal transplant, obstructive uropathy
2. Impaired renal sodium absorption: Addison disease, adrenal enzyme deficiency (21 hydroxylase corticosterone methyl oxidase), hyporeninemic hypoaldosteronism, angiotensin insensitivity, prostaglandin inhibitor (indomethacin, piroxicam, ibuprofen, aspirin, naproxen, sulindac), β-adrenergic antagonist
3. Drug induced: Potassium sparing diuretics, trimethoprim, pentamidine, spironolactone and cyclosporin
4. Reduced distal flow of low sodium: Acute or chronic renal failure, Addison disease, cirrhosis, intravascular volume depletion and pulmonary edema
5. Renal failure: Acute tubular necrosis, interstitial nephritis

B. Abnormal potassium distribution: Metabolic acidosis, insulin deficiency, aldosterone deficiency, adrenergic antagonist, hyperkalemic periodic paralysis, tissue damage, severe exercise, cardiac surgery, drugs (diazoxide, somatostatin), hypertonic solution (mannitol), succinyl choline, arginine hydrochloride, digitalis

excretion, high potassium intake is seldom a cause of hyperkalemia (Table 13.12).

When the cause of hyperkalemia is not apparent from history, spot urine and serum potassium, and urine and serum osmolality should be measured to calculate trans-tubular potassium gradient (TTKG) as per the following formula:

$$TTKG = \frac{Urine\ K/serum\ K}{Urine\ osmolality/serum\ osmolality}$$

TTKG more than 7 suggests normal renal sodium absorption and normal potassium excretion, and TTKG less than 7 suggests reduced potassium excretion due to hypoaldosteronism.

Clinical features

Hyperkalemia affects skeletal and cardiac muscles resulting in muscle weakness and cardiac conduction abnormality or cardiac failure. Mild to moderate hyperkalemia may be asymptomatic or may have nonspecific symptoms such as generalized weakness, nausea, vomiting, diarrhea or intestinal colic. Patients usually become symptomatic when serum potassium exceeds 6.5 mEq/l. The examination should include blood pressure, heart rate and rhythm. There is varying degree of muscle weakness with normal to reduced tendon reflexes. Respiratory paralysis is rare. Patients may have symptoms and signs of underlying comorbid conditions.

Investigations: ECG is an important investigation for severity and deciding treatment of potassium disorder. ECG is abnormal when serum potassium is more than 6.5 mEq/l and the abnormalities include tall and peaked T wave, prolongation of PR and QRS complex, loss of P wave, sine waves or asystole (Parham et al., 2006; Spodick, 2008). The other investigations include blood urea nitrogen, blood glucose, serum creatinine, acid-base analysis, and urinary electrolyte and creatinine. In selected patients, renin, aldosterone and cortisone may be measured.

Treatment

The aim of treatment is to prevent life-threatening arrhythmia and respiratory paralysis due to muscle weakness. This is possible by shifting potassium into the cell, augmenting excretion of potassium and managing the underlying etiology. Indications of urgent treatment are serum potassium more than 6.5 mEq/l, ECG changes, symptomatic patients and associated renal, heart or liver disease.

Three modalities of treatment are used in the management of hyperkalemia: (a) cardiac stabilization by IV calcium, (b) measures to shift potassium into the cell and (c) elimination of potassium from the body.

Cardiac stabilization: Intravenous calcium antagonizes the effect of potassium on heart without affecting serum potassium level. 10 ml of 10%

calcium gluconate is administered intravenously in 5–10 min with ECG monitoring. If ECG changes of hyperkalemia persist even after 5–10 min of calcium infusion, a second dose may be repeated. In patients on digoxin therapy, calcium infusion should be given in 100 ml 5% glucose over 20–30 min.

Intracellular shifting of potassium: For shifting potassium into the cell, glucose insulin drip, and β agonist may be used. Glucose insulin drip is given adding 10 unit of insulin in 25–50 g glucose. Serum potassium starts declining after 10 min and the effect peaks by 60 min and lasts for 2–6 h. In the patients with hyperglycemia (>250 mg/dl), insulin may be given without glucose, but glucose levels should be monitored. Beta agonists may be administered through nebulizer, in 4 times higher dose than that used for bronchospasm. The side effects of β agonist therapy are tachycardia, palpitation and tremors; therefore, it should be avoided in patients with heart disease. This treatment is ineffective in the patients receiving beta blockers. Sodium bicarbonate is only indicated in the patients with metabolic acidosis ($HCO_3 < 22$ mEq/l) and has no role in reducing the level and may result in hypernatremia, hypocalcaemia and metabolic alkalosis (Khitan et al., 2018).

Lowering total body potassium: The total body potassium can be lowered by enhancing excretion of potassium through gastrointestinal tract or kidney. Loop diuretic (furosemide or torsemide) may be useful in renal failure. Hyperkalemia due to hypoaldosteronism may be treated with fludrocortisone. Sodium polystyrene sulphonate helps to reduce serum potassium by exchanging sodium with potassium in large intestine. It may be given orally or as retention enema and is helpful in subacute or chronic hyperkalemia due to chronic renal failure. Sodium polystyrene sulphonate produces constipation, therefore, should be used with sorbitol. The patient with chronic hyperkalemia should be advised to take low potassium diet and adjust or discontinue the offending drugs.

Hemodialysis is indicated in severe hyperkalemia with rhabdomyolysis, oliguric acute or chronic renal failure with metabolic acidosis and those refractory to medical treatment. Post dialysis hyperkalemia is common and should be monitored and managed.

Conclusion: Both hypokalemia and hyperkalemia are important electrolyte abnormalities. 90% of daily intake of potassium is excreted by the kidney with the help of renin–angiotensin–aldosterone system; therefore dysregulation of potassium is mainly due to renal causes. Trans-membrane shift is regulated by genetic, insulin, glucose or β-adrenergic system. Both hypokalemia and hyperkalemia primarily affect cardiac and skeletal muscles. Acute onset, severe hypokalemia or hyperkalemia with clinical symptoms and ECG abnormality requires prompt management. Treatment of hyperkalemia is summarized in Table 13.13 and Figure 13.3.

MAGNESIUM

Magnesium is the fourth commonest cation in the body after calcium, potassium and sodium. It is the second commonest cation in the cell. Total body magnesium concentration is 25 g (2000 mEq) and only 1% of the total body magnesium is found in extracellular compartment, 60%–65% is in the bone, 20% in the muscle and 20% in other body tissues. The blood concentration of magnesium ranges between 1.5 and 1.9 mEq/l because serum contains only 0.3% of body magnesium. About 20% of serum magnesium is bound to protein and 80% is ultra-filterable. Magnesium acts as a cofactor in several enzymatic reactions of the body (Table 13.14). Both hypomagnesemia and hypermagnesemia affect parathormone secretion, hence influence calcium metabolism.

Magnesium homeostasis: Daily consumption of magnesium is 300 mg; 30% of which is excreted in urine and remaining in the feces. The daily requirement of magnesium is higher in pregnancy, lactation, debilitating illness and those with higher fat, calcium and phosphate containing diet or in stress. The food items rich in magnesium are nuts, legumes, cereals and green leafy vegetables. Dairy products are poor source of magnesium. Magnesium is lost during cooling and boiling. The intake and output balance of magnesium is maintained by GI tract and kidney. Dietary magnesium is absorbed mainly in jejunum and ileum by passive and active transport mechanism. Vitamin D helps in absorption of magnesium. Kidney filters about 2 g of magnesium daily, 95% of which is reabsorbed and 5% is excreted. The most of magnesium is absorbed in the ascending loop of Henle. In distal convoluted tubule, fine tuning of magnesium absorption is influenced by parathormone, TRPM6 and EGF (Dai et al., 2001; Schlingmann et al., 2002; Groenestege et al., 2007).

Table 13.13 Treatment of hyperkalemia

Drugs	Doses	Response	Duration of effect	Rate of K reduction	Side effect
Cardiac stabilization					
Calcium gluconate	10% , 30 ml iv in 5–10 min	Immediate	30–60 min	-	-
Calcium chloride	10% 10 ml iv 5–10 min				
Intracellular shift					
Insulin	10 unit insulin followed by 50 ml 50% glucose	10–20 min	2–6 h	0.1–1 mEq/l	Hypoglycemia. If blood sugar is >250 mg/dl glucose is not necessary
β agonist	Nebulization using four times the bronco dilator dose	3–5 min	1–4 h	0.5–1 mE/l	Palpitation, tremor, arrhythmia
Augmenting excretion					
Furosemide	40–80 mg iv	5–30 min	2–6 h	-	Hyponatremia, hypovolemia
Cation exchange resin	Oral 5 g, 1–4 times daily. Rectal 30–50 g 6 hourly	2–24 h	Variable	Variable	Constipation, intestinal necrosis
Hemodialysis		Immediate	?	1 mmol/l in 1 h, 2 mmol/l in 3 h	Rebound hyperkalemia, volume depletion

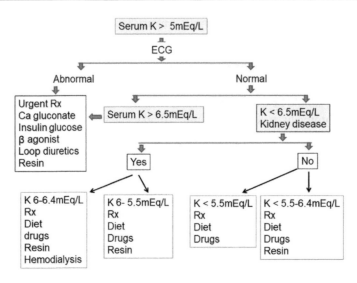

Figure 13.3 Schematic diagram showing management strategies of the patients with hyperkalemia.

Table 13.14 Physiological function of magnesium

Enzymatic reaction: Hexokinase, creatine kinase, protein kinase, Na^+-K^+-ATPase, Ca^+ ATPase, adenyl cyclase, guanylate cyclase

Enzyme activation: Creatine kinase, phosphokinase, 5-phosphosyl-pyrophosphate synthetase, adenylate cyclase, Na^+-K^+-ATPase

Membrane function: Cell adhesion, transmembrane electrolyte flux

Structural function: Polyribosomes, nucleic acids, multiple enzyme complexes, mitochondria, protein

Calcium antagonist: Muscle contraction and relaxation, action potential in nodal region, neurotransmitter release

Hypomagnesemia is commoner than hypermagnesemia. There is no simple and accurate method of measuring total body magnesium. For clinical practice, serum magnesium is measured, but is influenced by serum protein and calcium level. In hypoproteinemia, serum magnesium may be higher and in hyperproteinemia it may be lower. Measuring plasma magnesium concentration may be fallacious as magnesium binds to citrate. Hemolysis can spuriously increase the serum magnesium level. In elderly, serum magnesium may be higher and in the third trimester of pregnancy magnesium level may be lower. In a patient with hypomagnesemia, urinary excretion of magnesium more than 1 mmol/day suggests renal loss. Urinary magnesium below 0.5 mmol/l suggests magnesium deficiency.

HYPOMAGNESEMIA

Hypomagnesemia is a common electrolyte abnormality, which has been realized more recently. About 7%–11% of hospitalized patients have hypomagnesemia, and in critically ill patients, hypomagnesemia may be as common as 65% (Nadler et al., 1995; Noronha et al., 2002; Hayes et al., 1989; Ryzen, 1989). Hypomagnesemia is usually associated with other electrolyte abnormalities such as hypokalemia in 40%, hypophosphatemia in 30% and hypocalcemia in 22%–32% (Kingston et al., 1986; Boyd et al., 1983; Whang et al., 1984). Hypomagnesemia is associated with high mortality.

Etiology

Hypomagnesemia occurs due to redistribution of magnesium, poor intake, impaired absorption, GI loss and renal loss. Redistribution of hypomagnesemia refers to shift of magnesium into the cell which occurs during refeeding syndrome, treatment of metabolic acidosis, hungry bone syndrome

(parathyroidectomy, diffuse osteoblastic metastases), acute pancreatitis and increased catecholamine especially after cardiac surgery or congestive heart failure are important causes of hypomagnesemia (Yoshida et al., 2020). Chronic diarrhea is an important cause of hypomagnesemia, and occurs in Crohn's disease, coeliac diseases, and Whipple's disease. Inherited disorder of magnesium absorption occurs in TRPM-6 gene mutation, which manifests with hypocalcemia, hypomagnesemia, tetany and seizure. Because of the mutation, intestinal absorption of magnesium drops from 70% to 30%, because these genes encode ion channels for magnesium absorption in the small intestine. The clinical manifestation of this disease can be overcome by increasing magnesium intake.

Renal cause of hypomagnesemia includes prolonged saline infusion, chronic kidney diseases, peritoneal dialysis, acute renal failure in diuretic phase, and genetic disease like Bartter syndrome and Gitelman syndrome. Drugs such as antimicrobial, antifungal, β-adrenergic and proton pump inhibitors may also produce hypomagnesemia (Martin et al., 2009; Gile et al., 2020; Chrysant et al., 2019) (Table 13.15).

Clinical features

Hypomagnesemia remains asymptomatic unless serum magnesium is < 0.5 mEq/l. The clinical symptoms depend on the rapidity of hypomagnesemia and amount of total body magnesium loss. The clinical manifestations of hypomagnesemia also depend on associated dyselectrolytemia especially hypokalemia and hypercalcemia. The neurological manifestations of hypomagnesemia are neuromuscular and neuropsychiatric changes. The neuromuscular manifestation includes muscle cramps, carpopedal spasm, tremor, fasciculations, tetany, and weakness. In suspected patients,

Table 13.15 Causes of hypomagnesemia

Redistribution:
Refeeding syndrome, insulin therapy, correction of acidosis, massive blood transfusion, hungry bone syndrome (parathyroidectomy, diffuse osteoblastic metastasis), excess catecholamines
Loss of magnesium:
Gastrointestinal loss: chronic diarrhea, Crohn's disease, coeliac disease, ulcerative colitis, intestinal resection, TRMP6 gene mutation
Renal loss: reduced sodium absorption, saline infusion, diuretics, post obstructive, nephropathy, diuretic phase of acute renal failure, dialysis, Bartter syndrome, Gitelman syndrome
Reduced magnesium intake: low oxalate diet, cellular phosphate, magnesium free IV fluid
Endocrinal cause: diabetes mellitus, hyperthyroidism, hyperparathyroidism, hyperaldosteronism
Drug: Diuretics, chemotherapy, cisplatin, gallium nitrate, antimicrobial (aminoglycosides), cyclosporin, ritodrine, β-adrenergic agonist, amphotericin, foscarnet, pentamidine
Alcoholism and others

Chvostek's sign and Trousseau's sign may help to demonstrate neuromuscular hyper excitability. Increased neuromuscular excitability is due to impaired entry of calcium into the presynaptic nerve terminal and sarcolemma due to associated hypocalcemia and hypophosphatemia. Central nervous system manifestations include vertigo, seizure, depression, psychosis and choreoathetoid movement disorder. The exact mechanism of CNS dysfunction is not known but is attributed to over activity of excitatory neurotransmitters.

The cardiovascular manifestation of hypomagnesemia includes cardiac arrhythmias and increased sensitivity to digoxin. Chronic hypomagnesemia is associated with altered glucose homeostasis, hypertension, myocardial infarction, atherosclerosis, osteoporosis, chronic fatigue and reduced endurance (Table 13.16).

Treatment

In severe hypomagnesemia (<1 mEq/l) which is generally associated with neurological or cardiac manifestation should be urgently treated with infusion of 2 g magnesium sulfate in 100 ml of 5% dextrose over 5–10 min. This should be followed by magnesium sulfate 4–6 g daily for 3–5 days provided the renal function is normal. The underlying cause of hypomagnesemia should be treated. The maintenance therapy is magnesium oxide 400 mg or magnesium gluconate 500 mg twice or thrice daily.

Mild hypomagnesemia (1–1.5 mEq/l) is often detected in critically ill patients, diabetics, alcoholics and those on chemotherapy. The benefit of treatment of mild hypomagnesemia is not clear. If the patient is on diuretic therapy, potassium sparing diuretic (spironolactone) should be used.

Hypermagnesemia

Hypermagnesemia is less common and its prevalence is 5.7%–9.3% (Whang and Ryder, 1990). It has been reported following drowning in dead sea (Oren et al., 1987). The other causes of hypermagnesemia are drug toxicity, rectal magnesium enema, urethral irrigation, renal failure, rhabdomyolysis and endocrinal dysfunction such as hypothyroidism and Addison's disease (Table 13.17).

Clinical features: The symptoms of hypermagnesemia occur once serum magnesium is above 2 mEq/l. The neuromuscular symptom is the commonest and occurs due to impaired release of presynaptic acetylcholine resulting in neuromuscular blockade and cardiac conduction. Loss of tendon reflex is the earliest sign and occurs at 2–4.5 mEq/l, somnolence may occur at 2 mEq/l, muscle weakness

Table 13.16 Clinical features of hypomagnesemia

Neuromuscular: cramps, fasciculation, carpopedal spasm, tetany
Central nervous system: Vertigo; nystagmus, tremor, depression, delirium, choreoathetosis
Cardiovascular: Atrial tachycardia, atrial fibrillation, ventricular arrhythmia, Torsade-de pointes, sensitivity to digitalis, myocardial infarction, atherosclerosis
Others: osteoporosis; asthma, fatigue, low endurance and migraine

Table 13.17 Causes of hypermagnesemia

Excessive intake: antacid, laxative, salt water, magnesium enema, urethral irrigation, parenteral administration of magnesium sulphate
Renal: acute or chronic renal failure
Redistribution: acidosis
Others: rhabdomyolysis, hypothyroidism, Addison disease, milk alkali syndrome, familial hypocalciuric hypercalcemia, lithium

Table 13.18 Clinical features of hypermagnesemia

Neurological: Areflexia, weakness, respiratory paralysis, confusion
Gastrointestinal: Nausea, vomiting, paralytic ileus
Cardiac: Hypotension, bradycardia, heart block, cardiac arrest

and respiratory paralysis usually occur at serum magnesium >5 mEq/l. Hypocalcemia aggravates the symptoms and signs of hypermagnesemia. Serum magnesium above 2–3 mEq/l is associated with hypotension and symptomatic hypotension occurs at higher level. Serum magnesium more than 3 mEq/l may be associated with prolonged PR and QT interval and wide QRS complex. Serum magnesium more than 7 mEq/l is associated with bradycardia and heart block. There may be nausea and paralytic ileus (Table 13.18).

Management: Magnesium administration in any form should be stopped. Calcium gluconate 1 g IV may be administered in severe hypermagnesemia, which should be followed by 100–150 mg over 5–10 min. This results in prompt clinical improvement. Infusion of glucose and insulin also helps in shifting magnesium into the cell. If patient is on dialysis, low magnesium containing fluid for dialysis should be used. In neonate, severe hypermagnesemia may be treated by exchange transfusion (Swaminathan et al., 2003; eJIFCC, 1999).

CALCIUM

Calcium is an important element for bone mineralization, muscle contraction, transmission of nerve impulse, blood clotting and hormonal secretion. The daily requirement of calcium is mentioned in (Table 13.19) (Institute of Medicine, National Academy of Sciences, 2000). Dietary sources of calcium are mentioned in Table 13.20. Three hormones including parathyroid hormone, vitamin D and calcitonin play an important role in calcium homeostasis. Vitamin D helps in absorption of calcium in the intestine. Parathormone regulates calcium secretion in distal renal tubule,

and calcitonin acts on bone cells to increase the calcium level in the blood. Dietary deficiency, impaired homeostasis, renal, gastrointestinal and skeletal abnormalities result in hypercalcemia or hypocalcaemia (Fong and Khan, 2012).

HYPOCALCAEMIA

Hypocalcaemia is defined when serum calcium is less than 8.5 mg/dl (2.12 mmol/l). Serum calcium is bound to albumin; therefore, measurement of ionic calcium is important in the patients with hypoalbuminemia. For measuring ionic calcium, samples should be kept at 4°C, and should be measured within 2 h of sample collection (Ferrone et al., 2019).

Causes of hypocalcaemia: Hypocalcemia may occur due to vitamin D deficiency, parathyroid hormone deficiency, end stage renal disease, heavy metal toxicity, hypomagnesemia, hypermagnesemia, sclerotic metastasis, hungry bone syndrome, critical illness and phosphate or citrate infusion. The causes of hypocalcemia are mentioned in Table 13.21.

Table 13.19 Recommended daily calcium intake as per Institute of Medicine, National Academy of Sciences 2000

Age	Calcium (mg/day)
0–6 months	200
7–12 months	260
1–3 years	700
4–8 years	1000
9–18 years	1300
19–70 years	1000
51–70 years	1200

Table 13.20 Calcium content in dietary items

Dairy	Calcium (mg/100 g)
Whole milk	113
Fat free milk	122
Breast milk	32
Cottage cheese	83
American cheese	1045
Cheese cheddar	721
Goat cheese	298
Yogurt	110–150
Nuts	
Mixed	117
Cashew	37
Hazelnut	114
Pistachio	105
Almonds	250
Peanuts	92
Vegetables	25–50
Okra	82
Nonvegetarian	
Egg boiled	50
Poultry	138
Mutton, pork	<50

Clinical presentation: Hypocalcemia may be asymptomatic or may have severe clinical manifestations. The symptoms include muscle cramps, perioral paresthesia, tetany, seizure and heart failure. Children may have stridor. In chronic parathyroid disorder, there may be neuropsychiatric manifestations. Electrocardiogram changes reveal prolonged QT interval and may simulate myocardial infarction. Family history of hypocalcemia suggests familial hyperparathyroidism and genetic disease which is usually associated with mental retardation, congenital deafness, and skeletal abnormality. During clinical examination one should look for scar in front of neck, Chvostek's sign and Trousseau's sing. Chvostek's sign is elicited by taping the facial nerve 2 cm anterior to ear lobe below the zygomatic process. In hypocalcemeia, there is contraction of cheek and lip. Trousseau's sign is elicited by raising BP cuff above the systolic blood pressure for 3 min, and results in carpopedal spasm in hypocalcemic patient (Table 13.22). It is highly specific of hypocalcemia as only 1% of normal individuals may have similar response; whereas Chvostek's sign can be present in 25% of normal individuals (Bove-Fenderson and Mannstadt, 2018; Hujoel, 2016).

Diagnosis of hypocalcemia: Diagnosis of hypocalcemia is done by measuring the serum calcium below 8.5 mg/dl, which should be corrected for hypoalbuminemia. Serum phosphate, alkaline phosphatase, magnesium, electrolytes and serum creatinine, as well as blood glucose should be measured. Complete blood counts and erythrocyte sedimentation rate are important. Urinary excretion of phosphate, calcium, magnesium and 24 h urinary creatine is important to understand the role of kidney in producing hypocalcemia. Ultrasonography of abdomen should be performed to rule out nephrolithiasis. In the patient with central nervous system manifestation, CT or MRI may reveal calcification of basal ganglia and dentate nuclei (Figure 13.4; Kalita et al., 2010). In a patient with genetic or familial disease, biochemical assay of first degree relative and genetic sequencing are helpful (Table 13.23).

Treatment: Acute onset hypocalcemia is treated by IV calcium gluconate or calcium chloride if serum calcium is less than 7.6 mg/dl (1.9 mmol/l), ionized calcium less than 4 mg/dl (1 mmol/l) or if the patient is symptomatic. Large vein is used for calcium infusion because it is hyperosmolar. Calcium gluconate 1 g is equivalent to 93 mg of

Table 13.21 Cause of hypocalcemia

1. Vitamin D deficiency or resistance
2. Parathyroid disorders: parathyroidectomy, autoimmune or genetic parathyroid disorders, pseudo or pseudopseudohypoparathyroidism, infiltration, copper or iron toxicity, radiation of neck, metastasis
3. Renal disease: renal failure, Fanconi syndrome
4. Cirrhosis of liver
5. Hypo or hypermagnesemia
6. Osteosclerotic metastasis
7. Critical illness
8. Citrated blood transfusion or infusion of phosphate

Table 13.22 Clinical manifestations of hypocalcemia

1. **Neurological**: muscle cramps, tetany, seizure, movement disorder, neuropsychiatric (anxiety, depression), perioral paresthesia, pseudotumor cerebri
2. **Cardiovascular:** hypotension, heart failure, cardiomyopathy, QTc prolongation, AV block
3. **Respiratory**: stridor, bronchospasm
4. **Renal:** hypercalciuria, nephrocalcinosis, reduced glomerular filtration rate
5. **Ophthalmology:** cataract, corneal calcification, papilledema
6. **Skin and others**: alopecia, xeroderma, dental enamel hypoplasia

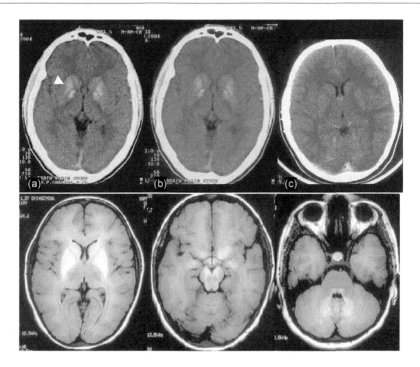

Figure 13.4 Pseudohypoparathyroidism in three patients with hypocalcemia and seizure. (a) and (b) Calcification of basal ganglia on CT scan in patient no 1 & 2. (c) CT scan of the patient 3 was normal but his MRI (lower panel) shows hyper intensity in basal ganglia, mid brain and dentate nuclei of the cerebellum in T1 sequence. (With permission from Kalita, J., Kumar, N., Maurya, P. K., Misra, U. K. 2010. A study of computed tomography scan and magnetic resonance imaging findings in pseudohypoparathyroidism. *Annals of Indian Academy of Neurology* 13(3):204–206.

Table 13.23 Baseline investigations in a patient with hypocalcemia

A. Serum chemistry: Serum calcium, albumin, phosphates, Mg, Na, K, creatinine, alkaline phosphatase, ionic calcium, and blood pH
B. Complete blood counts, ESR
C. Hormones: 25-OH vitamin D3, parathyroid hormone
D. Urine: 24 h urinary phosphate, calcium, magnesium, creatinine
E. X-ray abdomen, ultrasound abdomen, CT scan head
F. Family history if positive: biochemistry of first-degree relatives, DNA sequencing

elemental calcium, and that of 1 g calcium chloride is equivalent to 273 mg of elemental calcium. In an adult, the dose of elemental calcium is 100–300 mg which is infused in 100 ml glucose in 10–20 min. This is followed by continuous infusion of 0.5–1.5 mg/kg of elemental calcium per hour until serum calcium is normalized. Caution is needed in cardiac patient on digitalis because calcium infusion may precipitate cardiac arrhythmia (Murphy, 2008; Dickerson, 2009; Fong and Khan, 2012).

Long-term management of hypocalcemia is based on 1 g of dietary calcium daily. This dietary supplement is not sufficient in patients with hypoparathyroidism, pseudohypothyroidism and pseudopseudohypoparathyroidism, and in them, high dose of calcium and Vitamin D is needed. Associated hypomagnesemia should also be corrected (Liamis et al., 2009).

The side-effects of long-term calcium supplementation are calciuria, nephrolithiasis and soft tissue calcification. Biochemical and hormonal profiles need to be monitored 6 monthly.

HYPERCALCEMIA

The frequency of hypercalcemia is 1 in 500 patients in a general medical practice (Wermers et al., 1997). Hypercalcemia is associated with variety of underlying conditions; the commonest being malignancy and primary hyperparathyroidism accounting 90% of patients (Carroll and Schade, 2003). In asymptomatic individuals, isolated laboratory hypercalcemia is diagnosed in routine biochemical screening. The causes of hypercalcemia are mentioned in Table 13.24.

Clinical manifestations: Hypercalcemia leads to hyperpolarization of cell membrane leading to diverse clinical manifestations including renal, skeletal, gastrointestinal, neuromuscular, cardiovascular and dermatological. The patients with serum calcium of 10.5–12 mg/dl are usually asymptomatic, but a higher level results in multisystem involvement with a mnemonic "stones, bones, abdominal moans and psychic groans".

Neurological manifestation: The patient may have muscle weakness, fatigue, poor concentration, impaired memory, confusion, stupor or coma. Visual impairment may occur due to corneal calcification or band keratopathy.

Renal: Polydipsia and polyuria are the commonest symptoms of hypercalcemia due to nephrogenic diabetes insipidus and nephrolithiasis. The patients may have nephrocalcinosis, renal colic and dehydration due to polyuria.

Gastrointestinal: Nausea, vomiting, anorexia, constipation, abdominal pain, peptic ulcer and pancreatitis are associated with hypercalcemia.

Skeletal system: Often the patient complaints of bone pain which may be due to osteoporosis or underlying malignancy. There may be joint pain and bone cyst.

Cardiovascular: Hypercalcemia may result in hypertension, vascular calcification, cardiac arrhythmia and short QT interval.

Miscellaneous: The patient may complain of diffuse itching, keratitis, band keratopathy and conjunctivitis (Walsh et al., 2016).

Diagnosis: The diagnosis of hypercalcemia is based on serum calcium above 10.5 mg/dl. Mild hypercalcemia refers to serum calcium of 10.5–12 mg/dl (ionic calcium 5.6–8 mg/dl), moderate 12–14 mg/dl (ionic calcium 8–10 mg/dl) and severe above 14 mg/dl (ionic calcium >10 mg/dl which is life threatening and is also called as hypercalcemic crisis needing urgent treatment (Carroll and Schade, 2003).

The diagnosis of underlying cause of hypercalcemia begins with history, clinical examination and associated clinical findings. If there is history of use of over-the-counter drugs, it should be stopped. Serum intact parathormone and 24 h urinary calcium should be measured. A low urinary calcium suggests familial hypocalciuric hypercalcemia, but if urinary calcium is normal or high it suggest primary or tertiary hyperparathyroidism. If serum parathormone level is low, the patient should be investigated for malignancy such as adenocarcinoma or squamous cell carcinoma of lung in which parathyroid hormone related peptide is increased. If negative, other malignant conditions like breast cancer, myeloma or lymphoma should be investigated. Patients should also be investigated for serum TSH, free T4, cortisol and insulin like growth

Table 13.24 Causes of hypercalcemia

- **Common causes:** cancer, primary hyperparathyroidism
- **Rare causes:** thiazide diuretics, theophylline, lithium, immobilization, thyrotoxicosis, sarcoidosis, acute renal failure, during diuretic phase, hypervitaminosis of A & D, rhabdomyolysis
- **Very rare:** Addison's disease, familial hypocalciuric hypercalcemia, milk-alkali syndrome, nonsarcoid granulomatous disease

factor-I including cranial MRI depending on the clinical judgment.

Management: Acute severe hypercalcemia is a medical emergency, and patient should be rehydrated using 4–6 l of 0.9% saline in 24 h. Loop diuretics may be used to reduce the fluid volume and serum calcium. Zoledronic acid 4 mg in 15 min may be administered for reducing serum calcium level. Pamidronate or ibandronic acid may also be used. Glucocorticoid (prednisone 40 mg) is helpful if hypercalcemia is due to granulomatous disease like lymphoma. Glucocorticoids inhibit vitamin D thereby reduce serum calcium level. In patient with renal failure, dialysis should be done (Carroll and Schade 2003; Walsh et al., 2016). Hypercalcemia due to primary hyperparathyroidism refractory to medical treatment may require parathyroidectomy.

PHOSPHORUS

Phosphorus is an essential element, and is needed for ATP synthesis, signal transduction and bone mineralization. About 85% of body phosphorus is in the form hydroxyapatite in bone and teeth. About 14% of total body phosphorus is in intracellular space and 1% as an inorganic phosphate (Pi) is in the extracellular space. Phosphorus is also a component of DNA, RNA, ATP and creatinine phosphate. Phosphorus binds to organic molecules such as membrane phospholipid, phosphoprotein, inositol pyrophosphate and ribonucleic acid. Diet contains plenty of phosphorus, therefore abnormalities in phosphate level is attributed to impaired homeostasis rather than dietary deficit. Both low and high phosphate result in health hazards affecting musculoskeletal, cardiovascular, respiratory, and renal systems as well as ageing process.

Phosphate homeostasis: The daily requirement of phosphorus in adult males is 1500–1700 mg and in females 1000–1200 mg. The age wise requirement of phosphorus is mentioned in Table 13.25 (Institute of Medicine, 1997). Intestinal absorption of inorganic phosphorus is the maximum in infancy and childhood and declines with increasing age. About 50%–70% of dietary phosphorus is bioavailable (Carpenter et al., 2020); 60%–65% of phosphorus is absorbed in small intestine as inorganic phosphorus by two mechanisms.

Table 13.25 Recommended daily allowance of phosphorus in different age group (Institute of Medicine, 1997)

Age	mg/day
0–6 months	100
7–12 months	275
1–3 years	460
4–8 years	500
9–18 years	1250
>18 years	700

1. Passive paracellular (70%).
2. Trans-cellular absorption (30%).

Serum phosphate concentration ranges between 0.8 and 1.45 mmol/l, the level is the lowest in the morning and the highest in the evening (Christov and Juppner, 2018; Portale et al., 1987). Children have higher phosphate level than the adults due to higher absorption, rapid growth and increased requirement. Phosphorus hemostasis is maintained by a dynamic balance between renal loss, GI absorption and bone deposition or reabsorption (bone-kidney-intestine network). This network is regulated by a loop including parathyroid hormone, fibroblast growth factor-23 (FGF-23) with its co-receptor Klotho, and active form vitamin D (Blau and Collins, 2015). In elderly, there is a negative phosphorus balance due to bone loss. Vitamin D helps in absorption of phosphorus by augmenting expression of Na-P transport protein in the apical membrane of intestinal epithelium (Kido et al., 2013). High intake of glucose liberates insulin, which results in intracellular shift of phosphorus. Kidney reabsorbs 70% of filtered phosphorus in the proximal tubule. This rate of phosphorus absorption increases with reducing filtration until it reaches its peak. In the brush border, there are Na-phosphorus co-transporters (NPT2a, 2c). NPT2a is internalized and degraded by lysosome if there is high dietary phosphorus and serum parathormone, thereby phosphate absorption is reduced (Miyamoto et al., 2011; Lotscher et al., 1997). Vitamin D can stimulate NPT2a expression to increase phosphate absorption. Low phosphate diet and vitamin D augment NPT2c expression resulting in increase in phosphate absorption. FGF-23 can influence vitamin D metabolism, thereby contribute to phosphate homeostasis. In spite of so many regulatory mechanisms, serum phosphate concentration is not strictly maintained unlike calcium and other electrolytes. Disturbance in PTH, vitamin D and FGF-23 may result in hypophosphatemia. The main reasons of hypophosphatemia are reduction in intestinal absorption, increase in renal loss and redistribution of phosphate from extracellular to intracellular space. The causes of hypophosphatemia are mentioned in Table 13.26.

Clinical features: The clinical presentation of hypophosphatemia depends on the age, rapidity of onset, severity of hypophosphatemia and its underlying cause. Hypophosphatemia results in multiple organ dysfunctions. There is reduction in erythrocytes 2.3 di-phosphoglycerate leading to increased affinity of hemoglobin to oxygen, thereby resulting in tissue hypoxia. Skeletal muscles are also affected due to reduction in cellular ATP synthesis, abnormal signal transduction and phosphocreatine concentration.

Acute hypophosphatemia: In acute hypophosphatemia, there may be acute rhabdomyolysis (Amanzadeh and Reilly, 2006), hemolysis, leucocyte dysfunction and infection. Severe hypophosphatemia is associated with respiratory failure due to muscle weakness. The patients in intensive care, presence of hypophosphatemia may increase the duration of mechanical ventilation and mortality (Schiffl and Lang, 2013; El Shazly et al., 2017). There may be cardiomyopathy, cardiac arrhythmia and heart failure. The neurological manifestations include fatigue, weakness, paresthesia, tremor, encephalopathy, seizures, neuropsychiatric abnormalities and coma. Sometimes there may be Guillain-Barre syndrome like illness (Weintraub, 1976; Land and Schoenau, 2008).

Chronic hypophosphatemia: Chronic hypophosphatemia is associated with musculoskeletal manifestation due to sarcopenia and bone changes. There may be weakness, waddling gait, bone pain and osteomalacia. There is expansion of wrist and growth plate along with bone pain, fracture and bowing of legs in children, and vertebral fracture, enthesopathy and spinal canal stenosis in adults. The hereditary form of hypophosphatemia is associated with frontal bossing, mid-facial hypoplasia and Arnold-Chiari malformation. Children may have poor dentition, tooth decay, micro fracture and dental abscess

Table 13.26 Causes of hypophosphatemia

Acquired	Genetic
Dietary phosphate deficiency	FGF23-mediated hereditary hypophosphatemic diseases
Vitamin D deficiency	(X-linked,
Peptic ulcer	ARHR, ADHR, MAS and FD, CSHS)
Autoimmune gastritis	Hereditary hypophosphatemic rickets with Hypercalciuria
Pernicious anemia	Hypophosphatemic rickets with hyperparathyroidism
Reduced absorption	
Inflammatory bowel disease	
Drugs	
Proton pump inhibitor	
Parenteral iron	
Phosphonocarboxylase	
Arsenate	
Niacin	
Adriamycin	
Insulin	
Bisphosphonate	
Theophylline	
Foscarnet	
Renal	
Rental tubular acidosis	

XLH, X-Linked hypophosphatemia; ARHR, autosomal recessive hypophosphatemic rickets; ADHR, autosomal dominant hypophosphatemic rickets; MAS/FD, McCune Albright syndrome and fibrous dysplasia; CSHS, cutaneous skeletal hypophosphatemic rickets.

especially in genetic form of hypophosphatemia. There may be hearing loss due to fall out of spiral ganglion cells, cochlear involvement and endolymphatic hydrops (Megerian et al., 2008).

Diagnosis: Hypophosphatemia is considered if serum phosphate is less than 2.5 mg/dl, ideally in the fasting blood sample. Hypophosphatemia is categorized into mild (1.8–2.5 mg/dl), moderate (1.0–1.7 mg/dl) and severe (<1 mg/dl). Acute hypophosphatemia is usually due to redistribution in which total body phosphorus is not depleted, whereas in the chronic hypophosphatemia, there is depletion of total body phosphorus. The clinical history, pedigree chart and examination help in focused investigation. Vitamin D and parathormone assay along with clinical history may suggest disorder related to drug, known hereditary disease, vitamin D deficiency or hyperparathyroidism. Next step is to measure renal excretion of phosphate by calculating percentage of tubular phosphate reabsorption (TPR), and or rates of maximum renal tubular reabsorption (TmP) to glomerular filtration rate ratio (Tmp:GFR). In normal individual, 85%–95% glomerular filtered phosphate is reabsorbed; therefore TPR is 85%–95%. A lower value of TPR or TmP:GFR suggests renal phosphate wasting, and normal or higher value suggests decreased phosphate intake or GI absorption defect. In the patients with renal phosphate wasting, FGF-23 is measured. Low FGF-23 suggests hereditary hypophosphatemic rickets with hypercalciuria, hereditary or acquired form of Fanconi syndrome. Normal or elevated FGF-23 suggests X-linked hypophosphatemia, autosomal recessive or dominant hypophosphatemic rickets, McCune-Albright syndrome and fibrous dysplasia, cutaneous skeletal hypophosphatemic rickets, tumor induced osteomalacia or intravenous iron therapy. The specific genetic diagnosis is possible by DNA sequencing (Figure 13.5).

Treatment: The offending factors of hypophosphatemia should be removed if possible. Acute mild hypophosphatemia and chromic hypophosphatemia are treated with oral phosphate (sodium or potassium phosphate) thrice daily. In the patient with renal impairment, serum potassium should be monitored if potassium phosphate is used. The dose of phosphate should be modified depending on the response and side effect such as gastric, diarrhea, abdominal pain, secondary or tertiary hyperparathyroidism. In symptomatic and severe hypophosphatemia, infusion of sodium or potassium phosphate in a dose of 5 mg/kg slowly over 6h is given, which should be repeated till the serum phosphate is 1.5 mg/dl. Serum calcium should also be monitored. Patients with renal dysfunction may develop hyperphosphatemia following phosphate infusion unless closely monitored. In the developing countries, hypophosphatemia is a major problem in severely malnourished children. Correction of phosphorus has generally not been given due attention. If hypophosphatemia is due to tumor induced osteomalacia, removal of tumor is recommended. If removal is not possible, oral phosphate and vitamin D are helpful (Carpenter et al., 2011). The treatment choices in various causes of hypophosphatemia are summarized in Table 13.27. The age specific dose of oral phosphorus and vitamin D is presented in Table 13.28 (Florenzano et al., 2020).

HYPERPHOSPHATEMIA

Hyperphosphatemia is defined when serum phosphate level is more than 4.5 mg/dl in adults and 7 mg/dl in children. In hospitalized patients, hyperphosphatemia occurs in 12% patients excluding renal failure. In end stage renal failure, the prevalence of hyperphosphatemia ranges between 50% and 74% (Thongprayoon et al., 2018; Leaf and Wolf, 2013). Hyperphosphatemia may occur up to 45% children with malignancy receiving liposomal amphotericin (Knoderer and Knoderer, 2011).

Causes and pathophysiology: Hyperphosphatemia may occur due to phosphate overload, impaired renal excretion, hypoparathyroidism, pseudohypoparathyroidism and transcellular shift. Renal failure is the commonest cause of hyperphosphatemia. Since phosphorus is not bound to albumin, therefore all the phosphorus is filtered through the glomeruli. About 90% of daily phosphate load is excreted by kidneys; hence, in renal failure especially in end stage is associated with hyperphosphatemia. In the early stage of renal failure, hyperphosphatemia is prevented by elevated PTH and FGF-23. In the end of stage renal failure, there is reduced calcitriol (active form of vitamin D). Acidosis can also contribute to hyperphosphatemia in renal failure. Phosphate load may increase because of high dietary intake of phosphate containing diet, laxative, vitamin D intoxication and tumor lysis. Majority of phosphate is intracellular;

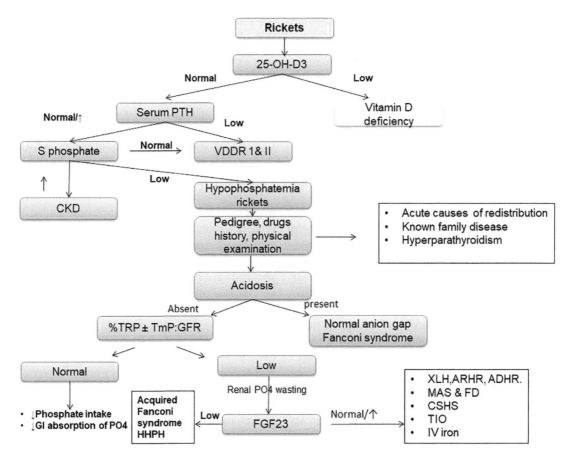

Figure 13.5 Evaluation of a patient with hypophosphatemic rickets. ARHR, autosomal dominant hypophosphatemic rickets; CSHS, cutaneous skeletal hypophosphatemic rickets; FGF-23, fibroblast growth factor 23; HHRH, hereditary hypophosphatemic rickets with hypercalciuria; MAS and FD, McCune-Albright syndrome and fibrous dysplasia; TRP, tubular phosphate reabsorption; Tmp: GFR, maximum renal tubular phosphate reabsorption per unit of glomerular filtration rate; XLH, X-Linked hypophosphatemic; TIO, tumor-induced osteomalacia.

Table 13.27 Treatment of hypophosphatemia

A. Acute symptomatic hypophosphatemia: IV sodium or potassium phosphate
B. Acute asymptomatic and chronic hypophosphatemia: oral sodium or potassium phosphate and active vitamin D
C. Treatment of underlying cause:
   1. FGF-23 mediated hypophosphatemia: oral phosphate and vitamin D
   2. Fanconi syndrome: oral phosphate and vitamin D
   3. Heredity hypophosphatemic rickets with hypercalciuria: oral phosphate
   4. X linked hypophosphatemia: burosumab (inhibits FGF-23)
   5. Vitamin D deficiency: vitamin D and calcium

therefore, cell lysis or cell turnover may result in rise of serum phosphate. Hyperphosphatemia can also occur in pseudohypoparathyroidism, which is characterized by hypocalcemia, hyperphosphatemia and inappropriately high level of PTH.

A number of hereditary disorders also result in hyperphosphatemia (Table 13.29).

Clinical manifestations: Hyperphosphatemia is generally asymptomatic, but patients may have seizures, symptoms of hypocalcemia and underlying

Table 13.28. Oral dose of phosphorus and vitamin D for the patients with hypophosphatemia

	Children	Adults
Phosphorus	20–40 mg/kg in 3–5 divided doses	75–1000 mg/day in 3–4 divided dose.
Active vitamin D (calcitriol)	20–30 ng/kg/day in 2–3 divided doses	0.5–0.75 µg/kg/day in 2 divided doses

Source: Modified from Schouten et al. (2009).

Table 13.29 Causes of hyperphosphatemia

A. Acquired causes:

- Chronic renal failure
- Low calcium high phosphate diet
- Reduced gastric pH
- Tumor lysis, bone metastasis
- Rhabdomyolysis
- Drugs: vitamin D, phosphate supplementation, FGF receptor inhibitors

B. Genetic causes:

- Hyperphosphatemic familial tumoral calcinosis type I, type 2 and type 3
- Idiopathic hyperphosphatemia
- Juvenile Paget's disease
- Pseudohypoparathyroidism
- Familial isolated pseudohypoparathyroidism
- Blomstrand disease

disorders. There may be hypertension and heart failure. Hyperphosphatemia may result in soft tissue calcification leading to pain, restricted joint mobility, atherosclerosis, hypertension, conjunctivitis, keratitis, band keratopathy and cataract. Hyperphosphatemia associated with short stature, short fourth metacarpal, and other bones of hands and feet, round face, dental hypoplasia, cognitive impairment and soft tissue calcification suggest Albright hereditary osteodystrophy.

Diagnosis: Serum phosphate more than 5 mg/dl in adults and 7mg/dl in children suggests hyperphosphatemia. Fasting morning sampling is necessary for serum phosphate measurement. Rise in serum phosphate in renal failure manifests only when GFR is below 30 ml/min/1.73 m². Renal function test, serum calcium, vitamin D, and PTH should be measured. Presence of high serum creatinine, BUN and PTH, and low calcium suggest renal etiology of hyperphosphatemia. Normal renal function with high vitamin D and elevated phosphate suggest vitamin D intoxication. Very high increase in phosphate, uric acid and potassium along with low calcium suggest

tumor lysis syndrome. In rhabdomyolysis, CK is very high whereas in tumor lysis it is normal or marginally elevated.

Radio diagnosis and ultrasonography of abdomen may reveal soft tissue calcification or renal stone suggesting pseudohypoparathyroidism. If renal failure, serum vitamin D level and parathyroid disorder are excluded, genetic cause should be considered and investigated.

Treatment: Acute hyperphosphatemia with normal renal function is treated by increasing intravascular volume with saline infusion and diuretics. Low phosphate diet is advisable to the patients with renal failure on dialysis. The recommended daily phosphate dose is 800–1000 mg with protein intake of 1.29 g/kg. High phosphate containing foods such as milk, meat, bean, fish and nuts should be avoided. Phosphate binders are used in the patient with serum phosphate more than 6 mg/dl. Aluminum based phosphate binders are most effective although there is possibility of aluminum toxicity including encephalopathy, anemia and premature death. Calcium based phosphate binders are also effective without much side effect. Magnesium carbonate also reduces serum phosphate and is well tolerated, and there is no risk of soft tissue calcification. Sevelamer is another phosphate binder which exchanges phosphate with HCl or carbonate in GI tract. Lanthamer carbonate, ferric citrate, sucrroferic oxyhydroxide are also phosphate binders.

Drugs which reduce intestinal phosphate transporter expression reduce phosphate absorption. Nicotinic acid and nicotinamide reduce NTP2b expression. These drugs however modestly reduce phosphate absorption. Tenapenor inhibits Na/OH ion exchange isoform 3 and plays an important role in reducing active phosphate absorption. In patients with renal failure, peritoneal or hemodialysis also help in reducing phosphate burden. The recommended phosphate level in renal failure is 3.5–5.5 mg/dl. Secondary hyperphosphatemia may be controlled by use of calcitriol.

CONCLUSION

Electrolytes are important element for cell function and are intricately maintained in a narrow physiological range through kidney, GI tract and neuroendocrine system. Elevated or low sodium results mainly central nervous system abnormality; whereas elevated or low potassium manifest with skeletal muscle, cardiac and GI tract dysfunction. In calcium, magnesium and phosphate abnormalities, both central and peripheral nervous system may be affected. Acute and rapidly developing symptomatic electrolyte abnormalities need urgent correction, whereas chronic and asymptomatic electrolyte abnormalities may be corrected slowly. Treatment of underlying cause is important.

REFERENCES

Adrogue, H. J., Madias, N. E. 2000. Hypernatremia. *The New England Journal of Medicine* 342:1493–1499.

Amanzadeh, J., Reilly, R. F., Jr 2006. Hypophosphatemia: An evidence-based approach to its clinical consequences and management. *Nature Clinical Practice. Nephrology* 2(3):136–148.

Blau, J. E., Collins, M. T. 2015. The PTH-vitamin D-FGF23 axis. *Reviews in Endocrine & Metabolic Disorders* 16(2):165–174.

Bove-Fenderson, E., Mannstadt, M. 2018 Hypocalcemic disorders. Best practice & research. The *Journal of Clinical Endocrinology and Metabolism* 32(5):639–656.

Boyd, J. C., Bruns, D. E., Wills, M. R. 1983. Frequency of hypomagnesemia in hypokalemic states. *Clinical Chemistry* 29(1):178–179.

Braun, M. M., Barstow, C. H., Pyzocha, N. J. 2015. Diagnosis and management of sodium disorders: Hyponatremia and hypernatremia. *American Family Physician* 91(5):299–307.

Carpenter, T. O., Imel, E. A., Holm, I. A., Jan de Beur, S. M., Insogna, K. L. 2011. A clinician's guide to X-linked hypophosphatemia. *Journal of Bone and Mineral Research: The Official Journal of the American Society for Bone and Mineral Research* 26(7):1381–1388.

Carpenter, T.O., Bergwitz, C., Insogna, K.L., 2020. Chapter 20—Phosphorus homeostasis and related disorders. In: Bilezikian, J.P., Martin, T.J., Clemens, T.L., Rosen, C.J. (Eds.) *Principles of bone biology*. 4th ed. Cambridge, MA: Academic Press, pp. 469–507.

Carroll, M. F., Schade, D. S. 2003. A practical approach to hypercalcemia. *American Family Physician* 67(9):1959–1966.

Carvounis, C. P., Nisar, S., Guro-Razuman, S. 2002. Significance of the fractional excretion of urea in the differential diagnosis of acute renal failure. *Kidney International* 62(6):2223–2229.

Chen, Z., Jia, Q., Liu, C. 2019. Association of hyponatremia and risk of short- and long-term mortality in patients with stroke: A systematic review and meta-analysis. *Journal of Stroke and Cerebrovascular Diseases: The Official Journal of National Stroke Association* 28(6): 1674–1683.

Christov, M., Jüppner, H. 2018. Phosphate homeostasis disorders. *Best Practice & Research. Clinical Endocrinology & Metabolism* 32(5):685–706.

Chrysant S. G. 2019. Proton pump inhibitor-induced hypomagnesemia complicated with serious cardiac arrhythmias. *Expert Review of Cardiovascular Therapy* 17(5):345–351.

Czupryna, P., Moniuszko, A., Garkowski, A., Pancewicz, S., Guziejko, K., Zajkowska, J. 2014. Evaluation of hyponatraemia in patients with tick-borne encephalitis: A preliminary study. *Ticks and Tick-Borne Diseases* 5(3):284–286.

Dai, L. J., Ritchie, G., Kerstan, D., Kang, H. S., Cole, D. E., Quamme, G. A. 2001. Magnesium transport in the renal distal convoluted tubule. *Physiological Reviews* 81(1):51–84.

Di, B., See, M. 2012. Direct Healthcare Professional Communication on the risk of increases in serum sodium with tolvaptan (Samsca) which are too rapid. Available from: http://www.mhra.gov.uk.

Dickerson R. N. 2007. Treatment of hypocalcemia in critical illness: Part 1. *Nutrition (Burbank, Los Angeles County, CA)* 23(4):358–361.

El Shazly, A. N., Soliman, D. R., Assar, E. H., Behiry, E. G., Gad Ahmed, I. (2017). Phosphate disturbance in critically ill children: Incidence, associated risk factors and clinical outcomes. *Annals of Medicine and Surgery 21*:118–123.

Ferrone, F., Pepe, J., Danese, V.C., et al. 2019. The relative influence of serum ionized calcium and 25-hydroxyvitamin D in regulating PTH secretion in healthy subjects. *Bone 125*:200–206.

Florenzano, P., Cipriani, C., Roszko, K. L., Fukumoto, S., Collins, M. T., Minisola, S., Pepe, J. 2020. Approach to patients with hypophosphataemia. *The Lancet. Diabetes & Endocrinology 8*(2):163–174.

Fong, J., Khan, A. 2012. Hypocalcemia: Updates in diagnosis and management for primary care. *Canadian Family Physician 58*:158–162.

Gankam-Kengne, F., Ayers, C., Khera, A., de Lemos, J., Maalouf, N. M. 2013. Mild hyponatremia is associated with an increased risk of death in an ambulatory setting. *Kidney International 83*(4):700–706.

Gile, J., Ruan, G., Abeykoon, J., McMahon, M. M., Witzig, T. 2020. Magnesium: The overlooked electrolyte in blood cancers? *Blood Reviews*, 44:100676. DOI: 10.1016/j.blre.2020.100676.

Groenestege, W. M., Thébault, S., van der Wijst, J., et al. 2007. Impaired basolateral sorting of pro-EGF causes isolated recessive renal hypomagnesemia. *The Journal of Clinical Investigation 117*(8):2260–2267.

Hayes, J. P., Ryan, M. F., Brazil, N., Riordan, T. O., Walsh, J. B., Coakley, D. (1989). Serum hypomagnesaemia in an elderly day-hospital population. *Irish Medical Journal 82*(3):117–119.

Hujoel, I. A. (2016) The association between serum calcium levels and Chvostek sign: A population-based study. *Neurology. Clinical Practice 6*(4):321–328.

Institute of Medicine (US) Panel on Dietary Antioxidants and Related Compounds. 2000. *Dietary reference intakes for vitamin C, vitamin E, selenium, and carotenoids.* Washington, DC: National Academies Press. Food and Nutrition Board, Institute of Medicine-National Academy of Sciences Dietary Reference Intakes: Recommended Intakes for Individuals. Available from: https://www.ncbi.nlm.nih.gov/books/NBK225472/.

Institute of Medicine, Food and Nutrition Board. 1997. *Dietary reference intakes for calcium, phosphorus, magnesium, vitamin D, and fluoride.* Washington, DC: National Academies Press.

Kalita, J., Kumar, N., Maurya, P. K., Misra, U. K. 2010. A study of computed tomography scan and magnetic resonance imaging findings in pseudohypoparathyroidism. *Annals of Indian Academy of Neurology 13*(3):204–206.

Kalita, J., Singh, R. K., Misra, U. K. 2017. Cerebral salt wasting is the most common cause of hyponatremia in stroke. *Journal of Stroke and Cerebrovascular Diseases: The Official Journal of National Stroke Association 26*(5):1026–1032.

Karandanis, D., Shulman, J. A. 1976. Recent survey of infectious meningitis in adults: Review of laboratory findings in bacterial, tuberculous, and aseptic meningitis. *Southern Medical Journal 69*(4):449–457.

Kardalas, E., Paschou, S.A., Anagnostis, P., Muscogiuri, G., Siasos, G., Vryonidou, A. 2018. Hypokalemia: A clinical update. *Endocrine Connections 7*(4):R135–R146.

Khitan, Z. J., Shweihat, Y. R., Tzamaloukas, A. H., Shapiro, J. I. 2018. Dietary potassium and cardiovascular profile. Results from the modification of diet in renal disease dataset. *Journal of Clinical Hypertension (Greenwich, CT) 20*(3):611–612.

Kido, S., Kaneko, I., Tatsumi, S., Segawa, H., Miyamoto, K. 2013. Vitamin D and type II sodium-dependent phosphate cotransporters. *Contributions to Nephrology 180*:86–97.

Kingston, M. E., Al-Siba'i, M. B., Skooge, W. C. 1986. Clinical manifestations of hypomagnesemia. *Critical Care Medicine 14*(11):950–954.

Knoderer, C. A., Knoderer, H. M. 2011. Hyperphosphatemia in pediatric oncology patients receiving liposomal amphotericin B. *The Journal of Pediatric Pharmacology and Therapeutics: JPPT: The Official Journal of PPAG 16*(2):87–91.

Land, C., Schoenau, E. 2008. Fetal and postnatal bone development: Reviewing the role of mechanical stimuli and nutrition. *Best Practice & Research. Clinical Endocrinology & Metabolism 22*(1):107–118.

Leaf, D. E., Wolf, M. 2013. A physiologic-based approach to the evaluation of a patient with hyperphosphatemia. *American Journal of Kidney Diseases: The Official Journal of the National Kidney Foundation 61*(2):330–336.

Lechner, S. G., Markworth, S., Poole, K., et al. 2011. The molecular and cellular identity of peripheral osmoreceptors. *Neuron 69*(2):332–344.

Leung, A. A., McAlister, F. A., Finlayson, S. R., Bates, D. W. 2013. Preoperative hypernatremia predicts increased perioperative morbidity and mortality. *The American Journal of Medicine 126*(10):877–886.

Liamis, G., Milionis, H. J., Elisaf, M. 2009. A review of drug-induced hypocalcemia. *Journal of Bone and Mineral Metabolism 27*(6):635–642.

Liamis, G., Rodenburg, E.M., Hofman, A., Zietse, R., Stricker, B.H., Hoorn, E.J. 2013. Electrolyte disorders in community subjects: Prevalence and risk factors. *The American Journal of Medicine 126*(3):256–263.

Liedtke, W., Choe, Y., Martí-Renom, M. A., et al. 2000. Vanilloid receptor-related osmotically activated channel (VR-OAC), a candidate vertebrate osmo-receptor. *Cell 103*(3):525–535.

Lippi, G., Favaloro, E.J, Montagnana, M., Guidi, G.C. 2010. Prevalence of hypokalaemia: The experience of a large academic hospital. *Internal Medicine Journal 40*(4):315–316.

Lötscher, M., Kaissling, B., Biber, J., Murer, H., Levi, M. 1997. Role of microtubules in the rapid regula-tion of renal phosphate transport in response to acute alterations in dietary phosphate content. *The Journal of Clinical Investigation 99*(6):1302–1312.

Mannesse, C. K., Vondeling, A. M., van Marum, R. J., van Solinge, W. W., Egberts, T. C., Jansen, P. A. 2013. Prevalence of hyponatremia on geriatric wards compared to other settings over four decades: A systematic review. *Ageing Research Reviews 12*(1):165–173.

Mapa, B., Taylor, B. E., Appelboom, G., Bruce, E. M., Claassen, J., Connolly, E. S., Jr 2016. Impact of hyponatremia on morbidity, mortality, and compli-cations after aneurysmal subarachnoid hemor-rhage: A systematic review. *World Neurosurgery 85*:305–314.

Martin, K. J., González, E. A., Slatopolsky, E. 2009. Clinical consequences and management of hypo-magnesemia. *Journal of the American Society of Nephrology: JASN 20*(11):2291–2295.

Megerian, C. A., Semaan, M. T., Aftab, S., et al. 2008. A mouse model with postnatal endolymphatic hydrops and hearing loss. *Hearing Research 237*(1–2):90–105.

Misra, U. K., Kalita, J., Kumar, M. 2018. Safety and efficacy of fludrocortisone in the treatment of cerebral salt wasting in patients with tuberculous meningitis: A randomized clinical trial. *JAMA Neurology 75*(11):1383–1391.

Misra, U. K., Kalita, J., Singh, R. K., Bhoi, S. K. 2019. A study of hyponatremia in acute encephalitis syndrome: A prospective study from a tertiary care center in India. *Journal of Intensive Care Medicine 34*(5):411–417.

Mistry, A. M., Mistry, E. A., Ganesh Kumar, N., et al. 2016. Corticosteroids in the management of hyponatremia, hypovolemia, and vasospasm in subarachnoid hemorrhage: A meta-analysis. *Cerebrovascular Diseases (Basel, Switzerland) 42*(3–4):263–271.

Miyamoto, K., Haito-Sugino, S., Kuwahara, S., et al. 2011. Sodium-dependent phosphate cotransport-ers: Lessons from gene knockout and mutation studies. *Journal of Pharmaceutical Sciences 100*(9): 3719–3730.

Murphy, E., Williams, G.R. 2009. Hypocalcaemia. *Medicine 37*(9):465–468.

Nadler, J. L., Rude, R. K. 1995. Disorders of magnesium metabolism. *Endocrinology and Metabolism Clinics of North America 24*(3):623–641.

Narotam, P.K., Kemp, M., Buck, R., Gouws, E., van Dellen, J.R., Bhoola, K.D. 1994. Hyponatremic natriuretic syndrome in tuberculous meningitis: the probable role of atrial natriuretic peptide. *Neurosurgery 34*(6):982–988; Discussion 988. DOI: 10.1227/00006123-199406000-00005. PMID: 8084408.

Noronha, J. L., Matuschak, G. M. 2002. Magnesium in critical illness: Metabolism, assessment, and treat-ment. *Intensive Care Medicine 28*(6):667–679.

Oren, S., Rapoport, J., Zlotnik, M., Brami, J. L., Heimer, D., Chaimovitz, C. 1987. Extreme hypermagnese-mia due to ingestion of Dead Sea water. *Nephron 47*(3):199–201.

Paice, B., Gray, J.M., McBride, D., Donnelly, T., Lawson, D.H. 1983. Hyperkalaemia in patients in hospital. *British Medical Journal (Clinical Research Ed.) 286*(6372):1189–1192.

Paice, B.J., Paterson, K.R., Onyanga-Omara, F., Donnelly, T., Gray, J.M., Lawson, D.H. 1986. Record linkage study of hypokalaemia in hospitalized patients. *Postgraduate Medical Journal 62*(725):187–191.

Parham, W., Mehdirad, A., Biermann, K.M., Fredman, C. 2006. Hyperkalemia revisited. *Texas Heart Institute Journal 33*(1):40–47.

Pfennig, C. L., Slovis, C. M. 2012. Sodium disorders in the emergency department: A review of hypona-tremia and hypernatremia. *Emergency Medicine Practice 14*(10):1–26.

Portale, A. A., Halloran, B. P., Morris, R. C., Jr 1987. Dietary intake of phosphorus modulates the circadian rhythm in serum concentration of phos-phorus. Implications for the renal production of 1,25-dihydroxyvitamin D. *The Journal of Clinical Investigation 80*(4):1147–1154.

Reynolds, R. M., Padfield, P. L., Seckl, J. R. 2006. Disorders of sodium balance. *BMJ (Clinical Research Ed.) 332*(7543):702–705.

Ryzen, E. 1989. Magnesium homeostasis in critically ill patients. *Magnesium 8*:201–212.

Schiffl, H., Lang, S. M. 2013. Severe acute hypophos-phatemia during renal replacement therapy adversely affects outcome of critically ill patients with acute kidney injury. *International Urology and Nephrology 45*(1):191–197.

Schlingmann, K. P., Weber, S., Peters, M., et al. 2002. Hypomagnesemia with secondary hypocalcemia is caused by mutations in TRPM6, a new mem-ber of the TRPM gene family. *Nature Genetics 31*(2):166–170.

Shemer, J., Modan, M., Ezra, D., Cabili, S. 1983. Incidence of hyperkalemia in hospitalized patients. *Israel Journal of Medical Sciences* 19(7):659–661.

Sood, L., Sterns, R. H., Hix, J. K., Silver, S. M., Chen, L. 2013. Hypertonic saline and desmopressin: A simple strategy for safe correction of severe hyponatremia. *American Journal of Kidney Diseases: The Official Journal of the National Kidney Foundation* 61(4):571–578.

Spasovski, G., Vanholder, R., Allolio, B., et al., 2014. Clinical practice guideline on diagnosis and treatment of hyponatraemia. *European Journal of Endocrinology* 170(3):G1–G47.

Spodick, D. 2008. Effects of severe hyperkalemia. *American Heart Hospital Journal* 6(1):68.

Sterns, R.H., Silver, S.M. 2008. Cerebral salt wasting versus SIADH: What difference? *American Society of Nephrology* 19(2):194e6.

Sterns, R. H., Nigwekar, S. U., Hix, J. K. 2009. The treatment of hyponatremia. *Seminars in Nephrology* 29(3):282–299.

Swaminathan, R. 2003. Magnesium metabolism and its disorders. *The Clinical Biochemist. Reviews* 24(2):47–66.

Thongprayoon, C., Cheungpasitporn, W., Mao, M. A., Sakhuja, A., Erickson, S. B. 2018. Admission hyperphosphatemia increases the risk of acute kidney injury in hospitalized patients. *Journal of Nephrology* 31(2):241–247.

Torres V.E., Chapman, A.B., Devuyst, O., et al. 2012. Tolvaptan in patients with autosomal dominant polycystic kidney disease. *New England Journal of Medicine* 367: 2407–2418. DOI: 10.1056/NEJMoa1205511.

U.S. Food and Drug Administration. 2013. FDA Drug Safety Communication: FDA limits duration and usage of Samsca (tolvaptan) due to possible liver injury leading to organ transplant or death. Available from: http://www.fda.gov.

Vaishya, R., Kaur, J., Seema, C., Jaswal, S. 2012. Mortality predictors in severe hyponatraemia in emergency inpatients. *Journal of the Indian Medical Association* 110(2):94–97.

Verbalis, J. G., Goldsmith, S. R., Greenberg, A., et al., 2013. Diagnosis, evaluation, and treatment of hyponatremia: expert panel recommendations. *The American Journal of Medicine* 126(10 Suppl 1):S1–S42.

Viera, A. J., Wouk, N. 2015. Potassium disorders: Hypokalemia and hyperkalemia. *American Family Physician* 92(6):487–495.

Walsh, J., Gittoes, N., Selby, P., Society for Endocrinology Clinical Committee 2016. Society for endocrinology endocrine emergency guidance: Emergency management of acute hypercalcaemia in adult patients. *Endocrine Connections* 5(5):G9–G11.

Wang, W. H., Giebisch, G. 2009. Regulation of potassium (K) handling in the renal collecting duct. *Pflugers Archiv: European Journal of Physiology* 458(1):157–168.

Weintraub, M. E. 1976. Hypophosphatemis mimicking acute Guillanin-Barré-Strohl syndrome. A complication of parenteral hyperalimentation. *JAMA* 235(10):1040–1041.

Wermers, R. A., Khosla, S., Atkinson, E. J., et al. 1997. The rise and fall of primary hyperparathyroidism: a population-based study in Rochester, Minnesota, 1965–1992. *Annals of Internal Medicine* 126(6):433–440.

Whang, R., Ryder, K. W. 1990. Frequency of hypomagnesemia and hypermagnesemia. Requested vs routine. *JAMA* 263(22):3063–3064.

Whang, R., Oei, T. O., Aikawa, J. K., Watanabe, A., Vannatta, J., Fryer, A., Markanich, M. 1984. Predictors of clinical hypomagnesemia. Hypokalemia, hypophosphatemia, hyponatremia, and hypocalcemia. *Archives of Internal Medicine* 144(9):1794–1796.

WHO 2012. *Guideline: Sodium intake for adults and children*. Geneva: World Health Organization (WHO). Available from: https://www.who.int/publications/i/item/9789241504836.

Yoshida, M., Izawa, J., Wakatake, H., et al. 2020. Mortality associated with new risk classification of developing refeeding syndrome in critically ill patients: A cohort study. *Clinical Nutrition (Edinburgh, Scotland)* S0261–5614(20):30399-X. Advance online publication.

14

Specific dietary management of certain neurological disorders

INTRODUCTION

Dietary management is an important component of treatment of several inborn errors of metabolism (IEM). It is important to diagnose these conditions at the earliest to start treatment including dietary management to prevent irreversible brain damage and poor outcome. The IEM have become more important because of neonatal screening programs. The management of these conditions requires a teamwork including an expert in metabolic disorders, pediatrician, neurologist and dietitian. This chapter presents an overview of disorders which require specific dietary management. Because of importance of ketogenic diet in refractory epilepsy, a section on the ketogenic diet has also been included.

PHENYLKETONURIA

Phenylketonuria (PKU) is an inborn error of phenylalanine metabolism, and is an important cause of hyperphenylalaninemia (HPA). Phenylketonuria is due to deficiency of phenylalanine hydroxylase resulting in impaired metabolism of phenylalanine or conversion of phenylalanine to tyrosine. Based on the concentration of phenylalanine in blood, phenyl alanine hydroxylase (PAH) deficiency is classified into classic PKU (phenylalanine > 1200 µM/l), moderate PKU (phenylalanine 600–1200 µM/l) and mild PKU (phenylalanine < 600 µM/l). Untreated PKU manifests with growth failure, seizure, microcephaly, intellectual impairment and high level of blood phenylalanine. Phenylketonuria is a rare disorder occurring in 1/10,000–15,000 live births in Caucasians (Guldberg et al., 1995; Okano et al., 1992).

Historical aspect

Phenylketonuria was first described by Norwegian physician Asbjorm Folling in 1924. The patients' mother consulted for possible association of mushy odor of urine and intellectual impairment of her twins. Extensive analysis of urine of these children revealed that urine contained phenyl pyruvic acid. This was followed by examination of 340 intellectually retarded patients, eight of whom had urinary phenyl pyruvic acid. The enzyme deficiency of PKU was described by Jervis (1947, 1953) and improvement following dietary management was reported by Robert Guthrie from Canada. After the birth of his son and niece with PKU, Guthrie changed his research interest and developed the screening test for PKU (Guthrie and Susi, 1963). Development of screening test and dietary management of PKU have improved the outcome of patients globally and was forerunner of the diagnosis and management of many other IEM.

Metabolic abnormality

L-Phenylalanine is an essential amino acid. Its sources are diet and endogenous recycling. Phenylalanine is utilized by its integration to proteins, oxidation to tyrosine or conversion to other metabolites, thereby balancing the blood level of phenylalanine. Conversion of phenylalanine to tyrosine takes place by the enzyme phenylalanine hydroxylase (PAH) and tetrahydrobiopterin BH4 (Figure 14.1). The reduction of tyrosine leads to deficiency of catecholamine and serotonin, and hyperphenylalaninemia resulting in a number of toxic

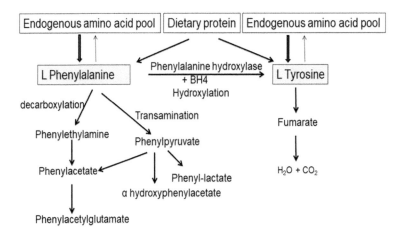

Figure 14.1 Metabolic pathway of phenylalanine.

effects. The human PAH gene is located on chromosome 12q23.2. Untreated PKU manifests with growth failure, intellectual impairment, seizure and microcephaly (Figure 14.2). These features are attributed to toxicity of phenylalanine and reduced tyrosine. Impaired production of tyrosine leads to reduced melanin, thyroxin and catecholamine synthesis. The mechanism of cognitive impairment in PKU is not well understood but hyperphenylalaninemia may result in delayed myelination or demyelination. The impaired neurotransmitter and hormonal synthesis may also contribute to cognitive decline (Williams et al., 2008).

Diagnosis

The screening test for PKU is done by Guthrie Card test, confirmed by phenylalanine hydroxylase enzyme assay and genetic testing. In a patient with hyperphenylalaninemia, it is important to look for biopterin (B4) deficiency.

Treatment

The aim of treatment is to reduce phenylalanine concentration in the blood by reducing dietary intake. The three dietary approaches are as follows:

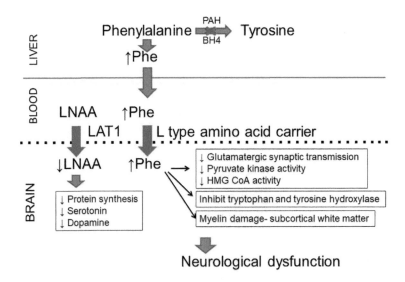

Figure 14.2 Mechanism of phenylketonuria and its effect on the nervous system. BH4, tetrahydrobiopterin; LAT1, L-type amino acid carrier; LNAA, large neutral amino acid; PHA, phenylalanine hydroxylase; Phe, phenylalanine.

1. Natural protein restriction
2. Phenylalanine free L-amino acid
3. Low protein food

The dietary items rich in phenylalanine are egg, meat, fish, milk, cheese, beans and legumes which should be avoided. Restriction of proteins in the diet results in deficiency of essential amino acids, trace elements and micronutrients, leads to growth failure, poor bone health and other nutritional disorders. These patients require supplementation of phenylalanine free amino acid formula, low protein diet, micronutrients and trace elements.

For dietary management of PKU, phenylalanine tolerance is important and is defined as amount of phenylalanine which maintains the blood phenylalanine in the target range. This may also be defined as natural protein tolerance expressed as gram per day. Treatment should be started within 10 days of life to prevent neurological damage. The target phenylalanine in different age is presented in Table 14.1 (van Wegberg et al., 2017).

Definite treatment of PKU may be enzyme replacement and gene therapy. Pegvaliase is a bacterially derived phenylalanine ammonia lyase and is an enzyme substitution therapy which metabolizes phenylalanine to transcinnamic acid and ammonia. Phase II trial of pegvaliase lyase has revealed substantial and sustained reduction of blood phenylalanine as well as improvement in mood and attention (Thomas et al., 2018).

MAPLE SYRUP URINE DISEASE

Maple syrup urine disease (MSUD) is a rare autosomal recessive IEM affecting branched chain amino acid (BCAA) metabolism, is a type of organic acidemia. The branch chain ketoacid dehydrogenase (BCKAD) deficiency is due to mutation of BCKDHA, BCKDHB and DBT gene. Deficiency of BCKD enzymes results in accumulation of BCAA namely leucine, isoleucine and valine and their corresponding ketoacids. The prevalence of MSUD in USA is 1/180,000 live births and in Austria 1/250,000 live births. In the communities with high consanguinity, its incidence may be 1 per 176 live births as in Nennonites in Pennsylvania and Amish (Chuang, 1998).

Historical aspects

In 1954, Menkes and his colleagues reported four patients in a family with progressive neurological disease including seizures, spasticity, respiratory irregularity, and respiratory arrest who had brain edema (Menkes et al., 1954). These patients were diagnosed as ketoacidosis in their first week of life and they died by three months of age. The

---

Table 14.1 The target blood phenylalanine (Phe) level in in phenylketonuria in different age groups

1. When to treat:
   <12 years: All untreated PKU patients with Phenylalanine > 360 μM/l
   >12 years: All untreated PKU patients with Phe > 600 μM/l
   Pregnancy: All untreated PKU patients with Phe > 360 μM/l
2. Target of treatment:
   <12 years: Phe 120–360 μM/l
   >12 years: Phe 360–600 μM/l
   Pregnancy: Phe < 360 μM/l
3. Monitoring Phenyl alanine:
   1 year : Weekly
   1–12 years: Fortnightly
   >12 years: Monthly
   Preconception: Weekly
4. Monitoring therapy:
   1) Annual review for weight, height, body mass index
   2) Laboratory: Hemoglobin, mean corpuscular volume, ferritin, amino acid homocysteine, methyl malonic acid and albumin
   3) Vitamin and hormone assay depending on clinical condition

urine of these children had a peculiar sweet smell (maple syrup); therefore it was named as maple syrup urine disease (MSUD). The offending agent was recognized as a BCAA by Dencis, Menkes and colleagues in 1959 (Westfall et al., 1957; Menkes et al., 1959). The disease is therefore also known as branch chain ketoaciduria or ketonuria. In 1960, same group reported metabolic block at decarboxylation of branch chain α-ketoacid (Dancis et al., 1960). In 1978, Bovine BCKDM complex was discovered by Reeds group (Pettit et al., 1978) and in 1980 cDNA of subunit of BCKAD complex was reported (Chuang et al., 1995, 1998).

Pathophysiology

Due to mutations in BCDKHA, BCKDHB and DBT genes, there is deficiency of BCKD complex leading to accumulation of leucine, isoleucine, valine and their ketoacids in the blood and urine which gives a sweet smell (maple syrup urine). Normally BCKAD complex breaks down leucine, isoleucine and valine through branched chain aminotransferase to corresponding α-ketoacid. In the next step, α-ketoacids are converted to acetoacetate, acetyl CoA and succinyl CoA through oxidative decarboxylation of respective ketoacid. There are four subunits of BCKAD complex E1α (chromosome 19), E1β (chromosome 6), E2 (chromosome 1) and E3 (chromosome 7). E3 subunit is also a component of pyruvate dehydrogenase complex and oxoglutarate dehydrogenase complex (Chuang et al., 1998). In MSUD, these genes are mutated giving rise to different proportion of enzyme deficiency. The elevated levels of BCAA especially leucine is responsible for clinical manifestations including brain edema.

Clinical features

The clinical phenotype of MSUD depends on the proportion of normal BCKD enzyme activity. The lower the proportion of normal enzyme, worse is the illness. Based on phenotypic expression MSUD is categorized into classic, intermediate, intermittent and thiamine responsive type. The proportion of normal BCKD enzyme activity in classic type is 0%–2%, intermediate type 3%–30%, intermittent 5%–20% and thiamine responsive type 2%–40% (Chuang and Shih, 2001; Strauss et al., 2020). The details of neurological manifestations in different sub types of MSUD are presented in Table 14.2.

In the classic type of MSUD, the newborn manifests with maple syrup odor in the cerumen and the blood concentration of BCAA and isoleucine are elevated. In 2–3 days, the newborn develops irritability, excessive sleepiness and poor feeding. The urine reveals branched chain α-ketoacids, acetoacetate and β-hydroxybutyrate along with elevated concentration of BCAAs and alloisoleucine. Urine has a sweet odor. If untreated for 4–6 days, the newborn develops encephalopathy, apnea, opisthotonus and various focal or generalized movement disorders including fencing or bicycling

Table 14.2 Different subtypes of maple syrup urine disease

Type	Age of onset	Clinical features	Laboratory findings
Classic	Neonatal	Sweet odor of cerumen, Irritability, lethargy, poor feeding, movement disorder (dystonia, opisthotonus, fencing, bicycling movement), respiratory arrest	↑BCAA in blood, and urine, ketonuria
Intermediate	Variable	Sweet odor in urine, poor growth and feeding, developmental delay, cognitive decline, crisis	Same as classic but lesser elevated
Intermittent	Variable	Normal growth and development in early life, intermittent decompensation	Normal BCAA during asymptomatic period Same as classical during crisis
Thiamine responsive	Variable	Similar to intermittent	Clinical improvement following thiamine

movements. By 7–10 days, untreated newborns further deteriorate with coma and respiratory failure because of brain edema.

Intermediate MSUD has partial deficiency of BCKD enzymes. The patient has a variable age of onset with milder clinical manifestations. Severe metabolic crisis may occur during the state of high metabolic demand. The child has poor growth and development and neurocognitive dysfunction.

Intermittent type of MSUD may have a normal growth and development in the initial stage of life. During episodic de-compensation, the patient may have encephalopathy and acidosis. Biochemical parameters during the asymptomatic period are normal and during crisis these are similar to the classic type.

Thiamine responsive MSUD can present at any age and the clinical presentation is similar to the intermediate type. The only difference is that the patient improves with thiamine (10–1000 mg daily) including the biochemical parameters.

The diagnosis of MSUD is an emergency especially the classic type because the delay in the diagnosis and treatment may result in irreversible brain damage. Urinary odor suggests different types of IEM (Table 14.3).

Differential diagnosis: The neonatal encephalopathy in MSUD should be differentiated from birth asphyxia, hypoglycemia, kernicterus, status epilepticus and meningoencephalitis. Moreover, the IEM producing neonatal encephalopathy such as hyperkeratosis syndrome, urea cycle defect, propionic acidemia, methylmalonic acidemia and hyperglycemic encephalopathy need to be differentiated.

Table 14.3 Odors typical of inborn error of metabolism

Inborn error of metabolism	Odor
Phenylketonuria	Mousy
Maple syrup urine disease	Sweet
Glutaric acidemia type II /Isovaleric acidemia	Sweaty feet
Tyrosinemia type I	Boiled cabbage
Cystinuria	Sulfur
Trimethyl aminuria /dimethyl glycine dehydrogenase deficiency	Old fishy
Multiple carboxylase deficiency	Cat urine

Diagnosis

The MSUD is suspected based on newborn screening test, which is confirmed by enzyme assay using fibroblast culture, lymphocyte or liver cells, and more recently by genetic studies demonstrating BCKDHA, BCKDHB or DBT gene mutation. In a family with a proband having MSUD, the diagnosis can be directly confirmed by genetic study. Mutation study not only helps in the diagnosis but also helps in predicting phenotypic expression and outcome.

Treatment

The treatment of MSUD starts with dietary restriction of leucine, BCAA free medical formula, and supplementation of calorie, fluid, micronutrient and vitamins. Frequent biochemical and clinical monitoring is essential. Most of the protein rich food such as dairy products, meat, fish, eggs, soy, nuts, whole grain, seeds, beans, pulses, avocado, algae and edible sea weeds have high amount of leucine and BCAA; therefore cannot be allowed especially in classic type of MSUD and during crisis. Once the patient is stabilized, isoleucine and valine may be prescribed.

Management of crisis in classic MSUD: The classical type of MSUD has severe illness at the time of diagnosis and all other types may also develop crisis during stress, such as infection, trauma or surgery. The management during crisis is aimed at achieving clinical and biochemical normalization, prevent catabolism and providing exogenous amino acid formula free of BCAA. For energy 150 kcal/kg and fluid 150 ml/Kg are prescribed. Though leucine is excluded, valine and isoleucine are prescribed judiciously once the patient stabilizes, to maintain anabolism and prevent epithelial damage of skin, eye and gastrointestinal tract. In very severe cases, hemodialysis or hemofiltration may be needed to remove the toxic products.

In the nonacute state, sick day guideline should be followed throughout the life. It includes calorie rich diet with isoleucine and valine but avoiding leucine. This is combined with frequent amino acid monitoring in blood and urine.

Thiamine responsiveness MSUD should be tested in all the patients as in partial enzyme deficiency patients. The clinical and biochemical parameters improve following thiamine treatment especially in the patients with E2 mutations. Thiamine pyrophosphate is a cofactor for mut subunit enzyme branch chain ketoacid dehydrogenase. Following 50–200 mg thiamine daily for one month, there may be clinical response. Higher dose of thiamine is unlikely to produce toxic effect as it is water soluble and the excess amount is excreted in urine.

Pregnancy and puerperium: During pregnancy, the protein and energy requirement is high because of cell proliferation and fetal growth. During this period, vitamin and nutrients should be supplemented and catabolism should be prevented by BCAA free amino acid supplementation. Special attention is needed during hyperemesis gravidarum. The goal of treatment is to achieve plasma leucine level of 75–200 μM/l during infancy and 75–300 μM/l during 1–5 years of age. The target level of valine and isoleucine at any age is 200–400 μM/l. The recommended nutrition intake during asymptomatic period of MSUD is given in Table 14.4.

Liver transplant: The role of liver transplantation is not clear. Liver transplant reduces the number of crisis but does not affect the existing neurological deficit. The risk benefit ratio of liver transplantation should be considered in an individual patient. The treatment of MSUD is presented in Table 14.4 and composition of diet in Table 14.5.

METHYL MALONIC ACIDEMIA AND PROPIONIC ACIDEMIA

Methyl malonic acidemia (MMA) and propionic acidemia (PA) are rare autosomal recessive IEM due to methyl malonyl CoA (MMCoA) mutase

and propionyl CoA carboxylase, respectively. In MMCoA mutase deficiency, there is excessive accumulation of MMA; and in propionyl CoA carboxylase deficiency, there is accumulation of propionic acid, propionyl carnitine, 3 methyl citrate and odd chain fatty acids. The integrity of these metabolic pathways is important for metabolism of amino acids (valine, isoleucine, threonine, methionine) and fatty acids (odd chain fatty acids and cholesterol side chain). With normal enzyme activity and their cofactors; biotin is needed for propionyl CoA carboxylase and adenosyl cobalamin for MMACoA mutase. The above mentioned amino acids and fatty acids are converted to succinyl CoA (Figure 14.3).

Methyl malonic acidemia is of two forms: (a) isolated MMA in which there is mutation in MMCoA mutase, and they have MMA in blood and urine. (b) Combined form in which MMA is associated with hyper homocysteineuria and is due to defect in coenzyme adenosyl cobalamin. The incidence of MMA is 1 in 48,000 to 1 in 61,000 live births, and that of PA is 1 in 50,000 to 1 in 500,000 live births. The incidence of PA is higher in Saudi Arabia, 1 in 2000–5000 live births (Shchelochkov, et al., 2012; Ozand et al., 1994).

Clinical features

The age and severity of presentation depends on the extent of enzyme deficiency. Complete enzyme deficiency manifests within seven days of life with metabolic acidosis, encephalopathy and hyperammonemia resulting in coma and death if untreated. Partial deficiency of enzymes manifests during infancy, childhood or in the later life. Like other

---

Table 14.4 Treatment during acute crisis maple syrup urine disease.

1. Energy provided should be 150% of usual requirement using carbohydrate, lipids and BCAA free amino acid. The fluid requirement is 150 ml/kg. Electrolyte and glucose should be monitored and if needed insulin and electrolyte are prescribed
2. Use parenteral nutrition alone or with enteral nutrition to meet calorie and fluid requirement
3. Hemodialysis or hemofiltration may be used to reduce BCAA and its toxic products
4. Monitor BCAA, keto-acids, acid–base balance, electrolyte, glucose, hemoglobin, albumin, kidney function, calcium and phosphorus
5. Add isoleucine and valine
6. Encourage breast milk and maintain growth and development chart
7. Mild illness: 50%–100% reduction of intact protein for 2 days
8. Reintroduce intact protein if plasma leucine is less than 200 μM/l in infants, and less than 300 μM/l in 1–5 years of age

Table 14.5 Recommended daily intake of nutrients in asymptomatic period in MSUD

Age	Calories (kcal/kg)	Fluid (ml/kg)	Protein (g/kg)	Leucine (mg/kg)	Isoleucine (mg/kg)	Valine (mg/kg)
0–6 months	95–145	125–160	2.5–3.5	40–100	30–90	40–95
7–12 months	80–135	125–145	2.5–3.0	40–75	30–70	30–80
1–3 years	80–130	115–135	1.5–2.5	40–70	20–70	30–70
4–8 years	50–120	90–115	1.3–2.0	35–65	20–30	30–50
9–13 years	40–90	71–90	1.2–1.8	30–60	20–30	25–40
14–18 years	35–70	40–60	1.2–1.8	15–50	10–30	15–30
>18 years	35–45	40–50	1.1–1.7	15–50	10–30	15–30

Source: Modified from Marriage (2010).

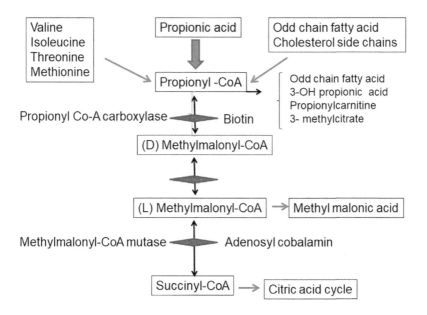

Figure 14.3 Propionic acid metabolic pathway.

IEM, there may be acute deterioration or crisis when metabolic demand increases. The clinical picture of both MMA and PA is characterized by involvement of multiple systems including nervous system, gastrointestinal, hematological, renal and cardiac. The details of clinical features are presented in Table 14.6.

Laboratory investigations

Laboratory investigations reveal metabolic acidosis with high anion gap, elevated serum lactate, hyperammonemia, ketone bodies in the urine and pancytopenia. These patients with acute encephalopathy should be differentiated from other IEM producing encephalopathy (Table 14.7).

Detection of organic acid in urine and acyl carnitine in blood are commonly used for the diagnosis of MMA and PA. In addition, plasma and urinary homocysteine levels help in the diagnosis of vitamin B12 responsiveness. The diagnosis can be confirmed by enzyme assay and genetic testing.

Antenatal diagnosis: Antenatal diagnosis is feasible in both MMA and PA. It should be undertaken if there is an index patient with biochemical or genetic diagnosis. Newborn screening is feasible but its long-term benefits are doubtful.

Treatment

The treatment of MMA and PA is an emergency and should start pending diagnostic confirmation. The

Table 14.6 Clinical features during acute and chronic presentation of methyl malonic acidemia and propionic acidemia

System	Acute	Chronic
Nervous system	Altered sensorium Seizure Movement disorder Stroke-like illness	Hypotonia Mental retardation Learning disability Seizure Psychosis Movement disorder Optic atrophy
Gastrointestinal	Vomiting Poor feeding	Vomiting Constipation Pancreatitis Abnormal feeding behavior
Cardiac	Heart failure Arrhythmia Cardiomyopathy	QTc prolongation Cardiomyopathy
Hematological	Neutropenia Anemia Thrombocytopenia	Neutropenia Anemia Thrombocytopenia Hemophagocytosis
Renal	-	Chronic renal failure in MMA
Others	-	Hearing loss Dermatitis

Table 14.7 Laboratory findings in acute encephalopathy due to inborn errors of metabolism

Parameters	MMA/ PA	UCD	MSUD	βKTD	β-Oxidation defect	HIHA	PC defect/ mito	PDH def	HMGCoA lyase def
Acidosis	+	+/-	-	++	+/-	-	+	+	+
Ketonuria	+++	-	++	+++	-	-	++	-	-
Ammonia ↑	+	++	-	-	+	+	+/-	-	+
Hypoglycemia	+/-	-	-	-	+	++	+/-	-	+
Lactic acidosis	+	-	-	+	+/-	-	++	++	+
↑AST/ALT	+/-	+	-	-	++	-	+/-	-	+/-
↑CK	-	-	-	-	++	-	+/-	-	-
↑Uric acd	+	-	+	+	+	-	+/-	+/--	+
↓RBC/WBC/Pl	+	-	-	-	-	-	+/-	-	-

Source: Modified from Haberle et al. (2012).
CK, creatine kinase; HIHA, hyperinsulinism hyperammonemia syndrome; HMGCoA, β-hydroxyl β-methyl gutaryl CoA; PC, pyruvate carboxylase; PDH, pyruvate dehydrogenase; MMA, methyl malonic acidemia; KTD+, ketothiolase deficiency; MSUD, maple syrup urine disease; PA, propionic acidemia; UCD, urea cycle defect.

Table 14.8 Treatment of acute hyperammonemia

1. IV glucose age adjusted
2. IV or IM L-carnitine: 10 mg/kg as bolus followed by 10 mg/kg/day
3. IV or IM hydroxycobalamin 1 mg/day
4. IV or oral biotin 10–40 mg/day
5. IV sodium benzoate 250 mg/kg in 10% glucose over 1.5–2 h, followed by 250 mg/kg/day
6. IV sodium phenyl butyrate in 10% glucose
7. L-Arginine hydrochloride in 10% glucose
8. N carbamyl glutamate 100 mg/kg per oral followed by 25–60 mg/kg 6 hourly

patient should receive IV glucose, protein restricted diet, stabilization of metabolic acidosis and hyperammonemia. Blood, plasma and urine should be collected periodically for monitoring and management. Hyperammonemia is a serious problem and needs special management, including IV glucose, L-carnitine, hydroxy cobalamin, sodium benzoate, sodium phenyl butyrate, L-arginine hydrochloride, carbamyl glutamate and biotin. The treatment of hyperammonemia is summarized in Table 14.8.

Once the diagnosis of PA is confirmed, the patient should be maintained on glucose and benzoate till hyperammonemia resolves. Parenteral nutrition is provided if there is feeding problem. Amino acids are gradually introduced to achieve safe amino acids levels and prevent catabolism. Vitamins, minerals and micronutrients should be supplemented. If ammonia level is more than 400 µMol/l extracorporeal detoxification by hemodialysis or hemofiltration is indicated. In MMA, forced diuresis and alkalinization of urine using sodium bicarbonate is useful to eliminate MMA.

Long-term management of these patients requires a team effort including metabolic experts, hematologist, gastroenterologist, nephrologist and neurologist (Baumgartner et al., 2014).

FATTY ACID OXIDATION DISORDERS

Fatty acid metabolism disorders are a group of autosomal recessive disorders in which β-oxidation of fatty acids is impaired due to deficiency of certain enzymes. Normally during fasting or hypoglycemia, fats are mobilized and converted to fatty acids in the liver. The fatty acids are transported to the target cells in which these are oxidized to produce energy. In fatty acid oxidation defect (FAOD), the fatty acids accumulate in the liver or other organs. The patients manifest with exercise intolerance or may go into crisis especially during fasting or hypoglycemic state. The different types of fatty acid oxidation disorder are mentioned in Table 14.9.

Table 14.9 Types or fatty acid oxidation disorder

Disorders	Prevalence	Gene
Medium chain acyl CoA dehydrogenase deficiency	1/20,000 live births	ACADMD
Long chain 3 hydroxy acyl CoA dehydrogenase deficiency	1/110,000–150,000	HADHA
Very long chain acyl Co A dehydrogenase deficiency	1/42,000–120,000	ACADVL
Tri functional protein deficiency	Rare	HADHA,HADHB
Carnitine palmitoyl transferase type 1 deficiency	1/500,000	CPT1A
Carnitine palmitoyl transferase type 2 deficiency	Rare	CPT2
Carnitine – acylcarnitine translocase deficiency	Rare	SLC25A20
Carnitine transporter deficiency	1/20,000–1,20,000	SLC22A5
Short chain acyl CoA dehydrogenase deficiency	1/35,000–50,000	ACADS
Multiple acyl CoA dehydrogenase deficiency	Rare	ETFA, ETFB, ETFDH
3-hydroxy acyl-CoA dehydrogenase deficiency	Rare	HADH

Epidemiology: Fatty acid oxidation disorders (FAOD) are more common than aminoaciduria. The incidence of some types of FAODs is 1 in 5000–10,000 live births. However it varies in different ethnicity (Merritt et al., 2018). Medium chain acyl CoA deficiency is the commonest FAOD. Its mortality has declined from more than 20% to 5% after newborn screening test and early intervention (Nennstiel-Ratzel et al., 2005; Grosse et al., 2006; Wilcken et al., 2007; Fauchtbaum et al., 2018).

Clinical features: The patient with FAOD may present acutely at any age. Newborns manifest within a few hours of fasting but adults and adolescents take up to 48 h. There are three clinical presentations

1. Neonatal onset
2. Infantile and childhood
3. Adolescent and adult form.

The neonatal onset type of FAOD manifests with severe cardiomyopathy, hypoketotic hypoglycemia and liver dysfunction. This is often fatal within a few days of life.

Infantile childhood type of FAOD manifests with intermittent lethargy, vomiting and infection leading to hepatic dysfunction, hypoketotic hypoglycemia and encephalopathy. These children may die suddenly.

Adolescent and adult-onset type of FAOD manifests with episodic muscle weakness, myalgia and rhabdomyolysis which may lead to renal failure.

Diagnosis: Newborn screening test helps in identifying the patients with FAODs. Laboratory tests of non ketotic hypoglycemia and hyperammonemia should raise the possibility of FAODs. Diagnosis is confirmed by genetic studies.

Dietary management: The dietary management of FAODs includes avoidance of fasting, aggressive treatment of crisis and avoidance of fat. The key issues in the management of FAODs are as follows:

1. Lifelong dietary management as per advice of metabolic physician
2. Avoidance of fasting: infants need feeding every 3 h for 4 months
3. Gradually the interval of feeding may be increased 1 h per month and by 12 months feeding schedule may be 8 h. Avoid 10–12 h of fasting after infancy

4. Aggressive treatment during stress
5. Providing oral or enteral carbohydrate rich fluid every 3–4 hourly in mild to moderate illness
6. 10% dextrose at 1.5 times more than required amount. Maintaining electrolyte, vitamins and minerals
7. Carnitine supplementation may be helpful in secondary carnitine deficiency
8. In medium acyl CoA enzyme deficiency, medium chain triglyceride oil such as coconut oil or MCT oil should be avoided but coconut in moderation may be allowed
9. In long chain FAOD with severe illness, long chain fats should be restricted to 10% and MCT to 30% of energy in infancy. In moderate to mild disease, 20% each of long chain and MCT as energy source may be prescribed. Before exercise, the patient should have MCT (0.2 g/kg) supplementation with glucose, and after exercise protein and carbohydrate in 1:3 ratio should be prescribed to prevent rhabdomyolysis. For details at different ages, appropriate sources may be consulted (Merritt et al., 2018).

GLYCOGEN STORAGE DISEASE

Glycogen storage disease (GSD) is a group of hereditary metabolic diseases of either defect in glycogen synthesis or glycogenolysis due to defect in several enzymes involved in this process (Figure 14.4). Glycogen storage disease was first described by a German physician, Edgar von Gierke in 1929 (von Gierke., 1929). Type I GSD is the commonest and is named after him. In 1952, Gerty and Carld Cori reported deficiency of glucose 6 phosphatase in liver cells as cause of von Gierke disease (Cori and Cori., 1952). This is the first inborn error of metabolism to be attributed to an enzyme defect. The cumulative incidence of GSD is one in 20,000 live births (Dambska et al., 2017).

Pathophysiology: Brain utilizes glucose as the main source of energy. Constant supply of glucose is essential for human survival. There are three main sources of glucose diet, glycogenolysis and gluconeogenesis. The dietary source of glucose is episodic as it depends on meal frequency. To maintain a constant supply of glucose, glycogenolysis and gluconeogenesis should be efficient. Glycogen is mainly stored in liver and muscles.

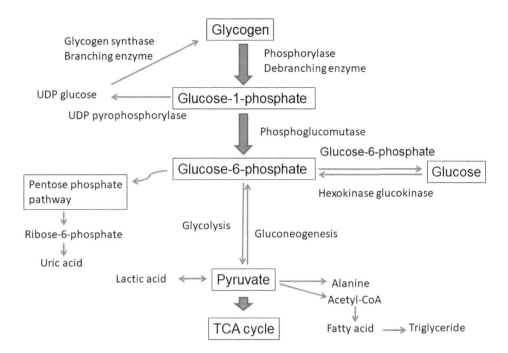

Figure 14.4 Glycogenolytic pathway. UDP, Uridy diphosphate; TCA, tricyclic acid cycle.

Glycogen is a branched chain homopolysaccharide synthesized from α D-glucose molecule. On fall of blood glucose, glycogen is broken down to glucose, whereas for maintaining muscle activity, the energy is supplied by glycogenolysis. If there is low or no glycogen store or there is defect in glycogenolytic pathway, there is gluconeogenesis in which glucose production takes place from protein (amino acid) or fat (lactate). In gluconeogenesis, there will be ketosis, hyperuricemia, hypertriglyceridemia and elevated lactate. Glycogen storage disease is broadly divided into hepatic and neuromuscular form. Glycogen synthesis is an ATP dependent process which occurs in liver cells. Glucose on entering the liver is rapidly phosphorylated to glucose 6 phosphate with the help of glucokinase. Glucose 6 phosphate is converted to glucose 1 phosphate by enzyme phosphoglucomutase. Glucose 1 phosphate is the starting point of glycogen synthesis. Glucose 1 phosphate is converted to uridine di phosphate (UDP) glucose with the help of UDP glucose phosphorylase in the presence of uridine tri-phosphate (UTP). The glucose fraction of UDP may be added to existing glycogen or protein glycogenin. With the formation of many long chains and branched points, glycogen molecule acquires a tree like structure with several branches. However, when needed, multiple glucose molecules may be detached thereby a steady glucose level is maintained during fasting. There are numerous glycogen storage disease discovered and these are described chronologically from GSD type I to GSD type XI. All the GSDs are autosomal recessive except IIa, IXa and IXd are X linked. These enzymatic defects manifest with dysfunction of liver, muscle or both. The different types of GSD are mentioned in Table 14.10.

Glycogen storage disease type I: GSD type I is due to deficiency of glucose 6 phosphatase complex. There are two subtypes, type Ia is due to deficiency of glucose 6 phosphatase α catalytic subunit and type Ib is due to glucose 6 phosphate transporter deficiency (Beyzaei et al., 2019). Glycogen storage disease type Ia accounts for 80% of GSD I defect. In GSD type 1a, there is accumulation of glycogen in liver, kidney and intestinal mucosa resulting in hepatomegaly and renomegaly. The patients usually manifest in the first year of life especially during the weaning period. The child has prominent symptoms of hypoglycemia such as sweating, irritability, drowsiness, weakness, and convulsions. There is growth retardation and developmental delay. Due to platelet dysfunction, easy bruising and epistaxis are common. Truncal obesity, short

Table 14.10 Different types of glycogen storage disease

GSD type	Gene	Chromosome	Enzyme/Protein	Hepatic/Muscle	Dietary management
GSD 0	GYS2	12p12.2	Glycogen synthase	Hepatic	Avoid fasting, high protein diet
GSD Ia	G6PC	17q21.31	Glucose 6 phosphatase – α catalytic subunit	Hepatic	
GSD Ib	SLC37A4	11q23.3	Glucose 6 phosphate transporter	Hepatic	
GSD II	GAA	17q25.3	α-1,4 glucosidase	Neuromuscular	High protein+BCAA
GSD IIb[a]	LAMP2	Xq24	LAMP-II protein	Neuromuscular	
GSD III	AGL	1p21.2	Glycogen debranching enzyme	Both	Protein 3–4 g/kg + corn starch
GSD IV	GBE	3p12.3	Glycogen branching enzyme	Both	Cornstarch
GSD V	PYGN	11q13.1	Glycogen phosphorylase (muscle)	Neuromuscular	Glucose, sucrose before exercise
GSD VI	PYGL	14q22.1	Glycogen phsphorylase (liver)	Hepatic	Cornstarch + protein supplement
GSD VII	PFKM	12q13.11	Phosphofructokinase (muscle)	Neuromuscular	Protein + B6 , worsening by CHO
GSD IXa[b]	PHKA2	Xp22.13	Phosphorylase kinase, α subunit (liver)	Hepatic	High Protein + corn starch
GSD IXb	PHKB	16q12.1	Phosphorylase kinase, β subunit	Hepatic	
GSD IXc	PHKG2	16p11.2	Phosphorylase kinase, ϒ subunit	Hepatic	
GSD IXd[b]	PHKA1	Xq13	Phosphorylase kinase α subunit (muscle)	Neuromuscular	
GSD XI	SLC2A2	3q26.2	GLUT2 transporter	Hepatic	High protein + corn starch

[a] X-linked dominant.
[b] X-linked recessive Rest are autosomal recessive.

stature and doll like face are striking. In second and third decade, these patients may have osteoporosis, hepatic adenoma and carcinoma, focal segmental glomerulosclerosis, interstitial nephritis and type II renal tubular acidosis. Laboratory tests reveal calciuria, hypoglycemia and high serum lactate, uric acid and triglyceride. Glycogen storage disease type Ib also has similar clinical and biochemical findings. The additional findings in GSD type Ib are neutropenia and inflammatory bowel disease of small intestine. Recurrent infection and oral ulcers may contribute to hypoglycemia. The diagnosis of GSD was initially based on muscle biopsy and enzyme assays. Genetic studies are now preferred because of noninvasive nature, better characterization and helps in prenatal diagnosis.

Treatment: The aim of treatment of GSD type I is to prevent hypoglycemia and to reduce neoglucogenesis, thereby reducing the metabolic consequences. Feeding may be started orally or through nasogastric tube. Uncooked corn starch is given periodically depending on the age. Corn starch therapy is started by 6 months of age when pancreatic amylase activity matures. In the children below 2 years of age feeding is given three hourly and in older children and adults 4–5 hourly. The dose is calculated as per standard formula (Chen et al., 2016). The dose of corn starch is adjusted based on blood glucose (>75 mg/dl) and lactate (<2.2 mM/l). Corn starch should be mixed with water in 1:2 ratio and glucose, fructose and galactose are avoided. Multivitamin, fish oil, vitamin E are supplemented, allopurinol is prescribed for hyper-uricemia, ACE inhibitor for proteinuria and calcium and vitamin D for preventing osteoporosis. With proper dietary treatment and supplementation, most patients do well till adulthood and complications are uncommon. During pregnancy and surgery, the patient may need intravenous glucose and measures to control bleeding. In GSD 1b recurrent infections due to neutropenia need attention in addition to above measures. Recombinant human granulocyte colony stimulating factor is prescribed if there is severe mouth ulcer or diarrhea. The starting dose is 2.5 µg/kg/day. A lower dose is preferred because colony stimulating hormone is associated with splenic sequestration, splenic rupture and portal hypertension. For inflammatory bowel disease in GSD Ib, the corticosteroid or immunosuppression is not preferred. Nonabsorbable salicylate may be used.

GALACTOSEMIA

Galactosemia is an inborn error of metabolism caused by impairment of any of the three galactose metabolizing enzymes: galactokinase (GLK), galactose 1 phosphate uridyl transferase (GLAT) and UDP galactose 4 epimerase (GAE) which may lead to hypergalactosemia. In 1917, Friedrich Goppert from Germany described galactosemia. The defect in galactose metabolism was reported in 1956 by Herman Kalckar (Goppert, 1917; Isselbacher et al., 1956). Luis Federico Leloir contributed to understanding of metabolism of galactose–Leloir pathway (Coelho et al., 2017). Galactosemia is a rare autosomal recessive disease with an incidence of 1/40.000–60,000 live births in Europe and USA. The incidence is higher in Irish traveler population, 1 in 480 live births (Murphy et al., 1999)

Pathology: Galactose is an aldohexose and is present in all living organisms. Dietary galactose is absorbed by enterocytes of small intestine and is actively transported by sodium glucose co-transporter (SGLT1). About 88% of ingested galactose reaches liver where it is internalized by the liver cells with the help of glucose transporter 2 (GLUT2). The remaining 12% of galactose is distributed to the other organs. In the cells, galactose is metabolized by Leloir pathway. There are three enzymatic reactions in Leloir pathway (Figure 14.5):

1. Galactose is converted to galactose 1 phosphate
2. Galactose 1 phosphate and UDP glucose are converted to UDP galactose and D-glucose 1 phosphate with the help of galactose 1 phosphate uridyl transferase (GALT)
3. UDP galactose is converted to UDP glucose with the help of UDP galactose 4-epimerase (GALE).

Defect in metabolism in these three processes results in accumulation of galactose or galactose 1 phosphate depending on the enzyme defect. If there is defective Leloir pathway, glucose is metabolized through alternative pathway leading to accumulation of metabolites galactitol and galactonate. The intracellular increase in galactitol leads to hyperosmotic state, oxidative stress and is responsible for cataract. In GALT and GALK

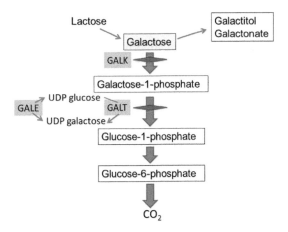

Figure 14.5 Leloir pathway of galactose metabolism. GALE, UDP-galactose 4-epimerase; GALK, galactokinase; GALT, galactose-1-phosphate uridylyltransferase.

deficiency, there is also reduction in myoinositol. Based on residual enzyme activity of GALT, it can be classified into classic (severe deficiency), childhood variant (residual deficiency in RBC and liver) and biochemical variant galactosemia (15%–30% of GALT activity).

Classic galactosemia: Classical galactosemia manifests during neonatal period with the features of poor feeding, growth retardation, hepatomegaly, jaundice, hypotonia, renal tubular dysfunction, cataract and *E. coli* septicemia. Restriction of galactose in early life reverses the symptoms; however neuropsychiatric, speech and autistic behavior may persist in 38%–88%. The patients may also have ataxia, tremor, dystonia and dysarthria (Kaufman et al., 1995; Waggoner et al., 1990; Berry et al., 2017). Periodic evaluation of the patients is important. Cranial MRI reveals cerebral and cerebellar atrophy. Gonadal failure occurs in nearly all the patients with classical galactosemia. These patients have delayed puberty, primary or secondary amenorrhea, infertility and premature menopause. In males, there is high incidence of cryptorchidism, reduced gonadal hormone and infertility. The diagnosis of classical galactosemia is suspected by clinical features, newborn screening test and confirmed by galactose 1 phosphate level and is RBC GALT enzyme activity or GALT gene mutation. Plasma galactose level is usually more than 10 mg/dl which is absent in normal individuals. Galactose 1 phosphate level is more than 120 mg/l in classical galactosemia ($N < 1$ mg/dl). The

other laboratory abnormalities are elevated serum bilirubin, transaminases and hypoglycemia, hyperchloremic metabolic acidosis, generalized aminoaciduria, hypophosphatemia and anemia. There are more than 300 mutations in classical galactosemia, the commonest being pq1 88 R (C563A-G) in Caucasians.

Clinical and biochemical variants of galactosemia: Clinical variant of galactosemia has minimal GALT activity in RBC, liver and intestinal cells. The patient presents like classical galactosemia during the neonatal period. On diet restriction, they do not have long-term effects. The RBC galactose 1 phosphate is more than 10 mg/dl which falls to less than 1 mg/dl on dietary restriction.

Biochemical variant of galactosemia is asymptomatic and is detected during newborn screening. Blood galactose is normal, but GALT activity is reduced. This variant does not require dietary restriction.

GALK deficiency: GALK deficiency is rare (less than 1 in 100,000 live birth) and occurs due to mutation in GALK 1 gene located in chromosome 17q 24. There is accumulation of galactose and galactitol. It is characterized by cataract within 1 month of age.

GALE deficiency: GALE deficiency is an autosomal recessive disorder due to GALE gene. It has 3 presentations, severe generalized galactosemia, intermediate and peripheral forms. The intermediate and peripheral forms usually remain asymptomatic, but the generalized form is similar to classical galactosemia.

Treatment: The treatment of classic galactosemia is galactose restricted diet lifelong which is mainly restriction of dairy products. The target level of RBC galactose 1 phosphate is 1–4 mg/dl and urinary galactitol 100–400 μM/mMol of creatinine.

UREA CYCLE DISORDERS (UCD)

Normally urea cycle is responsible for endogenous production of arginine, ornithine, and citrulline as well as clearing the waste nitrogen product during protein turnover especially ammonia to urea or uric acid. Urea cycle was first described by Hans–Krebs and Kurt Henseleit in 1932 (Krebs and Henseleit, 1932). There are five enzymes in urea cycle – carbamoyl phosphate synthetase (CPS1),

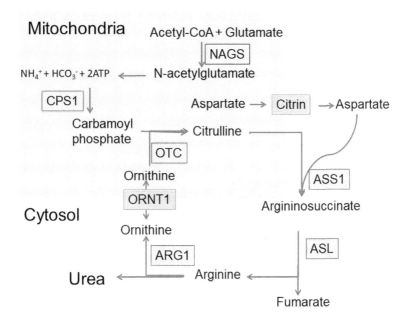

Figure 14.6 Urea cycle. Five enzymes: CPS1, carbamoyl phosphate synthetase (CPS1); OTC, ornithine transcarbamylase; ASS, argininosuccinic acid synthetase; ASL, argininosuccinic acid L-lyase and ARG1, arginase. One cofactor producing enzyme: NAGS, N Acetyl glutamate synthase and two amino acid transporter; ORNT1, Ornithine translocase and Citrin.

ornithine transcarbamylase (OTC), argininosuccinic acid synthetase (ASS), argininosuccinic acid L-lyase (ASL) and arginase (ARG1). There is one cofactor producing enzyme (N acetyl glutamate synthase, NAGS) and two amino acid transporter [ornithine translocase (ORNT1) and citrin]. Any of these enzymes or transporter defects may result in urea cycle disorder (UCD) leading to accumulation of ammonia and other metabolites proximal to the enzyme defects (Figure 14.6).

The incidence of USD is 1 in 8000 to 35,000 live births, OTC deficiency being the commonest. All the UCDs are autosomal recessive except OTC which is X linked. The accumulation of ammonia in the blood is the key feature of UCD. Chronic hyperammonemic state may result in impaired ion gradient, neurotransmitter and mitochondrial function, metabolite transport and α-ketoglutarate to glutamine ratio

Clinical features: The clinical presentation of UCD depends on the type and extent of enzyme defects. Severe deficiency of first four enzymes and cofactors is associated with marked accumulation of ammonia and other precursor metabolites within 1–2 days of birth. In UCD, a normal newborn at birth becomes lethargic rapidly, has poor

feeding, hypothermia, seizures, abnormal posturing, hypo or hyperreflexia and coma. Partial enzyme deficiency may lead to milder symptoms such as anorexia, vomiting, lethargy, neuropsychiatric abnormality, sleep disturbances or may be normal. The defect in the final enzyme of urea cycle ARG1 may have subtle clinical manifestations. The defects in amino acid transporter of urea cycle have similar manifestations as in those with enzyme deficiency. These patients may have additional features of chronic liver disease. All forms of UCDs may have acute crisis at any age. The acute and chronic manifestations of UCDs are presented in Table 14.11.

The clinical pictures of different types of UCDs are similar except spasticity in arginase deficiency and trichorrhexis nodosa (fragile hair) in ALSM deficiency. Any patient with unexplained acute encephalopathy or neuropsychiatric abnormality irrespective of age should be evaluated for plasma ammonia. High plasma ammonia (>150 μM/l), normal anion gap and normal blood glucose are suggestive of UCD. Quantitative amino acid measurement may suggest tentative enzyme defect. Urinary orotic acid measurement may help in differentiation of OTC deficiency (normal or low)

Table 14.11 Clinical features of UCD during acute and chronic presentations (Haberle et al., 2012)

Acute presentation
Central nervous system:
Drowsiness to coma
Seizure
Ataxia
Stroke like illness
Transient visual loss
Psychosis
Gastrointestinal:
Vomiting, anorexia, hepatic encephalopathy
Others: Multi-organ failure, peripheral circulatory failure
Neonates may have sepsis or encephalitis-like presentation and respiratory distress
Chronic presentation
Central nervous system: Learning disability, developmental delay, mental retardation, visual loss, chorea, tremor, asterexis, headache, dizziness, confusion
Gastrointestinal: Abdominal pain, vomiting, protein aversion, hepatomegaly, raised liver enzymes
Psychiatric: Hyperactivity, behavioral abnormality, autistic behavior, self-injury behavior
Others: Fragile hair, dermatitis, episodic worsening

from CPS1 or AGS deficiency (high). Newborn screening for UCD is not widely practiced. Genetic studies are confirmatory.

Management: The management of acute crisis is aimed at rapid lowering of plasma ammonia to near normal by dialysis, nitrogen restriction by using scavenging drugs like sodium phenyl acetate or benzoate, arginine infusion, or oral citrulline. In NAGS deficiency, N-acetyl glutamate and carbamyl glutamate may be curative. Complete restriction of dietary protein should not exceed 24 h to prevent catabolism. Daily measurement of plasma amino acid level and supplementation is required to prevent catabolism of insulin glucose drip is recommended during acute crisis. Attention should be paid to maintain fluid, electrolyte balance and control of seizures.

KETOGENIC DIET

Ketognic diet (KD) is a high fat low carbohydrate diet that increases ketone body formation through fat metabolism in the liver. It simulates the condition of fasting without depriving the body of calories to sustain growth and development. Normally dietary carbohydrate is converted to glucose which is circulated in the body and is the main source of energy for brain. In the absence of carbohydrate liver converts fat into fatty acids and ketone bodies. The brain uses ketone bodies as energy source instead of glucose. High ketone level in the blood "ketosis" reduces seizures and was an important treatment before modern anticonvulsants were available.

Fasting or water diet was a method of treatment of epilepsy by ancient Greek physicians as early as 400 BC. Erasis Tratus, the royal physician advised fasting without "mercy" for the treatment of epilepsy. Galen also recommended attenuating diet for the treatment of epilepsy. Scientific evaluation of fasting in treatment of epilepsy was conducted (Gulepa and Marrie, 1911). Henry Rawle and Geyelil reported the benefit of fasting in 36 patients with epilepsy. Rolling Turner–Wood Yatt in 1921 reported three water soluble compounds namely β-hydroxybutyrate, acetoacetate and acetone which are produced in the liver of starved subjects or those consuming high fat and low carbohydrate diet (Wheless, 2004). Russell Morse Wilder used the term "ketogenic diet" and also treated patients with epilepsy. For more than one decade, KD enjoyed the therapeutic preference in pediatric epilepsy when bromide and phenobarbital were the only anticonvulsants available. The interest in KD waned after 1940s, which has revived in 1990s for treatment of refractory epilepsy.

Composition of ketogenic diet: normal diet is composed of 55% carbohydrate, 30% protein and 15% fat. In KD, the main source of calories is fat, and carbohydrate is substantially reduced. The

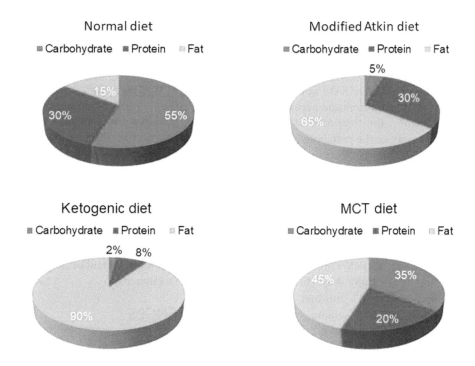

Figure 14.7 Composition of normal and different ketogenic diet.

CKD (classic ketogenic diet) comprises of 90% fat, 8% protein and 2% carbohydrate. This diet is very unpalatable and has side effects. For improving compliance it has been modified (Modified Atkins Diet, MAD) which includes 65% fats, 30% protein and 5% carbohydrate (Kossoff et al., 2008), subsequently using medium chain triglyceride (MCT) oil the proportion of fat is reduced to 45% and carbohydrate is increased to 35% and protein to 20% (Tanya et al., 2018, Zupec-Kania et al., 2008). In MCT variety KD the medium chain triglyceride is included by adding coconut or palm oil or both. The proportion of fat, carbohydrate and protein in different KD, is shown in Figure 14.7. Modified Ketogenic diet is advised based on age, tolerance, goal of ketosis and protein requirement (Zupec-Kania et al., 2008).

Mechanism of action: Ketones decrease synaptic transmission and have antioxidant and anti-inflammatory effect. At synaptic level, ketone reduces membrane excitability, alter neurotransmitter concentration and open ATP sensitive potassium channels. In MCT oil KD, acetoacetate and β-hydroxybutyrate increase GABA level. MCT oil also reduces AMPA receptors and glutamate levels. (Figure 14.8; Tanya et al., 2018; Ulamek-Koziol et al., 2019).

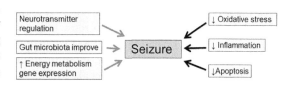

Figure 14.8 Mechanism of anti-seizure activity of ketogenic diet.

Ketogenic diet in epilepsy: KD is mainly used in drug resistant epilepsy in children and adults having generalized or focal epilepsy. In a study, 51 children with drug resistant epilepsy were treated with KD for 1 year, but only 47% could continue; 43% of whom were seizure free and 39% had seizure control by 50%–90%. Adverse events included dehydration, acidosis, infection, mood swing, lethargy, somnolence, vomiting and constipation (Vining et al., 1998). In another study on 150 children, KD resulted in seizure remission in 7% by 1 year, 90% seizure reduction in 27% and more than 50% reduction 50% children (Freeman et al., 1998; Wu et al., 2016). Randomized controlled trial in 145 children with drug resistant epilepsy, KD was useful in reducing frequency of seizures compared to control (75% vs 0%); 25% of these children had side effects (Neal et al., 2008). In a meta-analysis of

270 adults with drug resistant epilepsy, 168 of them received KD. The benefit of KD in different studies ranged between 13% and 70%, and pool benefit was present in 42% patients. This study suggested that MAD should be tried before KD (Ye et al., 2015). In GLUT deficiency, syndrome and pyruvate dehydrogenase deficiency, the treatment of choice is KD because it bypasses the metabolic defect and provides ketones as a source of energy to the brain (Kossoff et al., 2009). In myoclonic atonic epilepsy (Doose syndrome), and infantile myoclonic epilepsy (Dravet's syndrome), seizure control by KD has been reported. In infantile spasm, KD has been tried in vigabatrin and steroid resistant children. Seizure remission was 35% in the first month and 65% in the third month following KD in infantile spasm (Pires et al., 2013). A Cochrane review including 778 patients (712 children, 66 adults from 11 studies) reported seizure freedom in 0%–55% patients after 3 months. Seizure frequency was reduced in 85% patients. Gradual introduction of KD improved efficacy (Martin–McGill et al., 2018). A meta-analysis including children and adults revealed seizure reduction in 60% children at 3 months and 46% at 2 years. Classical KD and MAD have comparable efficacy in refractory epilepsy (Rezaei et al., 2019). Overall KD is effective in refractory generalized epilepsy, more in adults than in children (Ulamek-Koziol et al., 2019).

Adverse events of KD: KD diet is associated with a number of side effects which include cramps, bad breath, change in bowel habit, keto flu and loss of energy (Baranano et al., 2008). KD should be closely monitored once or twice a month for glucose, ketones, cardiac and other parameters (Shilpa and Mohan, 2018). Indian diet is rich in carbohydrate. STARCH study has revealed that Indians consume 65% of the calories from carbohydrate irrespective of their diabetic status (Joshi et al., 2014). PURE study revealed that consumption of carbohydrate more than 60% of total calorie is associated with high mortality whereas higher fat intake is associated with lower mortality, but not cardiovascular disease and cardiovascular disease mortality (Dehghan et al., 2017). An U-shaped curve on relationship between mortality and carbohydrate intake has been shown; more than 60% and less than 30% carbohydrate intake was associated with high mortality. The risk of mortality was lower when carbohydrate intake was between 50% and 55%, however, mortality was lower when

dietary carbohydrate was replaced by plant-based protein and fat, and higher with animal-based protein and fat (Seidelmann et al., 2018).

CONCLUSION

Dietary management is an integral part of IEM. The management of IEM requires high index of suspicion, and laboratory confirmation is possible by genetic testing. In view of urgency, prompt treatment and evaluation should go on simultaneously. Proper understanding of mechanism and rational management are key to success. The rarity of IEM, high cost of diagnostic confirmation and treatment requires social support. Ketogenic diet is also an useful treatment option in selected cases of refractory epilepsy.

REFERENCES

Barañano, K. W., Hartman, A. L. 2008. The ketogenic diet: Uses in epilepsy and other neurologic illnesses. *Current Treatment Options in Neurology* 10:410–419.

Baumgartner, M. R., Hörster, F., Dionisi-Vici, C., et al. 2014. Proposed guidelines for the diagnosis and management of methylmalonic and propionic acidemia. *Orphanet Journal of Rare Diseases* 9:130.

Berry, G. T. 2017. Classic galactosemia and clinical variant galactosemia. In: Adam, M. P., Ardinger, H. H., Pagon, R. A., Wallace, S. E., Bean, L. J. H., Stephens, K., Amemiya, A., (Eds.) *GeneReviews® [Internet]*. Seattle, WA: University of Washington, pp. 1993–2020.

Beyzaei, Z., Geramizadeh, B. 2019. Molecular diagnosis of glycogen storage disease type I: A review. *EXCLI Journal* 18:30–46.

Chen, M. A., Weinstein, D. A. 2016. Glycogen storage diseases: Diagnosis, treatment and outcome. *Translational Science of Rare Diseases* 1:45–72.

Chuang, D. T. 1998. Maple syrup urine disease: It has come a long way. *The Journal of Pediatrics 132*: S17–S23.

Chuang, D. T., Shih, V. E. 2001. Maple syrup urine disease (branched-chain ketoaciduria). In: Scriver, C. R., Beaudet, A. L., Sly, W. S., Valle, D., (Eds). *1971–2006. The metabolic and molecular bases of inherited disease*. New York: McGraw-Hill.

Chuang, J. L., Davie, J. R., Chinsky, J. M., Wynn, R. M., Cox, R. P., Chuang, D. T. 1995. Molecular and biochemical basis of intermediate maple syrup urine disease. Occurrence of homozygous G245R and F364C mutations at the E1 alpha locus of Hispanic-Mexican patients. *The Journal of Clinical Investigation* 95(3):954–963.

Coelho, A. I., Rubio-Gozalbo, M. E., Vicente, J. B., Rivera, I. 2017. Sweet and sour: An update on classic galactosemia. *Journal of Inherited Metabolic Disease* 40(3):325–334.

Cori, G. T., Cori, C. F. 1952. Glucose-6-phosphatase of the liver in glycogen storage disease. *Journal of Biological Chemistry* 199:661–667.

Dambska, M., Labrador, E. B., Kuo, C. L., Weinstein, D. A. 2017. Prevention of complications in glycogen storage disease type Ia with optimization of metabolic control. *Pediatric Diabetes* 18:327–331.

Dancis, J., Hutzler, J., Levitz, M. 1960. Metabolism of the white blood cells in maple-syrupurine disease. *Biochimica et Biophysica Acta* 43: 342–345.

Dehghan, M., Mente, A., Zhang, X., et al. 2017. Prospective Urban Rural Epidemiology (PURE) study investigators. Associations of fats and carbohydrate intake with cardiovascular disease and mortality in 18 countries from five continents (PURE): A prospective cohort study. *Lancet (London, England)* 390(10107): 2050–2062.

Feuchtbaum, L., Yang, J., Currier, R. 2018. Follow-up status during the first 5 years of life for metabolic disorders on the federal Recommended Uniform Screening Panel. *Genetics in Medicine* 20:831–839.

Freeman, J. M., Vining, E. P., Pillas, D. J., Pyzik, P. L., Casey, J. C., Kelly, L. M. 1998. The efficacy of the ketogenic diet-1998: A prospective evaluation of intervention in 150 children. *Pediatrics* 102(6): 1358–1363.

Goppert, F. 1917. Galaktosurie nach Milchzuckergabe bei angeborenem, familiaerem chronischem Leberleiden. *Klinische Wochenschrift* 54:473–477.

Grosse, S. D., Khoury, M. J., Greene, C. L., Crider, K. S., Pollitt, R. J. 2006. The epidemiology of medium chain acyl-CoA dehydrogenase deficiency: An update. *Genetics in Medicine: Official Journal of the American College of Medical Genetics* 8(4): 205–212.

Guelpa, G., Marie, A. 1911. "La lutte contre l'epilepsie par la desintoxication et par la reeducation alimentaire" [The fight against epilepsy by detoxification and by the reeducation about food]. *Rev Ther med-Chirurg* 78(1):8–13.

Guldberg, P., Henriksen, K. F., Sipilä, I., Güttler, F., de la Chapelle, A. 1995. Phenylketonuria in a low incidence population: Molecular characterisation of mutations in Finland. *Journal of Medical Genetics* 32(12):976–978.

Guthrie, R., Susi, A. 1963. A simple phenylalanine method for detecting phenylketonuria in large populations of newborn infants. *Pediatrics* 32:338–43.

Isselbacher, K. J., Anderson, E. P., Kurahashi, K., Kalckar, H. M. 1956. Congenital galactosemia, a single enzymatic block in galactose metabolism. *Science (New York, NY)* 123(3198): 635–636.

Jervis, G. A. 1947. Studies on phenylpyruvic oligophrenia: The position of the metabolic error. *Journal of Biological Chemistry* 169:651–656.

Jervis, G. A. 1953. Phenylpyruvic oligophrenia deficiency of phenylalanine-oxidizing system. *Proceedings of The Society for Experimental Biology and Medicine* 82:514–545.

Joshi, S. R., Bhansali, A., Bajaj, S., et al., 2014. Results from a dietary survey in an Indian T2DM population: A STARCH study. *BMJ Open* 4(10):e005138.

Kaufman, F. R., McBride-Chang, C., Manis, F. R., Wolff, J. A., Nelson, M. D. 1995. Cognitive functioning, neurologic status and brain imaging in classical galactosemia. *European Journal of Pediatrics* 154(7 Suppl 2):S2–S5.

Kossoff, E. H., Rowley, H., Sinha, S. R., Vining, E. P. 2008. A prospective study of the modified Atkins diet for intractable epilepsy in adults. *Epilepsia* 49(2):316–319.

Kossoff, E. H., Zupec-Kania, B. A., Amark, P. E., et al. International Ketogenic Diet Study Group. 2009. Optimal clinical management of children receiving the ketogenic diet: recommendations of the International Ketogenic Diet Study Group. *Epilepsia* 50(2):304–317.

Krebs, H. A., Henseleit, K. 1932. Untersuchungen uber die harnstoffbildungim tierkorper. *Hoppe-Seyler's Z Physiol Chem* 210:325–332.

Martin-McGill, K. J., Jackson, C. F., Bresnahan, R., Levy, R. G., Cooper, P. N. 2018. Ketogenic diets for drug-resistant epilepsy. *The Cochrane Database of Systematic Reviews* 11(11):CD001903.

McDonald, T., Cervenka, M. C. 2018. Ketogenic diets for adult neurological disorders. *Neurotherapeutics: The Journal of the American Society for Experimental NeuroTherapeutics* 15(4):1018–1031.

Menkes, J. H. 1959. Maple syrup disease: Isolation and identification of organic acids in the urine. *Pediatrics* 23:348–353.

Menkes, J. H., Hurst, P. L., Craig, J. M. 1954. A new syndrome: Progressive familial infantile cerebral dysfunction associated with an unusual urinary substance. *Pediatrics* 14:462–466.

Merritt, J. L. 2nd, Chang, I. J. 2019. Medium-chain acyl-coenzyme A dehydrogenase deficiency. In: Adam, M. P., Ardinger, H. H., Pagon, R. A.,

Wallace, S. E., Bean, L. J. H., Stephens, K., Amemiya, A., (Eds.) *GeneReviews® [Internet]*. Seattle, WA: University of Washington, pp. 1993–2020.

Murphy, M., McHugh, B., Tighe, O., et al. 1999. Genetic basis of transferase-deficient galactosaemia in Ireland and the population history of the Irish Travellers. *European Journal of Human Genetics: EJHG* 7(5):549–554.

Neal, E. G., Chaffe, H., Schwartz, R. H., et al. 2008. The ketogenic diet for the treatment of childhood epilepsy: A randomised controlled trial. *The Lancet. Neurology* 7(6):500–506.

Nennstiel-Ratzel, U., Arenz, S., Maier, E. M., et al. 2005. Reduced incidence of severe metabolic crisis or death in children with medium chain acyl-CoA dehydrogenase deficiency homozygous for c.985A>G identified by neonatal screening. *Molecular Genetics and Metabolism* 85(2):157–159.

Okano, Y., Hase, Y., Lee, D.H, et al. 1992. Frequency and distribution of phenylketonuric mutations in Orientals. *Human Mutation* 1:216–220.

Ozand, P. T., Rashed, M., Gascon, G. G., et al. 1994. Unusual presentations of propionic acidemia. *Brain & Development*, 16(Suppl): 46–57.

Pettit, F. H., Yeaman, S. J., Reed, L. J. 1978. Purification and characterization of branched chain alpha-keto acid dehydrogenase complex of bovine kidney. *Proceedings of the National Academy of Sciences of the United States of America* 75(10):4881–4885.

Pires, M. E., Ilea, A., Bourel, E., et al., 2013. Ketogenic diet for infantile spasms refractory to first-line treatments: An open prospective study. *Epilepsy Research* 105(1–2):189–194.

Rezaei, S., Abdurahman, A. A., Saghazadeh, A., Badv, R. S., Mahmoudi, M. 2019. Short-term and long-term efficacy of classical ketogenic diet and modified Atkins diet in children and adolescents with epilepsy: A systematic review and meta-analysis. *Nutritional Neuroscience* 22(5):317–334.

Seidelmann, S. B., Claggett, B., Cheng, S., et al., 2018. Dietary carbohydrate intake and mortality: A prospective cohort study and meta-analysis. *The Lancet. Public Health* 3(9):e419–e428.

Shchelochkov, O. A., Carrillo, N., Venditti, C., 2012. Propionic Acidemia. In: Adam, M. P., Ardinger, H. H., Pagon, R. A., Wallace, S.E., Bean, L. J. H., Stephens, K., Amemiya, A., (Eds.) *GeneReviews® [Internet]*. Seattle, WA: University of Washington, pp. 1993–2020.

Shilpa, J., Mohan, V. 2018. Ketogenic diets: Boon or bane? *Indian Journal of Medical Research* 148(3):251–253.

Strauss, K. A., Puffenberger, E. G., Carson, V. J. 2020. Maple syrup urine disease. In: Adam, M. P., Ardinger, H. H., Pagon, R. A., et al., (Eds.) *GeneReviews® [Internet]*. Seattle, WA: University of Washington, pp. 1993–2020.

Thomas, J., Levy, H., Amato, S., et al. 2018. Pegvaliase for the treatment of phenylketonuria: Results of a long-term phase 3 clinical trial program (PRISM). *Molecular Genetics and Metabolism* 124(1): 27–38.

Ułamek-Kozioł, M., Czuczwar, S. J., Januszewski, S., Pluta, R. 2019. Ketogenic diet and epilepsy. *Nutrients* 11(10):2510.

van Wegberg, A., MacDonald, A., Ahring, K., et al. 2017. The complete European guidelines on phenylketonuria: Diagnosis and treatment. *Orphanet Journal of Rare Diseases* 12(1):162.

von Gierke, E. 1929. Hepato-nephromegalia glykogenica (Glykogenspeicherkrankheit der Leber und Nieren). Beiträge zur Pathologischen Anatomie und zur Allgemeinen Pathologie. *Jena* 82:497–513.

Waggoner, D. D., Buist, N. R., Donnell, G. N. 1990. Long-term prognosis in galactosaemia: Results of a survey of 350 cases. *Journal of Inherited Metabolic Disease* 13(6):802–818.

Westfall, R. G., Dancis, J., Miller, S. 1957. Maple sugar urine disease [abstract]. *The American Journal of Diseases of Children* 94:571.

Wheless J. W. 2004. History and origin of the ketogenic diet. In: Stafstrom, C. E., Rho, J. M. (Eds.) *Epilepsy and the Ketogenic Diet. Nutrition and Health*. Totowa, NJ: Humana Press.

Wilcken, B., Haas, M., Joy, P., et al. 2007. Outcome of neonatal screening for medium-chain acyl-CoA dehydrogenase deficiency in Australia: A cohort study. *Lancet (London, England)* 369(9555):37–42.

Williams, R. A., Mamotte, C. D., Burnett, J. R. 2008. Phenylketonuria: An inborn error of phenylalanine metabolism. *The Clinical Biochemist. Reviews* 29(1): 31–41.

Wu, Y. J., Zhang, L. M., Chai, Y. M., et al. 2016. Six-month efficacy of the Ketogenic diet is predicted after 3 months and is unrelated to clinical variables. *Epilepsy & Behavior: E&B* 55:165–169.

Ye, F., Li, X. J., Jiang, W. L., Sun, H. B., Liu, J. 2015. Efficacy of and patient compliance with a ketogenic diet in adults with intractable epilepsy: A meta-analysis. *Journal of Clinical Neurology (Seoul, Korea)* 11(1):26–31.

Zupec-Kania, B. A., Spellman, E. 2008. An overview of the ketogenic diet for pediatric epilepsy. *Nutrition in Clinical Practice: Official Publication of the American Society for Parenteral and Enteral Nutrition* 23(6):589–596.

Index

Note: **Bold** page numbers refer to tables; *italic* page numbers refer to figures.

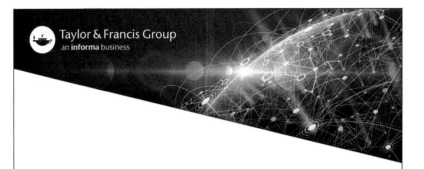